Principles of Healthcare Reimbursement

Anne B. Casto, RHIA, CCS

Elizabeth Layman, PhD, RHIA, CCS, FAHIMA

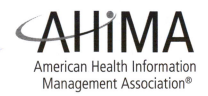

American Health Information
Management Association®

ISBN 1-58426-070-X
AHIMA Product No. AB202006

Ken Zielske, Director of Publications
Susan Hull, MPH, RHIA, CCS, CCS-P, Technical Reviewer
Marcia Loellbach, MS, Project Editor
Elizabeth Lund, Assistant Editor
Melissa Ulbricht, Editorial/Production Coordinator

All information contained within this book, including Web sites and regulatory information, was current and valid as of the date of publication. However, Web page addresses and the information on them may change or disappear at any time and for any number of reasons. The user is encouraged to perform his or her own general Web searches to locate any site addresses listed here that are no longer valid.

AHIMA strives to recognize the value of people from every racial and ethnic background as well as all genders, age groups, and sexual orientations by building its membership and leadership resources to reflect the rich diversity of the American population. AHIMA encourages the celebration and promotion of human diversity through education, mentoring, recognition, leadership, and other programs.

American Health Information Management Association
233 North Michigan Avenue, Suite 2150
Chicago, Illinois 60601-5800

http://www.ahima.org

Contents

About the Authors

Anne B. Casto, RHIA, CCS, is the program manager for the Health Information Management and Systems Division at Ohio State University in Columbus, Ohio. She teaches courses in ICD-9-CM and CPT coding, as well as healthcare reimbursement systems.

After earning her baccalaureate degree from Ohio State University in 1995, Anne was employed at Mount Sinai Medical Center and Beth Israel Medical Center in New York City managing several units including coding and abstracting, discharge processing, and DRG auditing.

In 1998, Anne moved into the healthcare financial arena and worked for the Center for Healthcare Performance Industry Studies as product manager of clinical information. She then served as vice president of clinical products for Cleverley and Associates.

Anne earned her CCS credential in 1998.

Elizabeth Layman, PhD, RHIA, CCS, FAHIMA, is professor and chair in the Department of Health Services and Information Management at East Carolina University, Greenville, North Carolina.

She previously worked at Hennepin County Medical Center and the University of Minnesota Hospitals, both in Minneapolis, Minnesota, from 1974 through 1990. She worked in several departments, such as third-party reimbursement, credit and collections, account auditing, outpatient registration, inpatient admissions, research studies, and quality management.

Elizabeth has her baccalaureate degree from the University of Minnesota. While working, she returned to school to earn her associate's degree in medical record technology. She completed St. Scholastica's progression program to earn her post-baccalaureate certificate in health information administration.

After earning her master's degree in organizational leadership from the College of St. Catherine's, Elizabeth joined the faculty of the Medical College of Georgia in Augusta, Georgia. She also consulted for the Physicians' Practice Group.

Elizabeth successfully sat for the first CCS examination in 1992. In 1995, she earned her doctorate in higher education from Georgia State University. In 2001, she was awarded the designation of Fellow of the American Health Information Management Association, one of the first two individuals in the country to receive this award.

Acknowledgments

The authors wish to thank
Eleanor Ann Joseph, MPA, RHIA, CHP, CPHQ, CCS, CCS-P, CPC,
and Leona Thomas, MHS, RHIA,
who served as external reviewers of the text
and provided excellent suggestions for its improvement.

Foreword

by William O. Cleverley, Ph.D.
Professor Emeritus, Ohio State University

I have taught healthcare financial management to graduate students for thirty years and have always believed that the critical area of understanding was reimbursement. When I first started teaching, the primary—perhaps exclusive—focus was on hospitals, but that has changed. Financing and organizational patterns have shifted over time to create large healthcare firms in other sectors, such as medical groups, nursing facilities, imaging centers, surgery centers, home health firms, and many others. The primary focal point of difference between healthcare firms and businesses in other industries is still, however, payment. Healthcare firms are very unique in the manner in which they receive compensation for the services that they provide. I could not find any other industry that had as complex a revenue function as healthcare firms when I started teaching thirty years ago, and that statement is still true today. In fact, the level of complexity for healthcare firms has increased exponentially over the last thirty years.

Noting that the revenue function, or reimbursement, is complex for a healthcare firm does not explain why this is critical. Let's examine the very basis of management in any business. Simply stated, management must control the difference between revenue and cost, which we define as profit. It makes little difference whether the firm is a taxable or tax-exempt entity. Viable businesses must manage that profit function. Although there are clearly differences in cost functions between healthcare firms and firms in other industrial sec-

tors, the differences are not all that significant. Generic principles for cost management might apply equally in a software firm or a hospital. The revenue function is, however, a completely different manner.

Why is the revenue function so different for healthcare firms compared to other industries? I believe there are at least four reasons. First, the vast majority of payment is not actually paid by the client (patient), but rather by a third party on behalf of the patient. Second, the level of payment for a set of identical services may vary dramatically based upon the actual third party payer. Third, the actual determination of payment for a specific third party payer is often complex, based upon preestablished or negotiated rules of payment that are frequently related to the codes entered upon a patient's bill or claim. Fourth, the government is often the largest single payer and does not negotiate payment but simply defines the rules for payment upon which it will render compensation for services provided to its beneficiaries.

To get a partial view of the complexity of reimbursement in the healthcare industry, let's describe a typical managed care contract with a hospital. Let's assume this payer pays for inpatient services on a per-diem basis, with separate rates for medical and surgical cases. In addition, carve-outs are present for cardiology DRGs. Finally, obstetrics and nursery care services are paid on case rates. To provide some additional risk protection to the hospital, a stop loss provision is also inserted after total charges exceed a certain limit. Outpatient services are paid on a mix of fee schedules and discounted billed charges. Outpatient surgical cases are paid on a fee schedule based upon designated ambulatory surgical groups. Emergency visits are also on a fee schedule, based upon level of service. Other fee schedules exist for specific imaging procedures, and everything else is paid on a discounted, billed-charge basis. Multiply this one payer by 100 to recognize other payers and throw in Medicare and Medicaid payment rules, and you have a nightmare in administration. It may be a nightmare, but it is very real to most healthcare firms; their very financial viability is contingent upon successful management of this complex revenue function.

Coding and billing issues are central to most of the present reimbursement plans. In fact, many healthcare firms can lose substantial sums of money because they are not coding their patients' claims in an accurate and complete manner. For example, failing to code an additional diagnosis can result in assignment of a lower DRG, and therefore lost revenue. While some healthcare executives may fail to understand the importance of the coding function, it would behoove them to acquire an appreciation of coding because so much of their revenue function is related to what is done by coders. Conversely, many people in health information management may understand the technical side of what they do, but they don't appreciate their role in the overall financial success of the health firm in which they work.

This background explains why I am so excited about the publication of this book. Anne Casto and Elizabeth Layman have put together a much-needed text on reimbursement that fills a void. I believe that this text is a first. It provides a comprehensive review of the reimbursement world for healthcare firms of multiple types. It also provides very specific material on the actual completion of claims and the rules for final payment determination. Medicare payment provisions are covered in great detail, but the text also includes other payers. It covers payment provisions for hospitals, but it also covers payment for other payers including managed care plans.

I believe this book is a must-read reference for healthcare executives who need a comprehensive reference on payment in the healthcare industry. It will be a fine supplement for healthcare management students who need to know how the firms they will manage will be paid and how coding and billing functions can impact results. It is also a critical text for health information managers and students. It is often easy to lose sight of the forest when you are engaged in tree cutting. This text provides a clear, concise description of the payment landscape for healthcare firms, which will enable health information managers to better integrate their functions into the overall organizational strategic position of the healthcare firms where they work. A large number of specific examples are also provided to help cement conceptual frameworks with operational reality. Another great feature of this text is its explanation of the myriad acronyms and jargon used in the healthcare industry. Short, concise definitions are given for everything from APCs to RBRVS.

This text met and exceeded the three R's that I use in evaluation. First, the text is very readable and easy to understand. Second, the text is especially relevant to all healthcare managers as they seek to improve financial performance. Third, the text is rich in detail and practical illustrations. This book will occupy a prominent position on my bookshelf and will be a great reference.

William O. Cleverley, Ph.D.
Professor Emeritus
Ohio State University

Preface

Health information management (HIM) professionals play a critical role in the delivery of healthcare services in the United States. To be fully effective in their roles, however, HIM professionals need an indepth understanding of healthcare reimbursement systems, reimbursement methodologies, and payment processes throughout the healthcare industry.

Principles of Healthcare Reimbursement integrates information about all U.S. healthcare payment systems into one authoritative source. It examines the complex financial systems within today's healthcare environment and provides an understanding of the basics of health insurance and public funding programs, managed care contracting, and how services are paid. Not only does the text provide step-by-step detail about how each payment system functions, but the history behind each is provided. This gives the reader an appreciation for the complexity of reimbursement systems and an understanding of the profound impact they have had on providers and payers, consumers, public policy makers, and the development of classification and information technology systems over the years.

Healthcare leaders and administrators often have to learn about healthcare payment systems on-the-job and on-the-fly. Other texts feature healthcare finance and healthcare economics, but not the bottom-line and nitty-gritty of the healthcare payment systems themselves. This book fills that gap.

Chapter 1, Healthcare Reimbursement Methodologies, introduces and explains the basic concepts and principles of healthcare reimbursement in step-by-step, simple terms. This introduction provides the reader with the solid foundation needed to understand the more detailed and complex discussions that follow in later sections of the book.

Chapter 2, Clinical Coding and Coding Compliance, presents baseline information about today's approved code sets and their functionality and explains the complex interrelationships between reimbursement, coded data, and compliance with the rules and regulations of public and private third party payers.

Chapter 3, Voluntary Healthcare Insurance Plans, explains private or commercial healthcare insurance plans and Blue Cross/Blue Shield plans, and provides the reader with a detailed understanding of the sections of a healthcare insurance policy.

Chapter 4, Government-Sponsored Healthcare Programs, differentiates among the various government-sponsored healthcare programs in effect today, explains the impact that these programs have had on the American healthcare system, and presents the history of Medicare and Medicaid programs in America.

Chapter 5, Managed Care Plans, describes the origins, evolution, and principles of managed care and discusses the numerous types of plans that have emerged through the integration of administrative, financial, and clinical systems to both deliver and finance healthcare services.

Chapter 6, Medicare-Medicaid Prospective Payment Systems (PPSs) for Inpatients, explains common models and policies of payment for inpatient

Medicare and Medicaid prospective payment systems and defines basic language associated with reimbursement under PPSs in acute care hospitals and inpatient skilled nursing, long-term care, rehabilitation, and psychiatric facilities.

Chapter 7, Ambulatory and Other Medicare-Medicaid Reimbursement Systems, explains common models and policies of payment for Medicare and Medicaid healthcare payment systems for physicians and outpatient settings, which include physician offices, ambulance services, ambulatory surgery centers, hospital outpatient services, and home health agencies.

Chapter 8, Revenue Cycle Management, explains the components of the revenue cycle, defines revenue cycle management, and describes the connection between effective revenue cycle management and providers' fiscal stability.

A complete glossary of reimbursement terminology is included at the end of the book. Throughout the text chapters, boldface type is used to indicate the first substantial reference to key terms included in the glossary. A detailed content index is also included at the conclusion of the text.

Notes to educators:

Each chapter contains "Check Your Understanding" questions for discussion and/or to help the reader in focusing on important points within the text. The answers to these questions are included at the end of the book.

Review quizzes also follow each chapter. The answer key for the review quizzes is available to instructors in online format from the individual book pages in the AHIMA Bookstore or through the Assembly on Education (AOE) Community of Practice (CoP).

Instructors who are AHIMA members can sign up for this private community by clicking on the help icon with the CoP home page and requesting additional information on becoming an AOE CoP member. An instructor who is not an AHIMA member or a member who is not an instructor may contact the publisher at publications@ahima.org. The instructor materials are not available to students enrolled in college or university programs.

Chapter 1
Healthcare Reimbursement Methodologies

Objectives

- To use basic language associated with health-care reimbursement methodologies

- To differentiate payment methods on unit of payment, timeframe, and risk

- To distinguish major payment methods in the United States

Key Terms

Allowable fee
Block grant
Capitation
Case-based payment
Cases
Charges
Claim
Copayments
CPR
Deductibles
Episode-of-care reimbursement
Fee
Fee schedule
Fee-for-service reimbursement
Global payment method
Guarantors
Insurance
Per-diem payment
Premium
Prospective payment method
Providers
Reimbursement
Resource-based relative value scale
Retrospective payment method
Risk pool
Self-insured plan
Third party payers
Third party payment
UCR

Introduction to Healthcare Reimbursement

The healthcare system of the United States (U.S.) is complex. New payment methods and rules contribute to the complexity. In 1999, this complexity was listed as one of five trends threatening the very future of medicine (Washburn 1999, 34). For example, a physician's office might have "at least a dozen separate contracts for providing healthcare services" (Washburn 1999, 35). Surely, if "insiders" find the system confusing, "outsiders," the patients, confront a veritable maze.

Health Insurance

Generally, reimbursement for healthcare services is dependent upon patients having health **insurance.** Insurance is a system of reducing a person's exposure to risk of loss by having another party (insurance company or insurer) assume the risk. In healthcare, the risk the healthcare insurance company assumes is the unknown cost of healthcare for a person or group of persons.

However, the insurance company that assumes the risk reduces its own risk by distributing the risk among a larger group of persons (insureds). This group of persons has similar risks of loss and is known as a **risk pool.** In healthcare, the variability of health statuses across many people allows the healthcare insurance company to make a better estimate of the average costs of healthcare.

The insurance company, though, receives a **premium** payment in return for assuming the insureds' exposure to risk of loss. The premium payments for all the insureds in the group are pooled. Insurers use actuarial data to calculate the premiums so that the pool is sufficiently large to pay losses of the entire group. Thus, specific to healthcare, the risk is the potential that a person will get sick or require health services and will incur bills (costs) associated with his or her treatment or services. The premium payments for health insurance are calculated

to pay for all the potential covered healthcare costs for an entire group of patients.

Historical Perspectives

Health insurance in the U.S. has been made available to help offset the expenses of the treatment of illness and injury. The first "sickness" clause was inserted in an insurance document in 1847. However, health insurance did not become established until 1929, when Blue Cross first covered school teachers in Texas. In 1932, a city-wide plan was begun in Sacramento, California. As an industry, health insurance became widespread after World War II (Longest, Rakich, and Darr 2000, 89–90).

Health Insurance and Employment

In the U.S. health insurance is usually tied to employment. Many larger employers as part of a package of employment benefits pay a portion of the health insurance premium. Employees may be required to pay extra for health insurance for their spouse or children (dependent coverage). Medicare is also considered insurance because payroll taxes, through both employers' and employees' contributions, finance one portion of Medicare coverage. Premiums paid by eligible individuals and matched by the federal government also finance Medicare's supplemental medical insurance program.

When people lose their jobs, they often lose their health insurance. Although people can continue their health insurance by paying for the insurance entirely by themselves, the payments are expensive, and people can only extend their health insurance for a limited period. Therefore, people without jobs are unlikely to have adequate health insurance.

For some employed people, the adequacy of the health insurance is an issue. Some health insurance plans require patients or their families to pay 20 percent or more of the costs of their healthcare. Healthcare costs can easily be in the thousands of dollars; 20 percent of $10,000 is $2,000—a sizable sum for many people. Other employees work for employers that do not offer health benefits. These persons must purchase their own insurance, at an extremely high rate, or have no health insurance. Obtaining and retaining adequate health insurance are problems for many U.S. workers.

Compensation for Healthcare

Reimbursement is the healthcare term that refers to the compensation or repayment for health-care services. Reimbursement is being repaid or compensated for expenses already incurred or, as in the case of healthcare, for services that have already been provided. In healthcare, services are often provided before payment is made. Unlike the car dealership, in which customers pay for a car or arrange a loan before driving the car off the lot, patients walk out of the hospital treated. Therefore, the physicians and clinics must seek to be paid back for services that they have already provided and for expenses, such as supplies, that they have already incurred. These physicians, clinics, hospitals, and other healthcare organizations and practitioners are requesting reimbursement for health services.

Third Party Payment

Experts in healthcare finance refer to **third party payment** or **third party payers.** Who or what are these parties? The first party is the patient himself or herself or the person, such as a parent, responsible for the patient's health bill. The second party is the physician, clinic, hospital, nursing home, or other healthcare entity rendering the care. These second parties are often called **providers** because they provide healthcare. The third party is the uninvolved insurance company or health agency that pays the physician, clinic, or other second party provider for the care or services to the first party (patient).

Characteristics of Reimbursement Methodologies

Three characteristics describe various methods of healthcare reimbursement. These characteristics are the unit of payment, the time orientation, and the degree of financial risk for the parties (Wouters, Bennett, and Leighton 1998, 3). The unit of payment can range from a payment for each service, such as a payment for each laboratory test, to a block payment for an entire population for a period of time, such as a governmental budget transfer to the state health department. The time orientation is retrospective versus prospective. In retrospective payment methods, the payer learns of the costs of the health services after the patient has already received the services. The provider also receives payment after the services have been provided. In a prospective payment method, the payments are preset before care is delivered. Financial risk refers back to the definition of health insurance. When the costs of health services are learned after the care is provided, the third party payer (health insurance entity) is at risk. When providers must project the costs of treating patients into the future and contract to provide all care for those estimated costs, the provider is at risk. Patients assume risk as they must pay higher and higher percentages of the costs as their share.

Types of Healthcare Reimbursement Methodologies

This chapter discusses the fundamental concepts in healthcare reimbursement methodologies. The chapter is organized by the two major types of unit of payment: **fee-for-service reimbursement** or **episode-of-care reimbursement.** Also briefly addressed are the other characteristics of healthcare payment methods—time frame and risk. The chapter concludes with a peek into the future of healthcare reimbursement.

Fee-for-Service Reimbursement

Fee-for-service reimbursement is a healthcare payment method in which providers receive payment for each service rendered. Fee-for-service is a common method of calculating healthcare reimbursement.

A **fee** is a set amount or a set price. Fee-for-service means a specific payment is made for each specific service provided ("rendered"). In the fee-for-service method, the provider of the healthcare service (the second party) charges a fee for each type of service, and the health insurance company pays each fee for a covered service. These fees or prices are known as **charges** in healthcare. Sometimes, there is little relationship between the actual costs to provide a service and its charge.

Typically, the physician, healthcare organization, or other practitioner bills for each service provided on a **claim** that lists the fees or charges for each service. The claim is sent to the third party payer (health insurance company or health agency). In healthcare, sending the claim to the third party payer is known as submitting a claim. Within the stipulations of the health insurance policy (contract) or the governmental regulations, the third party pays the claim. The majority of U.S. physicians use this method of billing.

People who have health insurance that reimburses on the basis of fee-for-service have the advantage of great independence. Their health insurance plans allow them to make almost all health decisions about which physician to see and about which conditions to have treated. The patient or the provider submits a claim to the health insurance company, and, if the service is covered in the health insurance policy, the patient or provider receives reimbursement. For the patient, the disadvantage of fee-for service is that fee-for-service plans often have higher **deductibles** or **copayments** than other types of health insurance, such as managed care plans.

For health insurance plans, fee-for-service has the disadvantage of uncertainty. The costs of reimbursing the providers are unknown because the services that patients will receive are unknown. Moreover, costs will increase if the providers increase the fees for each service, if patients receive more services than expected, and if more expensive services are substituted for less expensive services. Examples of fee-for-service reimbursement are self-pay, retrospective payment, and managed care.

Self-Pay

Self-pay is a type of fee-for-service because the patients or their **guarantors** (responsible persons, such as parents for children) pay a specific amount for each service received. The patients or guarantors make such payments themselves to the providers, such as physicians, clinics, or hospitals, that rendered each service. The patients or guarantors then seek reimbursement from their private health insurance or the governmental agency that covers their health benefits.

As previously discussed, some patients and guarantors do not have health insurance. These patients have not made advanced payments via an insurance premium. For these individuals, self-pay results because they lack health insurance or benefits under governmental health programs.

In self-pay, patients pay for all the costs of their healthcare themselves. Some may seek recompense from a third party payer and others may bear the burden of the costs of their healthcare themselves.

A related concept is the **self-insured plan.** A self-insured plan is one in which the employer eliminates the "middle-man." The employer administers its own health insurance benefits. Rather than shift the risk to a health insurance entity, the employer (or other entity, such as a professional association) assumes the costs of healthcare for its employees or members and their dependents.

Traditional Retrospective Payment

The **retrospective payment method** of reimbursement pays providers after the services have been rendered. Retrospective reimbursement is a type of fee-for-service because the providers are reimbursed for each service rendered. Third party payers reimburse providers for costs or charges previously incurred. The reimbursement payments are based on the charges for the services provided.

This method has historically been the traditional method of reimbursement.

Fee Schedules

In a fee-for-service environment, third party payers establish a **fee schedule.** A fee schedule is a predetermined list of fees that the third party payer allows for payment for all healthcare services. The **allowable fee** represents the average or maximum amount the third party payer will reimburse providers for the service.

Discounted Fee-for-Service Payments

To begin to control costs, the third party payers negotiated reduced fees for their members or insureds. The payment method using these reduced fees is known as discounted fee-for-service. Versions of the discounted fee-for-service payment method are the **UCR,** the **CPR,** and the **resource-based relative value scale** (RBRVS) (Blount and Waters 2001, 6).

UCR stands for usual, customary, and reasonable. "Usual" is for usual in the provider's practice; "customary" is for customary in the community; and "reasonable" is for reasonable for the situation. CPR stands for customary, prevailing, and reasonable. The UCR and the CPR were methods of payment within the type of traditional retrospective payment. Both methods were based on data from past claims. Private insurance companies used the UCR method. Medicare prior to the implementation of its current payment methods employed CPR.

Established in 1992, the resource-based relative value scale (RBRVS) is a discounted fee schedule that Medicare uses to reimburse physicians. The RBRVS is a payment method that classifies health services based on the cost of providing physician services in terms of effort, practice expenses (overhead), and malpractice insurance.

Uncertainty for Third Party Payers

For third party payers, the retrospective fee-for-service payment method has the disadvantage of great uncertainty. The payers have no way of knowing the total charges that will be incurred and for which they must reimburse the providers.

Managed Care Methods

In managed care reimbursement methods (discussed fully in Chapter 5), third party payers "manage" both the costs of healthcare and the outcomes of care. In managed care plans, the third party payer has implemented some provisions to control the costs of healthcare while maintaining quality care.

Features of Managed Care

Common features of managed care include:

- Comprehensiveness
- Coordination and planning
- Education of patients and providers
- Assessment of quality
- Control of costs

Purposes of Managed Care

The two purposes of the management or control are to (1) reduce the costs of healthcare for which the third party payer must reimburse the providers and (2) ensure continuing quality of care.

Managed care payers have instituted many means to control the costs and quality of healthcare. One example of a provision is the requirement that patients obtain prior approvals for surgeries. Another example is a hybrid of the discounted fee-based system in which the payer reimburses the provider up to a percentage of the allowable fee and the insured must pay the remaining percentage (Koch 2002, 109). Finally, having one primary care provider to coordinate all aspects of healthcare supports the quality of healthcare by reducing fragmentation and enhancing integration.

Forms of Managed Care

There are numerous forms of managed care. These forms include health maintenance organizations (HMOs), exclusive provider organizations (EPOs), point-of-service plans (POSs), and preferred provider organizations (PPOs). One can imagine these forms as a continuum of control with the HMOs representing the most controlled and the PPOs representing the least controlled.

Criticisms of Managed Care
Some critics of managed care argue that managed care too severely limits the following capabilities:

- Patients' access to care and their freedom to choose healthcare providers

- Providers' ability to order diagnostic tests and therapeutic procedures

These critics contend that administrators rather than medical and health personnel are making decisions about patients' health futures.

In general, in a fee-for-service environment, providers are reimbursed for each service they provide. In a fee-for-service environment, the more services a provider renders, the more reimbursement the provider receives. Some experts contend that fee-for-service reimbursement inappropriately inflates the costs of health care because the payment method rewards providers for more services, whether or not these services are warranted.

Episode-of-Care Reimbursement

Episode-of-care reimbursement is a healthcare payment method in which providers receive one lump sum for all the services they provide related to a condition or disease. In the episode-of-care payment method, the unit of payment is the episode, not each individual health service. Therefore, the episode-of-care payment method eliminates individual fees or charges. The episode-of-care payment method is an attempt to correct perceived faults in the fee-for-service reimbursement method. Thus, the episode-of-care reimbursement method controls costs on a grand or systematic scale.

An episode of care is the health services that a patient receives:

- For a particular health condition or illness

- During a period of relatively continuous care from a provider

In the episode of care, one amount is set for all the care associated with the condition or illness. Forms of episode-of-care reimbursement are **capitation,** global payment, and prospective payment.

Occasionally, an episode of care is defined as a specific number of days. The federal government's payment method for home care services is an example. The per-episode home health payment covers all home care services and nonroutine medical supplies delivered to the patient during a 60-day period.

Capitated Payment Method
Capitation is a method of payment for health services in which the third party payer reimburses providers a fixed, per capita amount for a period. "Per capita" means "per head" or "per person." A common phrase in capitated contracts is "per member per month" (PMPM). The PMPM is the amount of money paid each month for each individual enrolled in the health insurance plan. Capitation is characteristic of health maintenance organizations.

In capitation, the actual volume or intensity of services provided to each patient has no effect on the payment. More services do not increase the payment, nor do fewer services decrease the payment. If the provider contracts with a third party payer to provide services to a group of workers for a capitated rate, the provider receives the payments for each member of the group regardless of whether all the members receive the provider's services. There are no adjustments for the complexity or extent of the health services.

Example:
Z Company has a health insurance plan for its workers and their families through Wellness Health Maintenance Organization (HMO). Wellness HMO has contracted with Dr. T to provide health services (care) to

members of the Z Company group for the capitated rate of $15 per month ($15 PMPM).

Dr. T is under contract to receive $15 per month for every member of the Z group. The members of the Z group total 100. Each month Dr. T receives $1,500 ($15 × 100 members) from Wellness HMO for the Z group. Dr. T receives $1,500 whether no members of the group see him in clinic or all the members of the group see him in clinic. Dr. T receives $1,500 whether all the members receive complex care for cancer or all the members receive simple care for preventive flu shots.

The advantages of capitated payment are that (1) the third party payer has no uncertainty and (2) the provider has a guaranteed customer base. The third party payer knows exactly what the costs of healthcare for the group will be and the providers know that they will have a certain group of customers. However, for the provider, there is also great uncertainty because the patients' usage of provider services is unknown and the complexity and cost of the services are unknowns.

Global Payment Method

In the **global payment method,** the third party payer makes one combined payment to cover the services of multiple providers who are treating a single episode of care. Thus, this payment method consolidates payments. A **block grant** is a fixed amount of money given or allocated for a specific purpose. For example, in a block grant there is a transfer of governmental funds to cover health services. In the global payment method, there is no additional payment for higher volumes of services or more expensive or complex services.

Medicare's payment system for home health services is an example of a global payment method. Various types of home health services are consolidated into the single payment. These services include all speech therapy, physical therapy, and occupational therapy; skilled nursing visits; home health aide visits; medical social services, and nonroutine medical supplies.

The most comprehensive version of the global payment system is the total-episode-of-care. For an episode of care, the total-episode-of-care payment rate is a single price that covers costs across the continuum of care, which could include all of the following:

- Facility costs across the continuum of care, such as hospital, nursing home, clinic, and outpatient rehabilitation

- Technical and professional components of procedures in radiology, pathology, and the laboratory

- Physician professional fees for anesthesia, surgery, and consultation

- Home care costs

Less comprehensive versions of the global payment method exist. For example, some global payment methods include only ambulatory costs or only inpatient costs. These methods are termed ambulatory-episode-of-care and inpatient-episode-of-care, respectively. Another less comprehensive version is a global surgical package. The global surgical package encompasses the operation, local or topical anesthesia, a preoperative clinic visit, immediate postoperative care, and usual postoperative follow-up. In the special-procedure package, all the costs associated with a diagnostic or therapeutic procedure are included in the payment. Examples include extracorporeal shock wave lithotripsy and vasectomy. An ambulatory-visit package includes all ambulatory services, including the physicians' charges, laboratory tests, x-rays, and other ambulatory services associated with one clinic visit. The per-episode home health payment is also a less comprehensive global payment rate. The single payment covers all home care services and nonroutine medical supplies that a patient receives during a 60-day period.

As can be seen, third party payers and providers have created multiple variations of the global payment method. The multiple variations, however, have added to the complexity of healthcare reimbursement.

Prospective Payment Methods

In the **prospective payment method,** payment rates for healthcare services are established in advance for a specific time period. The predetermined rates are based on average levels of resource use for certain types of healthcare. It is important to note that prospective payment methods are based upon averages. On individual patients, providers can lose money or make money, but, over time, providers should come out even. Payment is determined by the resource needs of the average patient for a (a) set period of time or (b) given set of conditions or diseases. Prospective payment methods representing these two situations are **per-diem payment** and **case-based payment,** respectively.

Providers are paid the pre-established rates regardless of the costs they actually incur. Therefore, prospective payment is another method in which the actual number or intensity of the services does not affect a pre-established compensation. The intent of prospective payment methods is to reduce the likelihood that charges or costs will increase because limits on payments are pre-set for the future time period.

Per-Diem Payment

Per diem or per day (daily rate) is a limited type of prospective payment method. The third party payer reimburses the provider a fixed rate for each day a covered member is hospitalized. The Indian Health Service and some supplemental health insurance plans use per-diem methods. Traditionally, the per-diem payment method has been used to reimburse providers for inpatient hospital services.

Third party payers set the per-diem rates using historical data. For example, to establish an inpatient per diem, the total costs for all inpatient services for a population during a period are divided by the sum of the lengths of stay in the period. To determine the payment, the per-diem rate is multiplied by the number of days of hospitalization. In the absence of

historical data, third party payers and providers must consider several factors to establish per-diem rates. These factors include costs, lengths of stay, volumes of service, and patients' severity of illness.

Critics of the per-diem payment method contend that the method encourages providers to increase the number of inpatient admissions, to extend the lengths of stay, or both. These strategies would result in increased reimbursements. Another prospective payment method, case-based reimbursement, corrects the flaws perceived in the per-diem payment method.

Case-Based Payment

In the case-based payment method, providers receive a fixed, preestablished payment for each case. **Cases** are patients, residents, or clients who receive health services for a condition or disease. Third party payers reimburse providers for each case rather than for each service (fee-for-service) or per diem.

Example:

Two patients were hospitalized with pneumonia. One patient was hospitalized for three days and the other patient was hospitalized for thirty days. Each patient is a case. The third party payer has established a payment rate for cases with pneumonia. The hospital would receive two payments, exactly the same, for the two cases.

The payment is determined by the historical resource needs of the average patient for a given set of conditions or diseases. Case-based payment can be one flat rate per case or can be multiple rates that represent categories of cases (sets of conditions or diseases).

An example of the case-based payment system built on categories of cases is Medicare's method of payment for inpatient hospital services (prospective payment system; PPS). This method of payment is based on categories of payment called "diagnosis related groups" (DRGs). Each DRG categorizes patients who are homogeneous in terms of clinical profiles and requisite resources. Thus, patients classified to the same group have similar diagnoses and treatments, consumption of resources, and lengths of stay. Each DRG has a payment rate called a "weight." Weights are relative to one another. Higher weights are associated with groups in which patients require more resources for care and treatment. Higher resource consumption is related to higher intensity of services due to the severity of illness or the types of services needed for care and treatment, such as expensive equipment or medications. Higher weights translate into higher payments.

Several U.S. federal payment methods are case-based prospective payment methods. (See table 1.1 for a comparison of federal prospective payment systems.)

In summary, the relatively weighted group is the basic unit of payment. Higher relative weights link to higher payment rates.

Criticisms of Episode-of-Care Reimbursement

The impact of the case-based payment method is that it rewards effective and efficient delivery of health services and penalizes ineffective and inefficient delivery. The case-based payment rates are based on averages of costs for patients within the group. Generally, costs for providers that treat patients efficiently and effectively are beneath the average costs. The providers make money in this situation. On the other hand, providers that typically exceed average costs lose money. Inefficiencies include duplicate laboratory work, scheduling delays, and lost reports. Many healthcare organizations have implemented procedures to streamline the delivery of health services to offset inefficiencies. Poor clinical diagnostic skills are an example of ineffectiveness. Thus, the more efficiently and effectively a provider delivers care, the greater its operating margin will be.

Some consumer advocates have voiced concerns about episode-of-care reimbursement. These advocates have noted that the payment method creates incentives to substitute less expensive diagnostic and therapeutic procedures and laboratory and radiologic tests and to delay or deny proce-

Table 1.1.   Federal prospective payment systems

Site	System	Relative Weighted Group	Abbreviation	Effective Date
Ambulatory Surgery Center	Ambulatory surgery center (ASC) payment method	Ambulatory surgery center group	ASC group	1980
Inpatient Acute Care Hospital	Prospective payment system (PPS)	Diagnosis related group	DRG	October 1, 1983
Skilled Nursing Facility	Skilled nursing facility prospective payment system (SNF PPS)	Resource utilization group, version III	RUG III	July 1, 1998
Home Health Agency	Home health prospective payment system (HHPPS)	Home health resource group	HHRG	October 1, 2000
Outpatient Hospital Service	Outpatient prospective payment system (OPPS)	Ambulatory payment classification group	APC group	October 1, 2001
Inpatient Rehabilitation Facility	Inpatient rehabilitation facility prospective payment system (IRF PPS)	Case mix group	CMG	January 1, 2002
Long Term Care Hospital	Long term care hospital prospective payment system (LTCH PPS)	Diagnosis related group	DRG	October 1, 2002

dures and treatments. Healthcare analysts, on the other hand, point out the savings associated with eliminating wasteful or unnecessary procedures and tests and that volume and expense do not necessarily define quality.

Check Your Understanding 1.1

1. Insurers pool premium payments for all the insureds in a group, then use actuarial data to calculate the group's premiums so that:
    a. Premium payments are lowered for insurance plan payers
    b. The pool is large enough to pay losses of the entire group
    c. Accounting for the group's plan is simplified
    d. All of the above are reasons for using the data

2. Where and when did health insurance become established in the U.S.?

3. All of the following are types of episode-of-care reimbursement **except:**
    a. Global payment
    b. Prospective payment
    c. Capitation
    d. Self-insured plan

4. What discounted fee schedule does Medicare use to reimburse physicians?

5. Name and describe some versions of the global payment method.

Future of Healthcare Reimbursement Methodologies

The prospective payment system (PPS) for inpatient hospital services that Medicare implemented in 1983 proved to be very successful. Based on that success, many future healthcare reimbursement methodologies are refinements and derivations of the PPS. This section addresses three of these future payment methods: physician care groups, refinements in case-based payment methods, and clinical risk groups.

Physician Care Groups

Physician care groups (PCGs) is a prospective payment method for physician services in ambulatory settings. This method classifies patients into similar, homogenous categories (groups). PCGs are visit-based and classify services according to clinical similarity and setting (Averill et al. 1999). Proponents of the PCG payment method emphasize that the basis of payment is the purpose of the visit, necessitating clear definition of the patient's problem (Averill et al. 1999). The various ambulatory settings included in this payment method are "physician offices, hospital outpatient departments, hospital emergency rooms, ambulatory surgical centers, community mental health centers, comprehensive outpatient rehabilitation facilities, state or local public health facilities, and rural health clinics" (Averill et al. 1999, 4).

The payment method accounts for resource use in terms of (1) physician's (professional) services, (2) technical services (equipment and technicians), (3) interpretation (by the same physician or another physician), (4) facility overhead, and (5) ancillary services (laboratory tests) (Averill et al. 1999, 4–5). It is important to note the payment method also accounts for differences in resource use across ambulatory settings. Averill and colleagues explain that settings vary in terms of consuming the five components (1999, 4–5).

Example:

Patient A is seen in a hospital outpatient department for pneumonia. The hospital bills the third party payer for the facility overhead, technical services, interpretation, and ancillary services. The PCG for the physician's services include only the physician's professional services. However, if the same physician sees Patient A in her clinic instead of the hospital outpatient department, the PCG needs to account for resources for all five components (physician's services, technical services, interpretation, facility overhead, and ancillary services; Averill et al. 1999, 4–5).

The PCGs simplify payments to physicians for ambulatory services because there are about 400 PCGs compared to the more than 4,000 types of health services in the RBRVS payment method (Averill et al. 1999, 12). Each PCG has a predetermined relative weight. For ambulatory services, it is envisioned that PCG payment method could replace the federal government's RBRVS payment method.

Refined Case-Based Payment

Refined case-based payment methods enhance case-based payment methods to include patients from all age groups and from regions of the world with varying mixes of diseases and differing patterns of healthcare delivery. In the U.S., projects investigated means to enhance the inpatient PPS, the diagnosis related groups (DRGs). In its enhanced versions, the payment system is applicable to all types of patients, not the mostly elderly patients as covered by the DRGs. For international use, researchers created a classification method that, independent of coding system, measured patients' severity of illness and consumption of resources (Mullin et al. 2002).

Pediatric Modified Diagnosis Related Groups

In the mid-1980s, the National Association of Children's Hospitals and Related Institutions developed pediatric modified diagnosis related groups (PM-DRGs). This classification had classifications for neonates and pediatric patients (Averill et al. 2002, 46).

All-Patient Diagnosis Related Groups

In the late 1980s, the New York State Health Department contracted with researchers at 3M Health Information Systems (3M HIS) to develop a DRG payment method for non-Medicare patients. Including the PM-DRGs, the researchers developed the all-patient DRGs (AP-DRGs; Averill et al. 2002). AP-DRGs included classifications for neonatal patients, pediatric patients, high-risk obstetrical patients, multiple trauma patients, organ transplant patients, and ventilator-dependent patients. In addition, groups were created for patients with the following conditions or diseases: human immunodeficiency virus (HIV), cystic fibrosis, nutritional disorders, acute leukemia, hemophilia, and sickle cell anemia. Some Medicaid programs and Blue Cross plans adopted AP-DRGs. The Centers for Medicare and Medicaid Services (CMS) also later modified and adopted some of these refinements (Averill et al. 2002) for the inpatient PPS.

All-Patient Refined Diagnosis Related Groups

In the mid-1990s, continuing research and refinement by the 3M HIS team resulted in all-patient refined DRGs (APR-DRGs). The refinement is the inclusion of adjustments for severity of illness and risk of mortality. These adjustments result in 1,422 APR-DRGs. The classification method allows accurate comparisons of patients in terms of length of stay, resource consumption, and outcomes. "Through APR-DRGs, hospitals, consumers, payers, and regulators can gain an understanding of the patients being treated, the costs incurred, and within reasonable limits, the outcomes expected" (Averill et al. 2002, 50). Developers of the classification system suggest that, through APR-DRGs, organizational leaders can increase organizational efficiency and effectiveness as well as quality of care.

International Refined Diagnosis Related Groups

At the global level, the 3M HIS researchers developed a classification system that could be used within countries to describe patients' resource use and around the world to compare patients from one country to another (Mullin et al. 2002, 1). The international refined DRGs (IR-DRGs) are an inpatient classification system designed specifically to become the basis for payment, "budgeting, outcomes analysis, benchmarking, profiling, and utilization assessment" of international healthcare (Mullin et al. 2002, 3). There are 939 IR-DRGs reflecting severity of illness and resource consumption. The classification system provides healthcare decision makers with "a means of making relative comparisons of the resources patients consume and their associated clinical courses" (Mullin et al. 2002, 2).

Clinical Risk Groups

The methodology of clinical risk groups (CRGs) is a prospective payment system that predicts future healthcare expenditures. It is a capitated payment system for healthcare services for populations (Averill et al. 2001, 8). Its developers state that the methodology is a means to administer clinical pathways, product line management, and case management (Averill et al. 2001).

The payment method adjusts for risk and supports the clinical management of patients (Averill et al. 2001). CRGs classify patients into categories that account for the severity of the patient's illness or condition and that predict the costs of future medical care, debility, or death (Averill et al. 2001). To predict future healthcare expenditures, CRGs are assigned prior to health services being rendered. Moreover, CRGs predict costs for "an extended period of time" (Averill et al. 2001, 2).

CRGs include all age groups and cover the continuum of care. There are 1,075 CRGs (Averill et al. 2001, 8). These 1,075 CRGs are organized into the following nine statuses:

- Catastrophic conditions

- Dominant and metastatic malignancies

- Dominant chronic disease in three or more organ systems

- Significant chronic disease in multiple organ systems

- Single dominant or moderate chronic disease

- Minor chronic disease in multiple organ systems

- Single minor chronic disease

- History of significant acute disease

- Healthy

The 1,075 CRGs are not distributed evenly across the nine statuses. The status with the fewest CRGs is "Healthy" with one; the status with the most CRGs is "Single dominant or moderate chronic disease" with 398. Within these statuses, the severity-of illness level can range from none (healthy) to 6 (catastrophically ill) (Averill et al. 2001, table 1.1). According to Averill, "The severity level describes the extent and progression of the disease. A high level of severity is indicative of a high degree of treatment difficulty and a need for substantial future medical care" (Averill et al. 2001, 6).

Research has supported the ability of CRGs to identify patients who will require interaction with the health care system (Neff et al., 2002; 2004). Neff et al. found that CRGs were a useful tool to identify, classify, and stratify children with chronic health conditions. Thus, CRGs were found to support patient tracking, case management, utilization, and cost prediction (Neff et al., 2002; 2004).

To facilitate decision making, the CRGs can be collapsed into three hierarchical tiers of aggregate groups. Each tier of aggregate clinical risk groups (ACRGs) has fewer groups and less clinical precision. Thus, ACRG1 has the greatest number of CRGs, with 413, and ACRG3 the fewest, with 37 (Averill et al. 2001, 8). However, each tier of aggregation maintains clinical meaningfulness and severity levels. Thus, the classification system supports the various levels of detail needed by payers and providers (Averill et al. 2001).

The payment weights are calculated based on two years of historical data. The first year's data serves to classify the patient into a CRG. Averages of the second year's data are computed to set the weights of the CRGs. The second year's data predicts healthcare expenditures for patients in the CRG (Averill et al. 2001, 9). Higher weights correspond to higher severity levels. As a payment method, CRGs predict future consumption of healthcare resources. Their clinical precision and meaningfulness enable them to be used to manage care and their categorical nature serves as a means of reporting and communication. Finally, research has demonstrated that CRGs are able to predict payments comparable to other risk adjustment systems (Hughes et al. 2004).

Summary

The U.S. healthcare system is complex, partially because health insurance and employment are closely linked. Multiple methods exist to reimburse hospitals, physicians, and other health providers for the healthcare they render patients. Because recompense occurs after the healthcare has been provided, the term used is reimbursement. Two major types of payment methodologies—fee-for-service reimbursement and episode-of-care reimbursement—are based upon the unit of payment. Other descriptive characteristics of healthcare payment methods are time frame and bearer of risk. Important contemporary reimbursement methods are retrospective fee-for-service, managed care, capitation, global payments, and prospective payment systems. Researchers and government health agencies continue to develop and advance payment methods, both in the U.S. and internationally. Healthcare professionals need to monitor the continuing evolution of healthcare reimbursement methodologies.

Chapter 1 Review Quiz

1. Who are the first, second, and third parties in healthcare situations?

2. Compare the UCR and CPR payment systems.

3. Describe the two purposes of managed care.

4. Why have many insurers replaced retrospective health insurance plans with group plans such as HMOs and PPOs?

5. What are advantages of capitated payments for providers and payers?

6. How do third party payers set per-diem payment rates?

7. Describe the major benefits of episode-of-care reimbursement according to its advocates and the major concerns about episode-of-care reimbursement expressed by its critics.

8. How does the payment method used by physician care groups (PCGs) account for resources used in patient care?

9. In the episode-of-care reimbursement approach, providers are reimbursed a lump sum for all provided services related to a patient's condition or disease. True or false?

10. How do clinical risk groups (CRGs) manage healthcare costs?

References and Bibliography

Averill, R. F., J. Eisenhandler, N. I. Goldfield, J. S. Hughes, D. E. Gannon, B. V. Shafir, and L. W. Gregg. 1999. The development of a prospective payment system for ambulatory professional services. 3M HIS Research Report 3–99. Available online from www.3m.com/us/healthcare/his/pdf/reports/pcg-article399.pdf.

Averill, R. F., N. I. Goldfield, J. Eisenhandler, J. S. Hughes, and J. Muldoon. 2001. Clinical risk groups and the future of healthcare reimbursement. In *Reimbursement Methodologies for Healthcare Services* [CD-ROM], edited by L. M. Jones. Chicago: American Health Information Management Association.

Averill, R. F., N. I. Goldfield, J. Muldoon, B. A. Steinbeck, and T. M. Grant. 2002. A closer look at all-patient refined DRGs. *Journal of American Health Information Management Association* 73 (1): 46–50.

Blount, L. L., and J. M. Waters. 2001. *Managing the Reimbursement Process.* 3rd ed. Chicago: AMA Press.

Hughes, J. S., R. F. Averill, J. Eisenhandler, N. I. Goldfield, J. Muldoon, J. M. Neff, and J. C. Gay. 2004. Clinical risk groups (CRGs): A classification system for risk-adjusted capitation-based payment and health care management. *Medical Care* 42 (1): 81–90.

Koch, A. L. 2002. Financing health services. In *Introduction to Health Services.* 6th ed., edited by S. J. Williams and P. R. Torrens. Albany, N.Y.: Delmar.

Longest, B. B., J. S. Rakich, and K. Darr. 2000. *Managing Health Services Organizations and Systems.* 4th ed. Baltimore: Health Professions Press.

Mullin, R., J. Vertrees, R. Freedman, R. Castioni, and A. Tinker. 2002. Case-mix analysis across patient populations and boundaries: A refined classification system defined specifically for international use. 3M HIS Research Report 5–98. Available online from www.3m.com/us/healthcare/his/pdf/reports/ir_drg_whitepaper_09_02.pdf.

Neff, J. M., V. L. Sharp, J. Muldoon, J. Graham, J. Popalisky, and J. C. Gay. 2002. Identifying and classifying children with chronic conditions using administrative data with the clinical risk group classification system. *Ambulatory Pediatrics* 2 (1): 71–79.

Neff, J. M., V. L. Sharp, J. Muldoon, J. Graham, and K. Myers. 2004. Profile of medical charges for children by health status group and severity level in a Washington state health plan. *Health Services Research* 39 (1): 73–89.

Washburn, E. R. 1999. The coming medical apocalypse. *Physician Executive* 25 (1): 34–39.

Wouters, A., S. Bennett, and C. Leighton. 1998. Alternative Payment Methods: Incentives for Improving Health Care Delivery. *PHR Primer for Policymakers.* Available online from www.phrplus.org/Pubs/pps1.pdf.

Chapter 2
Clinical Coding and Coding Compliance

Objectives

- To differentiate the different code sets approved by the Health Insurance Portability and Accountability Act of 1996

- To describe the structure of approved code sets

- To examine coding compliance issues that influence reimbursement

Key Terms

Abuse
AHA Coding Clinic for HCPCS
AHIMA Standards of Ethical Coding
Ambulatory payment classification (APC)
Average length of stay (ALOS)
Balanced Budget Act of 1997 (BBA)
Benchmarking
Case mix index
Centers for Medicare and Medicaid Services (CMS)
Classification system
Coding Clinic for ICD-9-CM
Coding compliance plan
Comorbidity
Compliance
Compliance officer
Compliance program guidance
Complication
CPT Assistant
Current Procedural Terminology (CPT)
Current Procedural Terminology Category I Code
Current Procedural Terminology Category II Code
Current Procedural Terminology Category III Code
Diagnosis related group (DRG)
False Claims Act
Fraud
Health Care Procedure Coding System (HCPCS)
Health Insurance Portability and Accountability Act of 1996 (HIPAA)
Health information technology (HIT)

Hospital Outpatient Prospective Payment System (HOPPS)
Hospital Payment Monitoring Program (HPMP)
International Classification of Diseases, 9th Revision, Clinical Modification (ICD-9-CM)
ICD-9-CM Coordination and Maintenance Committee
Length of stay (LOS)
Local Coverage Determination (LCD)
Local Medical Review Policy (LMRP)
Major diagnostic category (MDC)
Modifier
Mortality
National Center for Health Statistics (NCHS)
National Correct Coding Initiative (NCCI)
National Coverage Determination (NCD)
Office of Inspector General (OIG)
Office of Inspector General Workplan
Operation Restore Trust
Outpatient Service Mix Index (SMI)
Payment Error Prevention Program (PEPP)
Program for Evaluation Payment Patterns Electronic Report (PEPPER)
Quality Improvement Organization (QIO)
Scope of work
Third party payer
Utilization Review Committee
World Health Organization (WHO)

The Clinical Coding–Reimbursement Connection

Simply put, reimbursement is payment to healthcare providers and facilities for services rendered to patients. Communication of the services provided is transmitted from the provider to the **third party payer,** public or private, via coded information. Using standardized coding systems allows for a stable and efficient payment process. Payment methodologies and systems used to determine coverage of services and supplies vary, but the code sets used remain constant across all the different healthcare settings.

One need not be a coding expert per se to be able to understand healthcare reimbursement. However, just using the designated code set is not enough. Physicians and healthcare facilities will receive accurate reimbursement for the services they render to patients only if claims submitted comply with the guidelines and conventions published for the various clinical coding sets. In order to fully understand the intricate workings of the various Medicare prospective payment systems (PPSs) and private payer systems, baseline knowledge of the approved code sets and their functionality is essential. The **Health Insurance Portability and Accountability Act of 1996 (HIPAA)** designated the code sets for healthcare services reporting to public and private insurers. The HIPAA compliant code sets are listed in table 2.1.

The International Classification of Diseases

HIPAA designates the International Classification of Diseases, 9th Revision, Clinical Modification, to report diagnoses in all healthcare settings and procedures for inpatient encounters. (See table 2.1.) The International Classification of Diseases (ICD) coding and **classification system** is used throughout the world for **mortality** reporting. ICD is maintained by the **World Health Organization (WHO)** and is updated approximately every 10 years.

Table 2.1.   HIPAA designated code sets

Provider	Inpatient		Outpatient	
	Diagnosis	Procedure	Diagnosis	Procedure
Physician	ICD-9-CM	CPT	ICD-9-CM	CPT
Facility	ICD-9-CM	ICD-9-CM	ICD-9-CM	HCPCS (CPT and HCPCS Level II)

ICD-10

The current international version of ICD is in the 10th revision and is referred to as ICD-10. The United States, however, adopted the 9th revision of ICD (ICD-9), modified it clinically, and continues to use it as the method for communicating diagnoses and inpatient procedures for public and private reimbursement systems.

ICD-9-CM

This clinical modification (CM) of ICD-9 was developed by the **National Center for Health Statistics (NCHS)** and has been in use since 1979. Although the international version of ICD focuses on acute illnesses and mortality, **ICD-9-CM** was expanded to include morbidity or chronic conditions and procedure reporting.

ICD-9-CM has several uses (AHA Central Office 2004):

- Classifying morbidity and mortality information for statistical purposes

- Classifying diagnosis and procedure information for epidemiological and clinical research

- Indexing of hospital records by disease and surgical procedure

- Reporting information to various healthcare reimbursement systems

- Analyzing resource consumption patterns

- Analyzing adequacy of reimbursement for health services

Providers use ICD-9-CM coding to determine payment categories for various PPSs, including the following:

- Hospital inpatient: Diagnosis related groups (DRGs)

- Hospital rehabilitation: Case mix groups (CMGs)

- Long-term care: Long-term care diagnosis related Groups (LTC-DRGs)

- Home health: Home health resource groups (HHRGs).

Structure of ICD-9-CM
ICD-9-CM contains three volumes:

- The Tabular List of Diseases and Injuries

- The Alphabetic Index to Diseases

- The Classification for Procedures

Table 2.2 lists the contents of each volume.

ICD-9-CM diagnosis codes vary in character length from three to five digits, with a decimal point placed after the third digit. The first three characters are a category code. The fourth and fifth digits are subcategory and subclassification codes that provide the specificity necessary to

accurately describe a patient's clinical condition. (See figure 2.1.)

Procedure codes also vary in length from two to four digits, with the decimal point placed after the second digit. The first two digits for procedures compose the category code and the third and fourth digits are the subcategory and subclassification codes indicating specific details about diagnostic and surgical procedures. (See figure 2.2.) Table 2.3 lists the top 10 diagnosis codes and top 10 procedure codes reported to Medicare for inpatient services in 2003.

Maintenance of ICD-9-CM
The **ICD-9-CM Coordination and Maintenance Committee,** composed of NCHS and the **Centers for Medicare and Medicaid Services (CMS),** is responsible for maintaining the U.S. clinical modification version of the code set. NCHS makes determinations regarding diagnosis issues, whereas CMS maintains the procedures. Advisory in nature, the committee was created in 1985 to discuss possible updates and revisions to ICD-9-CM. Final determinations are made by the director of the NCHS and the administrator of the CMS.

The committee holds public meetings every year in April and December, and suggestions for new codes, modifications, and deletions are submitted

Table 2.2.   ICD-9-CM codebook structure

Volume One—Tabular List of Diseases and Injuries	Volume Two—Alphabetic Index to Diseases	Volume 3—Classification for Procedures
Classification of Diseases and Injuries	Index to Diseases and Injuries	Alphabetic Index to Procedures
Supplementary Classifications	Table of Drugs and Chemicals	Tabular List for Procedures
Appendices	Alphabetic Index to External Causes of Injury and Poisoning	

Figure 2.1.   ICD-9-CM diagnosis code structure

250.41	
250	Diabetes mellitus
250.4	Diabetes with renal manifestations
250.41	Diabetes with renal manifestations, type 1, not stated as uncontrolled

Figure 2.2.   ICD-9-CM procedure code structure

36.01	
36	Operations on vessels of heart
36.0	Removal of coronary artery obstruction and insertion of stent(s)
36.01	Single vessel percutaneous transluminal coronary angioplasty (PTCA) or coronary atherectomy without mention of thrombolytic agent

Table 2.3.   ICD-9-CM codes

Medicare Top 10 Diagnoses by Volume FY 2004		Medicare Top 10 Procedures by Volume FY 2004	
Code	Description	Code	Description
428.0	Congestive heart failure	36.01	PTCA
486	Pneumonia, unspecified	99.04	Transfusion of packed cells
414.01	Coronary atherosclerosis	37.22	Left heart cardiac catheterization
491.21	COPD with exacerbation	81.54	Total knee replacement
V57.89	Encounter for rehabilitation	45.16	Esophagogastroduodenscopy
410.71	Subendocardial infarction	38.93	Venous catheterization
599.0	Urinary tract infection	39.95	Hemodialysis
427.31	Atrial fibrillation	45.13	Esophagogastroduodenscopy
786.59	Chest pain	81.51	Total hip replacement
276.5	Dehydration	88.72	Diagnostic ultrasound of heart

by members of both public and private sectors. Proposals for code changes are submitted prior to the semiannual meetings and include a description of the diagnosis or procedure and rationale for the requested modification. Supporting references, literature, statistics, and cost information may also be submitted. Requests must follow industry-accepted ICD-9-CM coding conventions. Each year after the December meeting the committee determines code modifications that become effective October 1 of the following year. Minutes and proposals for diagnosis issues are located on the NCHS portion of the Centers for Disease Control and Prevention Web site (www.cdc.gov). Minutes and Proposals for procedure issues are located on the CMS Web site (www.cms.hhs.gov).

ICD-9-CM Coding Guidelines

Because ICD-9-CM codes serve as the communication vehicle between providers and insurers, it is vital to follow ICD-9-CM guidelines at all times. Accurate reimbursement is dependent upon timely, accurate, and complete coding of the services and procedures provided to beneficiaries. The Coop-

erating Parties—NCHS, CMS, American Hospital Association (AHA) and American Health Information Management Association (AHIMA)—and the Editorial Advisory Board are responsible for publishing coding guidelines for ICD-9-CM. The coding guidelines are published by the AHA in ***Coding Clinic for ICD-9-CM,*** the only official publication for ICD-9-CM coding guidelines and advice. *Coding Clinic* is published quarterly and includes the following information (AHA Central Office 2004):

- Official coding advice and official coding guidelines

- Correct code assignments for new technologies and newly identified diseases

- Articles and topics which offer practical information and improve data quality

- Coding changes and/or corrections

- "Ask the Editor" questions with practical examples

Coding Clinic should be a component of all coding education and **compliance** programs for healthcare provider and facility coding units.

Healthcare Common Procedural Coding System

The *Healthcare Current Procedural Coding System (HCPCS)* is a two-tiered system of procedural codes used primarily for ambulatory care and physician services. A third tier, pertaining to codes developed by local payers, was eliminated as of December 31, 2003, in compliance with HIPAA standard procedure code requirements. HCPCS codes are frequently attached to inpatient and outpatient charge description masters (CDMs) for convenience and to facilitate communication between providers and payers about services and supplies included in the CPT or HCPCS Level II system.

CPT (HCPCS Level I)

Current Procedural Terminology (CPT®) is used throughout the United States to report diagnostic and surgical services and procedures. Created and first published by the American Medical Association (AMA) in 1966, CPT was designed to be a means of effective and dependable communication among physicians, patients, and third party payers (LaTour/Eichenwald 2002, 264). The terminology provides a uniform coding scheme that accurately describes medical, surgical, and diagnostic services. The CPT coding system is used by physicians to report services and procedures performed in the hospital inpatient and outpatient setting and by facilities for outpatient services and procedures (table 2.1). CPT has several uses:

- Communication vehicle for public and private reimbursement systems

- Development of guidelines for medical care review

- Basis for local, regional, and national utilization comparisons

- Medical education and research

The code set was adopted into the Healthcare Common Procedure Coding System in 1985 and became the HCPCS Level I code set for Medicare reporting. Therefore, CPT is referred to as HCPCS Level I as well as CPT in the coding and reimbursement communities.

Structure of CPT

The terminology is divided into six main sections, known as **Category I codes,** plus two types of supplementary codes (**Category II** and **Category III codes),** and **modifiers.**

Category I CPT codes comprise the following six sections:

- Evaluation and Management

- Anesthesia

- Surgery

- Radiology

- Pathology and Laboratory

- Medicine

The Surgery Section is further divided as follows:

Integumentary System	10021 to 19499
Musculoskeletal System	20000 to 29999
Respiratory System	30000 to 32999
Cardiovascular System	33010 to 39599
Digestive System	40490 to 49999
Urinary System	50010 to 53899
Male Genital System	54000 to 55980
Female Genital System	56405 to 58999
Maternity Care and Delivery	59000 to 59899
Endocrine System	60001 to 60699
Nervous System	61000 to 64999
Eye and Ocular Adnexa	65091 to 68899
Auditory System	69000 to 69979
Operating Microscope	69990

Table 2.4 contains a listing of the top 10 CPT codes reported to Medicare in 2003.

Table 2.4.   CPT codes

Medicare Top 10 Procedures by Unit of Service—CY 2004	
Code	**Description**
85025	Automated hemogram
93005	Electrocardiogram, tracing
71020	Chest x-ray
80048	Basic metabolic panel
80053	Comprehensive metabolic panel
85610	Prothrombin time
99213	Office/outpatient visit, established
88305	Tissue exam by pathologist
99283	Emergency department visit
90784	Injection, IV

Each of the three code categories in the CPT coding system serves a different and unique purpose.

Category I codes describe a procedure or service that is consistent with contemporary medical practice and is performed by many physicians in clinical practice in multiple locations (Beebe 2003, 84). The specific use of devices and drugs for all services in this category must be approved by the Food and Drug Administration (FDA). Category I codes are represented by a five-digit numeric code.

Within Category I codes there are "unlisted" codes. Unlisted codes are used to report services and procedures that are not represented by an existing code. Typically unlisted codes are used for new or innovative procedures that have not been added to the CPT coding system. When an unlisted code is reported, supporting documentation should be submitted to the third party payer to establish correct coding and medical necessity for that service.

Category II codes were created to facilitate data collection for certain services and/or test results that contribute to positive health outcomes and quality patient care (Beebe 2003, 84). This category of codes is a set of optional tracking codes for performance measurement. The services included in this category are often part of the Evaluation and Management service or other component part of a service. Category II codes have been implemented to help medical practices and facilities reduce operational costs by replacing time-consuming medical record documentation reviews and surveys with this streamlined code tracking system (Beebe 2003, 84). Use of Category II codes is optional, and they may not be used as substitutes for Category I codes. Category II codes are represented by a five digit alphanumeric code with the alpha character F in the last position: (1234F).

Category III codes represent emerging technologies. This category of codes was created to help facilitate data collection and assessment of new services and procedures (Beebe, 2003, 85). In order to qualify for inclusion in this category, a service or procedure must have relevance for research, either ongoing or planned. Like Category II codes, Category III codes are represented by an alphanumeric five-digit code with the alpha character T in the last field: (1234T).

In addition to the three categories of codes, CPT contains modifiers for use by physicians and other healthcare providers. A modifier is a two-digit numeric or alphanumeric character designed to give Medicare and other third party payers additional information needed to process a claim. A physician or facility uses a modifier to flag a service provided to a patient that has been altered by some special circumstance(s) but for which the basic code description itself has not changed. Following are common reasons to use a modifier (AMA 2005, xiv):

- A service or procedure has been increased or reduced.
- Only part of a service was performed.
- A bilateral procedure was performed.
- A service or procedure was performed more than once.

- Unusual events occurred during a procedure or service.

Medical record documentation must support the use of a modifier because the modifier may change the reimbursement for the service or procedure. For example, modifier 91 is used to indicate that a clinical laboratory test was repeated. Rules governing the usage of this modifier specify that it may not be used when an equipment or testing failure has occurred, but only when the test has been reordered to determine whether a change in the result has occurred. Therefore, using modifier 91 relays to the third party payer that the duplicate code reporting was not accidental or fraudulent but instead was correct and that the physician ordered the test twice based on medically necessary foundations. However, failure to have supporting documentation in the medical record that establishes medical necessity can result in claim denials and **fraud** or **abuse** penalties.

Maintenance of CPT

The CPT Editorial Research and Development Department supports the modification process for the code set. A sixteen-member CPT Editorial Panel meets four times per year to consider proposals for changes to CPT. The Editorial Panel is supported by the CPT Advisory Committee, which is composed of representatives of more than 90 medical specialty societies and other healthcare professional organizations. To stay current with new technologies and pioneering procedures, CPT is revised each year with changes effective the following January 1.

Requesting a Code Modification for CPT

CPT coding modifications are submitted to the CPT Editorial Research and Development Department at the AMA. The Coding Change Request Form found on the AMA Web site (www.ama-assn.org) must be used and submitted along with supporting documentation and clinical vignettes. A coding modification may be requested for all three categories of codes. Once the Coding Change Request Form is received,

it is reviewed for completeness by the AMA staff. If the form is complete, Coding Charge Request Forms for Category I and Category III codes are forwarded to the CPT Advisory Committee for a detailed review.

Coding Change Request Forms for Category II CPT Codes are sent to the Performance Measurement Advisory Group for review. These requests must receive a two-thirds majority opinion from the advisory group before they are passed on to the CPT Advisory Committee. The AMA established the Performance Measurement Advisory Group to help create and maintain the performance measurement codes (Beebe 2003, 84). The group comprises representatives from various organizations, AMA's CPT and clinical quality improvement staffs, the CPT Editorial Panel, health services researchers, and other knowledgeable experts.

After review by the CPT Advisory Committee, those requests that warrant final review are submitted to the CPT Editorial Panel responsible for final decisions on all coding modifications (AMA 2004). A calendar of regular meetings for the CPT Advisory Committee and the CPT Editorial Panel is posted in the AMA Web site.

CPT Coding Guidelines

The AMA provides several resources regarding the appropriate use of CPT. The official publication for CPT coding issues and guidance is *CPT Assistant* (AMA 1989–2005). *CPT Assistant* contains the following helpful features:

- Coding communication that provides up-to-date information on codes and trends

- Clinical vignettes that offer insight into confusing coding and modifier usage scenarios

- Coding consultation that covers the most frequently asked questions

All coding education and compliance programs should include the use of *CPT Assistant.*

HCPCS Level II

The Healthcare Common Procedure Coding System (HCPCS) was developed by CMS in the 1980s to report services, supplies, and procedures that are not represented in the CPT (HCPCS Level I) code set but are submitted for reimbursement (CMS 2004a). The descriptions identify items or services rather than specific brand names and do not endorse any manufacturer. This alphanumeric code set is a standardized coding system that provides an established environment for claims submission and processing. The system is managed by both private and public health insurers. The existence of a particular code does not guarantee or indicate coverage/reimbursement by Medicare, Medicaid, or other third party payers. There are two types of codes within the HCPCS Level II system: permanent and temporary.

HCPCS Level II Permanent Codes

HCPCS Level II permanent codes may be used by all public and private health insurers. Permanent codes are alphanumeric with five digits with an alpha character in the first position (A2345). The alpha character designates the category to which the code is classified. Table 2.5 lists the categories of permanent HCPCS codes.

Within the permanent codes are "miscellaneous/not otherwise classified" codes. These codes enable suppliers and healthcare providers to report items/services that have not been incorporated into the coding system but nonetheless have been approved for marketing by the Food and Drug Administration (FDA) (CMS 2004a). Miscellaneous codes are manually reviewed and must be submitted with accompanying pricing and medical necessity documentation.

Current Dental Terminology (CDT4) commonly known as "dental codes," comprises a separate category of national permanent codes. The codes are copyrighted and maintained by the American Dental Association (ADA). Dental codes are easily identified because they begin with the letter D.

HCPCS Level II Temporary Codes

HCPCS Level II temporary codes are used to meet the immediate and short-term operational needs of individual insurers, public and private (CMS 2004a).

Table 2.5.   Permanent HCPCS codes

Permanent Code Categories	Covers	Insurers
A codes	Ambulance and transportation services, medical and surgical supplies, administrative, and miscellaneous and investigational services and supplies	All payers
B codes	Enteral and parenteral therapy	All payers
D codes	Dental	All payers
E codes	Durable medical equipment	All payers
J codes	Drugs that cannot ordinarily be self-administered, chemotherapy, immunosuppressive drugs, inhalation solutions	All payers
L codes	Orthotic and prosthetic procedures and devices	All payers
M codes	Office services and cardiovascular and other medical services	All payers
P codes	Pathology and laboratory services	All payers
R codes	Diagnostic radiology	All payers
V codes	Vision hearing and speech-language pathology services	All payers

Temporary codes are also alphanumeric, with five digits and an alpha character in the first position. Like permanent codes, the alpha character designates the category to which the code is classified. Table 2.6 lists the categories of temporary HCPCS codes. Temporary codes may remain as such for an indefinite period of time. However, if deemed necessary, a permanent code will be created to replace the temporary code and the temporary code will be deleted. The top 10 HCPCS codes reported to Medicare in 2003 are found in table 2.7.

HCPCS Level II Modifiers

Like CPT, HCPCS Level II allows for modifiers. HCPCS Level II modifiers are two-digit alpha or alphanumeric codes. A modifier is designed to give Medicare and other third party payers additional information needed to process a claim. Many HCPCS Level II modifiers indicate body areas that allow for specific information to be provided to third party payers. Table 2.8 provides examples of HCPCS Level II modifiers.

Maintenance of HCPCS Level II Coding System

Permanent codes are maintained jointly by America's Health Insurance Plans (AHIP), the Blue Cross and Blue Shield Association (BCBSA), and the Centers for Medicare and Medicaid Services (CMS). Together these organizations compose the National Panel (CMS 2004a). Permanent National Codes are updated annually every January 1. Temporary codes, which compose 35 percent of Level II HCPCS codes, are maintained by the individual members of the National Panel rather than the group (CMS 2004a). For example, the HCPCS workgroup, a part of the CMS workgroup, makes the decisions about temporary codes for Medicare. Temporary codes can be added, changed, or deleted on a quarterly basis.

Requesting a Code Modification for HCPCS Level II

There are three types of coding modifications to HCPCS Level II codes that users can request: a code may be added to the code set, the language used to describe an existing code may be changed, and an existing code may be deleted. The HCPCS Level II coding review process is a continuous process. The review cycle runs from April 2 through the following April 1.

Requests for code changes may be submitted at any time throughout the year. The proper request format can be found on the CMS Web site

Table 2.6.   Temporary HCPCS codes

Temporary Code Categories	Covers	Insurers
C codes	Items that may qualify for pass-through payment under HOPPS	Medicare hospital outpatient claims
G codes	Professional health care procedures and services	Medicare hospital outpatient claims
Q codes	Drugs, biologicals, medical equipment	Medicare hospital outpatient claims
K codes	Durable medical equipment	DMERCs—durable medical equipment regional carriers
S codes	Drugs, services and supplies	BCBSA and AHIP and Medicaid
H codes	Mental health services	State Medicaid agencies
T codes	Items for which there are no permanent national codes	State Medicaid agencies and private insurers

Table 2.7.   HCPCS Level II codes

Medicare Top 10 Service, Procedures, or Supplies by Unit of Service—CY 2004	
Code	**Description**
G0001	Drawing blood for specimen
Q0136	Non ESRD epoetin alpha injection
Q0137	Darbepoetin alfa, Non ESRD
J2250	Injection midazolam hydrochloride
J0256	Alpha1 proteinase inhibitor, 10mg
Q0081	Infusion therapy other than chemotherapy
J1564	Immune globulin 10 mg
J3010	Fentanyl citrate injection, .1
J1785	Imiglucerase, unit
J2405	Ondansetron hcl injection 1 mg

Table 2.8.   HCPCS Level II modifier examples

LT	Left side
RT	Right side
E1	Upper left, eyelid
F1	Left hand, second digit

(www.cms.hhs.gov). Requests for coding modifications are submitted to the Alpha-Numeric HCPCS Coordinator at the CMS. Once a request is submitted, it is reviewed by the CMS HCPCS Workgroup at one of its regular monthly meetings. After considering the request, the HCPCS Workgroup will make a recommendation to the HCPCS National Panel. The HCPCS Workgroup may also create a temporary Medicare national code pending the National Panel action. The HCPCS Workgroup's recommendations usually fall into one of the following categories:

- Add a Code
- Use an Existing Code that Describes the Item or Service
- Use an Existing Code for Miscellaneous Items or Services
- Revise an Existing Code
- Delete an Existing Code

The National Panel is responsible for approving all coding modifications. All three members of the National Panel must agree on all requests before a change may be made. Once the decision is made regarding a request, the Panel will send a decision letter to the requester. If the requestor is unsatisfied with the decision, a new request with new supporting information may be submitted for reconsideration and evaluation (CMS 2004a).

HCPCS Level II Coding Guidelines
AHA Coding Clinic for HCPCS is a resource newsletter that provides coding advice for the users of HCPCS Level II. This quarterly newsletter was first introduced in March of 2001 and is published by the Central Office of ICD-9-CM. The newsletter includes an "ask the editors" section with actual examples, correct code assignment for new technologies, articles, and a bulletin of coding changes and/or corrections (AHA 2004). Although this is not "official" coding guidance, it is expert. There is no "official" coding resource for HCPCS Level II other than coverage determinations issued by CMS and its fiscal intermediaries.

Coding Systems as Communication Facilitators

Clinical coding systems serve as the communication vehicle between healthcare providers and public and private third party payers. This solid and reliable communication enables providers and facilities to be accurately reimbursed in a timely manner. Understanding the basics of clinical coding systems enables coding, billing and reimbursement professionals to fully grasp reimbursement principles and concepts.

Check Your Understanding 2.1

1. The code sets to be used for healthcare services reporting by both public and private insurers were designated by what legislation?

2. The first three characters in an ICD-9-CM diagnosis code represent its:
   a. Subclassification
   b. Subcategory
   c. Category
   d. Modifier

3. What organizations maintain the ICD-9-CM code set?

4. Where are the ICD-9-CM coding guidelines published?

5. What code set was incorporated into the Healthcare Common Procedure Coding System as HCPCS Level I?

Coding Compliance and Reimbursement

For coding, billing, and reimbursement professionals, being compliant means to perform one's job functions according to the laws, regulations, and guidelines set forth by Medicare and other third party payers. Today, being compliant with the rules and regulations is just one component of being proficient at a healthcare professional's job, but it is an indication that, as a professional, the person is able to perform at an acceptable skill level and ethical standard. It is the responsibility of coding, billing, and reimbursement professionals to perform their jobs with integrity at all times. The appendix to this chapter, *AHIMA Standards of Ethical Coding,* sets forth guidelines that all coding, billing, and reimbursement professionals should understand and ponder during ethical decision making.

Fraud and Abuse

Medicare defines *fraud* as "an intentional representation that an individual knows to be false or does not believe to be true and makes, knowing that the representation could result in some unauthorized benefit to himself/herself or some other person" (CMS 2004b). An example of fraud is billing for a service that was not rendered.

Abuse occurs when a healthcare provider unknowingly or unintentionally submits an inaccurate claim to for payment. Abuse generally results from unsound medical, business, or fiscal practices that directly or indirectly result in unnecessary costs to the Medicare program. An example of abuse involves inadvertently reporting a procedure code that describes a service that was more extensive that the procedure performed. In Medicare, the most common forms of fraud and abuse include (CMS 2004b):

- Billing for services not furnished

- Misrepresenting the diagnosis to justify payment

- Soliciting, offering, or receiving a kickback

- Unbundling or "exploding" charges

- Falsifying certificates of medical necessity, plans of treatment, and medical records to justify payment

- Billing for a service not furnished as billed, known as upcoding

The mid-1980s through late-1990s brought about a wave of legislation targeted at fighting Medicare and Medicaid fraud and abuse.

Legislative Background

It is important to explore and understand the legislative history of fraud and abuse. In an effort to eliminate erroneous healthcare spending for the Medicare and Medicaid programs, Congress passed several acts targeting fraud and abuse. Not only did the revamped and newly created legislation show a commitment to protecting the Medicare Trust Fund by Congress, but it gave CMS the resources and penalties necessary to battle fraud and abuse. Several target areas introduced in the legislation are still under review by **Quality Improvement Organizations (QIOs)** in the 8th **Scope of Work.**

False Claims Act

The **False Claims Act** was passed during the Civil War in order to prohibit contractors of any kind from knowingly filing a false or fraudulent claim, using a false record or statement, or conspiring to defraud the U.S. government (Schraffenberger 2005, 200). Today, the False Claims Act provides the support for the federal government to rebuke abusers of the Medicare and Medicaid systems. The Medicare and Medicaid Patient and Program Protection Act of 1987 supports the use of civil monetary penalties for acts of fraud and abuse against the Medicare and Medicaid programs. This act allows for fines up to $10,000 per violation and exclusions from Medicare participation.

Office of Inspector General (OIG)
Compliance Program Guidance

In 1991, the **OIG** released seven elements which the office believed should serve as the foundation of an effective corporate compliance plan (OIG 1991). These elements are:

1. Written policies and procedures

2. Designation of a **compliance officer**

3. Education and training

4. Communication

5. Auditing and monitoring

6. Disciplinary action

7. Corrective action

In response to numerous laboratory investigations for improper coding and billing, *Compliance Program Guidance for Clinical Laboratories* was released in February 1997 and then revised in February of the following year. The guidance provides principles for compliant documentation and coding practices in laboratories. For example, laboratories were instructed that they may not use diagnostic information from earlier dates of service on current laboratory testing orders. At the time, this was common practice and is a compliance risk because a patient's condition warranting a procedure may change from visit to visit.

In February of 1998, the OIG released *Compliance Program Guidance for Hospitals.* This document highlighted several coding and billing areas that were at risk for noncompliance. Some examples are: upcoding services, unbundling services, and reporting incorrect discharge destination.

Since 1998, numerous other *Compliance Program Guidance* documents have been released for various healthcare settings, including: hospice, home health, physician practices, and skilled nursing facilities.

Several years have passed since the *Compliance Program Guidance for Hospitals* was released. In January 2005 CMS released the *Supplemental Compliance Program Guidance for Hospitals* in the *Federal Register.* Because hospitals' operations and reimbursement systems have changed since 1998, the OIG decided to revise the Program Guidance. Though expanded, the original seven elements continue to be the basis for an effective hospital compliance plan (DHHS 2005, 4874–4876):

1. Designation of a Compliance Officer and compliance committee

2. Development of compliance policies and procedures, including standard of conduct

3. Developing open lines of communication

4. Appropriate training and education

5. Internal monitoring and auditing

6. Response to detected deficiencies

7. Enforcement of disciplinary standards

The *Supplemental Compliance Program Guidance for Hospitals* provides further detail about compliance risk areas for outpatient procedure coding, admissions and discharge criteria, supplemental payment considerations and use of information technology (*Federal Register* 2005, 4860–4862). A copy of the *Supplemental Compliance Program Guidance for Hospitals* can be found on the OIG Web site (www.oig.hhs.gov).

Operation Restore Trust

A joint effort of the Department Health and Human Services (DHHS), OIG, Centers for Medicare and Medicaid Services (CMS) and Administration on Aging (AOA), **Operation Restore Trust** was released in 1995 to target fraud and abuse among healthcare providers. The program originally focused on five states—California, Illinois, Florida, New York, and Texas—where 1/3 of the Medicare and Medicaid population resided. Within the first two years, Operation Restore Trust spent 7.9 million dollars and recovered 188 million dollars—a 24 to 1 return on investment. This major push for accurate coding and billing eventually spread to be a nationwide effort. In addition to fraud and abuse investigations, Operation Restore Trust paved the way for implementation of a national toll-free fraud and abuse hotline, the Voluntary Disclosure Program, and Special Fraud Alert documents.

Health Insurance Portability and Accountability Act of 1996

Although the Health Insurance Portability and Accountability Act (HIPAA) is widely known for its security and privacy provisions, a large portion of the Act focused on fraud and abuse prevention. The key fraud and abuse areas targeted by HIPAA are:

- Medical necessity
- Upcoding
- Unbundling
- Billing for services not provided

In addition to highlighting these key areas, HIPAA created the Medicare Integrity Program. Not only did Medicare continue to review provider claims for fraud and abuse, but the focus expanded to cost reports, payment determinations and the need for on-going compliance education (Schraffenberger 2005, 201).

Balanced Budget Act of 1997

One objective of the **Balanced Budget Act (BBA) of 1997** was to improve program integrity for Medicare. The provisions within the BBA attempted to educate Medicare beneficiaries on their role in preventing and reporting fraudulent acts. Beneficiaries were advised to review Medicare Summary Notices (formerly Explanations of Medicare Benefits or EOMBs) for errors and to report errors to the secretary of DHHS. Additionally, they were notified of their right to request copies of detailed bills for healthcare services and informed of the implementation of a toll-free fraud and abuse hotline. The BBA also initiated a data collection program to collect fraud and abuse information in the healthcare sector as mandated by HIPAA.

As legislation regarding healthcare fraud and abuse became more prevalent, the need for a stronger workforce behind the laws was inevitable. Personnel were added to the Department of Justice (DOJ) and Federal Bureau of Investigation (FBI) in order to keep up with the warranted reviews. Likewise, the focus of the quality improvement organizations, or QIOs (formerly peer review organizations, or PROs) shifted from the quality focus of the early 1990s to a payment error prevention role.

Quality Improvement Organizations

Quality improvement organizations (QIOs) have worked with Medicare for more than twenty years to improve the quality of care provided to its beneficiaries. Individual QIOs contract every three years with Medicare to monitor hospital performance on a state or regional basis. The QIOs are guided by Medicare's Scope of Work. In 1999, the

6th Scope of Work (SOW) introduced CMS' **Payment Error Prevention Program (PEPP).** Working under the assumption that most payment errors were caused by simple mistakes, not fraudulent or abusive acts (KePRO 2004), PEPP instructed the QIOs to reduce the number of payment errors in their states or regions through awareness, education, and training. PEPP focused on several coding and billing areas that have historically contributed to payment errors:

- Medically unnecessary admissions and/or procedures

- Incorrect DRG assignment

- Readmission to facility

- Inappropriate Transfers

QIOs used public data from CMS to identify abnormal payment patterns at hospitals in their contracted region or state. Those facilities were be targeted for review and if payment errors were identified, education and training was provided. If the deviation from normal reporting rates were due to fraud or abuse, those cases would be passed on to the OIG for further investigation.

7th Scope of Work

During the 7th Scope of Work, QIOs continued to focus on payment errors at Medicare participating facilities. The 7th Scope of Work had three goals (Estrella 2003, 47):

- Improve the quality of care for beneficiaries by ensuring that beneficiary care meets professionally recognized standards of healthcare

- Protect the integrity of the Medicare Trust Fund by ensuring Medicare pays only for services and items that are reasonable, medically necessary, and provided in the most appropriate setting

- Protect beneficiaries by expeditiously addressing individual cases such as beneficiary complaints, hospital-issued notices of noncoverage (HINNs), Emergency Medical Treatment and Active Labor Act (EMTALA) violations, and other statutory responsibilities

Several tasks were created to assist QIOs with achieving the 7th SOW goals. Task 3, improving the Medicare beneficiary protection program, includes the **Hospital Payment Monitoring Program (HPMP),** which expanded and replaced the PEPP.

Clinical Data Abstraction Centers (CDACs) have contracted with Medicare to provide encounter screening and validation services for QIOs across the nation. CDACs use random selection to review cases for Medicare participating hospitals in the various states and regions. Encounters that cannot be validated by the CDACs are passed on to the QIOs for further review. When a coding error is identified, it is corrected. If an overpayment has been made to the hospital, it is recouped by the fiscal intermediary. Underpayment resulting from coding errors is made to the hospital. All coding errors are entered into a QIO database for further analysis (Ohio KePRO 2004).

First-Look Analysis Tool for Hospital Outlier Monitoring Software

QIOs use Medicare's First-look Analysis Tool for Hospital Outlier Monitoring (FATHOM) software to identify hospitals with outliers. Target areas include (Estrella 2003, 44):

- One-day stays

- Same-day readmissions

- Against Medical Advice discharges

- Historically problem DRGs

- Case Mix Index Creep

- DRG Relationship Groups

QIO's analyze data from FATHOM to identify hospitals that perform outside of the state norm. QIOs look not only at current data but at data trends over a period of time to identify sudden shifts in reporting patterns. Sudden shifts can be caused by various issues, including:

- Coder turnover

- Increase or decrease of education and training

- Implementation of new information systems

- Implementation of a documentation improvement program

- Expansion or establishment of a service area

- Inaccurate advice received from healthcare consultants

Program for Evaluation Payment Patterns Electronic Report (PEPPER)

QIOs are also provided with hospital-specific data from the Hospital Payment Monitoring Program (HPMP) Quality Improvement Organization Support Center (QIOSC), which is the Texas Medical Foundation (TMF).

TMF provides hospital data for fourteen target areas on a quarterly basis to the QIOs via the **Program for Evaluation Payment Patterns Electronic Report (PEPPER)** v. 5.0. (KePRO 2004, 1) For a listing of the PEPPER target areas, see table 2.9. QIOs determine which of these fourteen reports to share with the hospitals in their contracted state or region. If a facility is at or above the 75th percentile or at or below the 10th percentile the facility may be targeted for an intensive medical record review. If fraud or abuse is suspected, the case is forwarded on to the OIG for further investigation.

8th Scope of Work

The 8th Scope of Work (in effect from August 1, 2005 through July 31, 2008) emphasizes quality care with particular attention at nursing homes, home health agencies, hospitals, and physician offices. The SOW includes a plan that addresses five major areas (CMS 2005):

- Promote dramatic improvements in the quality of healthcare so that every beneficiary receives the right care every time

- Promote the adoption and effective use of **healthcare information technology (HIT)**

- Work with prescription drug plans and providers to ensure quality care by creating improvement projects to monitor issues such as inappropriately prescribed drugs and harmful drug interactions

- Improve healthcare access for disadvantaged populations

- Work to improve provider-patient communication during beneficiary complaints regarding quality of care issues

Even though heavy emphasis is being placed on quality and HIT in the 8th SOW, the Hospital Payment Monitoring Program is still in effect. Groundwork laid during the 7th SOW for the HPMP will continue during the 8th SOW. In order to lessen the chance of a payment error investigation, coding and billing units should include preventive measures in their coding compliance plans.

Coding Compliance Plan

Every coding unit should have a **coding compliance plan,** which is a component of the HIM department compliance plan and the overall corporate compliance plan at its facility. The plan should focus on the unique regulations and guidelines with which coding professionals must comply. As discussed previously, the Department of Health and Human Services has released several versions of the *Compliance Program Guidance* for various healthcare settings. The model provided by the OIG guidance is also applicable to individual coding units. Building a complete compliance plan is essential for establishing a solid coding team. The core areas of the coding compliance plan are policies and procedures, education and training, and auditing and monitoring.

Policies and Procedures

Well-designed and complete policies and procedures provide employees with consistent guidance to perform their assigned tasks. Without such guidance, employees may complete their tasks in different ways causing major confusion, inefficiencies, and possibly noncompliance. Managers should perform a job analysis to assure that every task has an established policy or procedure to govern it. Because coding has so many rules and official guidelines, it is critical that this section

Table 2.9.   PEPPER target areas

Target Area	Focus
One-day stays excluding transfers	Site of service—was an inpatient admission warranted or could the patient been treated more efficiently as an outpatient?
One-day stay transfers	Site of service—was an inpatient admission warranted or could the patient been treated more efficiently as an outpatient?
DRG 127 one-day stays	Site of service—was an inpatient admission warranted or could the patient been treated more efficiently as an outpatient?
DRG 143 one-day stays	Site of service—was an inpatient admission warranted or could the patient been treated more efficiently as an outpatient?
DRGs 182 and 183 one-day stays	Site of service—was an inpatient admission warranted or could the patient been treated more efficiently as an outpatient?
DRGs 296 and 297 one-day stays	Site of service—was an inpatient admission warranted or could the patient been treated more efficiently as an outpatient?
DRG 014	Correct assignment of principal diagnosis
DRG 079	Correct assignment of principal diagnosis—under close review are ICD-9-CM codes: 507.x, 482.83, and 482.89
DRGs 239, 243, and 253	Site of service—was an inpatient admission warranted or could the patient been treated more efficiently as an outpatient?
DRG 416	Correct assignment of principal diagnosis—under close review is ICD-9-CM code 038.9
DRG 475	Correct assignment of principal diagnosis
Seven-day readmit to same facility or elsewhere	Inappropriate admission or discharge, quality of care issues, or coding and/or billing errors. Under close review for billing errors are discharge destination codes
Same-day readmit elsewhere	Inappropriate admission or discharge, quality of care issues, or coding and/or billing errors. Under close review for billing errors are discharge destination codes
Same-day readmit to same facility	Inappropriate admission or discharge, quality of care issues, or coding and/or billing errors. Under close review for billing errors are discharge destination codes

of the coding compliance plan be methodically compiled. Following is a far from exhaustive list of issues that should be included in a coding compliance plan:

- Physician query process
- Coding diagnoses not supported by medical documentation
- Upcoding (reporting services at a higher level than warranted)
- Unbundling (reporting multiple codes when only one is necessary)
- Coding medical records without complete documentation
- Assignment of discharge destination codes
- Correct use of encoding software
- Complete process for using scrubber software

Education and Training
A good education plan is essential to succeeding as a coding team. In order to be compliant, coding, billing, and reimbursement professionals must continuously participate in their education. Rules and regulations for public and private payers are released almost daily. Recognized means of communication of this vital information must be established in the coding compliance plan. A sample of issues that should be placed on the continuous education schedule includes:

- Public and private payer guidelines
- **Local Medical Review Policies (LMRPs)** and **Local Coverage Determinations (LCDs)**
- National Coverage Determinations (NCD)
- Official Coding Guidelines for ICD-9-CM, CPT, and HCPCS Level II codes

- Quarterly and yearly code changes
- Quarterly and yearly prospective payment system changes
- OIG Workplan issues
- National Correct Coding Initiative (NCCI)

Special attention should be paid to the work of new coders. Every coding manager must assess a new employee's compliance level and degree of understanding. Education must be provided to bring deficient coders up to speed with expected guidelines. Completion of required educational sessions should be built into annual evaluations/reviews for all coding, billing, and reimbursement employees.

Auditing and Monitoring
Managers must be diligent at auditing and monitoring compliance in the coding unit. During the auditing phase, the coding manager gathers information on the department's compliance with policies and procedures. Incorporating internal and external auditing into the coding compliance plan has proven to be the best strategy. Internal auditing enables managers to see first-hand where their unit's strengths and weaknesses lie. External auditing provides an unbiased view of the department's performance. Together, internal and external audits help the coding manager build an effective education plan for their unit.

Two forms of **benchmarking** can help a manager determine the staff's level of compliance: internal and external benchmarking. Internal benchmarking or trending allows the manager to examine reporting rates over a period of time. This exercise enables the manager to pinpoint the specific time period within which a compliance issue arose. External benchmarking or peer comparison helps a manager to know how his or her team has performed compared to their peers. Issues revealed, for example, include whether its **case mix index (CMI)** level puts the facility at risk. Benchmarking will help establish reasonable parameters to follow. Target areas for internal and external benchmarking should correlate with those highlighted in the policies and procedures and education and training sections of the coding compliance plan along with problem areas identified during routine internal and external audits.

Focus Areas

Establishing good focus areas takes a considerable amount of research by the coding manager. Managers must stay up-to-date on compliance issues that are published and discussed in various government and other third party payer documents. For example, the OIG Workplan should be reviewed each year. This document provides insight into the directions the OIG is taking as well as highlighting hot areas of compliance. Below are four case studies that show how a manager can use auditing results along with internal and external benchmarking to monitor compliance.

Case Mix Index Analysis

Analyzing the growth or decline of a facility's case mix index (CMI) is the beginning phase for assessing the quality of its coding and billing practices. Managers begin by comparing the CMI of the facility to that of its peers and the state or nation for the last three years. Questions posed include:

- Is the CMI steady?

- Does it increase steadily or drastically?

- Is there a sharp or sudden decline?

To explore the analysis issues, consider data for a medium size (250–400 beds), not-for-profit facility (Hospital A), its peer facilities, and the nation. Peer facilities included in this example are local hospitals with which this facility competes for market share. Figure 2.3 displays CMI trend from 2001 to 2003.

Clearly, this facility's CMI has increased at a much greater rate than the national average or that of its peers. Additionally, figure 2.4 shows that hospital A's CMI is greater than the nation and its peers. So not only has its CMI increased at a fast pace but it is also the highest in this data set. What has caused this major shift? The facility can now drill down to the **major diagnostic category (MDC)** level in order to pinpoint noteworthy changes at the service area level.

Figure 2.3.   CMI percent change—2001–2003

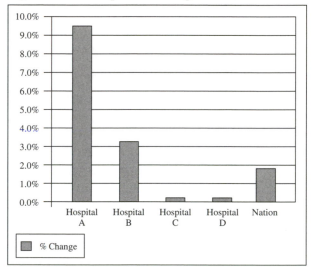

Figure 2.4.   CMI—2001–2003

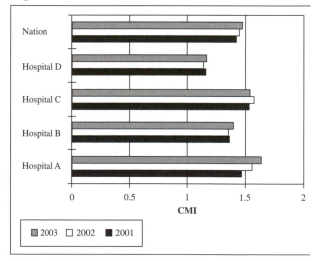

Figure 2.5 shows that the CMI for MDC 05, Diseases of the Circulatory System, increased greatly between years 2001 and 2003 (15.7 percent). What has caused this increase? One cannot tell from the data alone. However, by performing a thorough investigation the issue(s) can be identified. Several areas to consider include:

- Coding and billing errors

- Changes in DRG assignments

- Equipment purchases

- New or expanded service areas

- Acquisition of new facilities

- Changes in physician personnel

Regardless of the root cause of the data deviations, compliance with established rules and regulations must be verified. If coding practices are questionable, a medical record review should be completed to identify whether a compliance infraction has occurred. Managers should follow established procedures for correcting and reporting a compliance lapse. This exercise can also be completed for the facility's outpatient **service mix index (SMI).**

Figure 2.5.   MDC 05 CMI trend—2001–2003

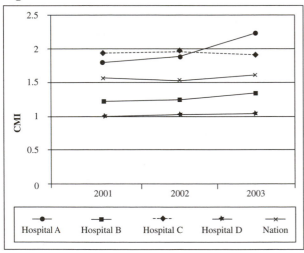

DRG Relationships Reporting

Within the DRG system, there are DRGs that have a relationship or similar grouping methodology to other DRGs. For example, DRG pairs exist where the listings of diagnoses used to drive the grouping are the same, but the presence or absence of a **complication** or **comorbidity** diagnosis assigns the case to a higher or lower DRG. These are known as "with and without CC pairs." These DRG relationships and pairs pose a compliance concern because the medical record documentation used to support the coding of principal diagnosis, complications, and comorbidities may not always be clear or used appropriately by the coder. Therefore, inaccurate coding can lead to incorrect DRG assignment and thus inappropriate reimbursement.

Example:

Included in the PEPPER reports is the DRG relationship comparing the DRG 079 reporting rate to those of DRGs 080, 089 and 090. DRG 079, Respiratory Infections and Inflammations, Age Greater than 17, with CC, has a higher relative weight than the other DRGs in this relationship and should be closely monitored. (See table 2.10.) In addition to the differences in relative weight, the rules and regulations concerning principal diagnosis assignment for pneumonia can be confusing and unclear for beginner coders, therefore leaving these DRGs at a greater risk for incorrect assignment. Reporting DRG 079 at a higher rate than warranted will cause the facility to receive reimbursement of which it is not entitled, creating noncompliance.

Again, hospital A is a medium size, not-for-profit facility and the peer facilities are local hospitals. Figure 2.6 compares hospital A's reporting rate for the DRG 079 relationship group to its peers and nation for 2003. Hospital A's reporting rate, 50.77 percent, is much higher than the nation average and that of all of its peers. In this situation, the coding manager may want to gather some more information. Did this reporting variation just "pop up" this year, or has this DRG been reported at higher rates in the past? The manager can look at a trend analysis for the past three or four years.

Figure 2.7 provides a yearly reporting trend of DRG 079 for hospital A. The trend shows that the reporting rate for DRG 079 has steadily increased between 2001 and 2003. It is clear that a medical record review is warranted to determine if inaccurate coding practices have contributed to or caused this trend. Medical records assigned to DRG 079 should be reviewed to determine whether the assignment of this DRG is supported through documentation in the medical record. Again, established procedures for compliance issues should be followed.

Poor documentation identified during the intensive medical record review should be addressed with the medical staff and incorrect code assignments should be immediately discussed with the coding staff.

Site of Service: Inpatient versus Outpatient
The following example illustrates the concept of a site-of-service review focused on DRGS prone to compliance problems.

Example:

Several DRGs are under a site-of-service review by QIOs. Documentation and admission criteria are reviewed to determine whether the inpatient setting is the most efficient and effective treatment area for patients. PEPPER data focuses on three DRGs (KePRO 2004, 2):

- DRG 239, Pathological Fractures and Musculoskeletal and Connective Tissue Malignancy
- DRG 243, Medical Back Problems
- DRG 253, Fractures, Sprains, Strains, and Dislocations of Upper Arm and Lower Leg except Foot, Age Greater than 17 with CC

Compliance investigators examine the reporting rates for DRG 243 at one facility. Hospital A is a medium size, not-for-profit facility. Analysis of figure 2.8 shows the reporting rate for DRG 243 or the percent of DRG 243 cases to total discharges for the facility in 2003. Hospital A reported DRG 243 at a much higher rate than its peers and the nation.

Table 2.10. DRG 079 relationship grouping

DRG Number	DRG Title	FY 2005 Relative Weight
079	Respiratory Infections and Inflammations, Age Greater than 17, with CC	1.5872
080	Respiratory Infections and Inflammations, Age Greater than 17, without CC	0.8497
089	Simple Pneumonia & Pleurisy, Age Greater than 17, with CC	1.0479
090	Simple Pneumonia & Pleurisy, Age Greater than 17, without CC	0.6172

Figure 2.6. Percent assigned to DRG 079

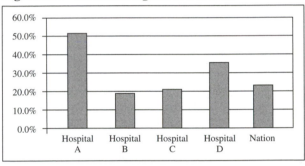

Figure 2.7. Hospital A reporting trend DRG 079

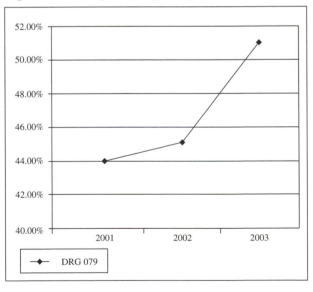

Compliance investigators next examine whether this is a trend or a new risk area. Figure 2.9 displays the reporting rate for DRG 243 from 2001 to 2003 for hospital A. The data shows that DRG 243 has been reported at a significantly high level for the past three years, peaking in 2002.

Because this DRG is under close review due to site-of-service questions, the coding manager should also review the **length of stay (LOS)** for this DRG. Do the majority of cases follow the **average length of stay (ALOS)** for this DRG or is there a much lower LOS? A lower LOS could indicate that the patients could have been treated as outpatients rather than inpatients. The average length of stay for DRG 243 at hospital A in 2003 was 4.73. The national ALOS for DRG 243 is 4.6. The data shows the hospital A's LOS is consistent with what is expected for patients grouping to this DRG.

However, examiners look more deeply and examine the frequency of LOS values for DRG 243. Figure 2.10 displays the LOS distribution for DRG 243 in 2003. Again, the data shows that the LOS reporting for this DRG is consistent with the national expected ALOS. Investigators review encounters in the one-day stay category to verify that admission criteria and medical necessity were met. After drill-down analysis, it appears that this DRG is being appropriately reported at this facility. However, if other DRGs show deviation, they should be investigated by a **Utilization Review Committee** consisting of representatives from HIM, Quality, Utilization, and Medical Staff. Together this interdisciplinary team can determine whether the site or service was appropriate for the encounters under review.

Evaluation and Management Facility Coding in the Emergency Department

The implementation of the **Hospital Outpatient Prospective Payment System (HOPPS)** has brought about new compliance challenges for hospitals. One area under review is Evaluation and Management (E/M) coding. Since the CPT code reported on a Medicare outpatient claim drives the **ambulatory payment classification (APC)** assignment and hence the level of reimbursement, the code assignment should be closely monitored. (See table 2.11.)

Figure 2.8.   DRG 243 reporting rate—2003

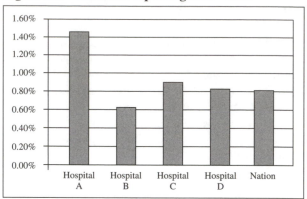

Figure 2.9.   Hospital A reporting trend DRG 243

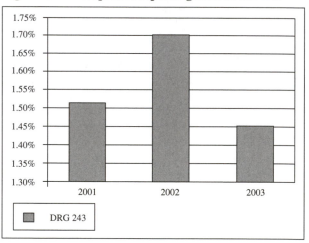

Figure 2.10.   Hospital A LOS distribution for DRG 243—2003

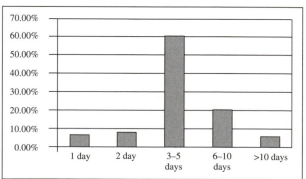

Table 2.11.   E/M Emergency department CPT codes and APC groupings (CY 2005)

	99281	99282	99283	99284	99285
APC Group	0610—Low Level ED Visit	0610—Low Level ED Visit	0611—Mid Level ED Visit	0612—High Level ED Visit	0612—High Level ED Visit
APC Relative Weight	1.3544	1.3544	2.3926	4.1139	4.1139
APC Payment (unadjusted)	$77.18	$77.18	$136.34	$234.42	$234.42

Example:

Code distribution may be compared among a medium size not-for-profit hospital, two peer facilities, and the nation. Figure 2.11 shows the E/M code distribution in 2003. The data shows that hospital A reported codes 99284 and 99285 (high-level emergency department visits) at a much higher percentage than hospital C and the nation. CMS has suggested that Emergency Department APC distribution should follow somewhat of a bell-curved shape. Clearly, hospital A deviates far from this configuration.

Again, it is important to examine the trend for hospital A. Figure 2.12 displays a trending graph for years 2000 to 2003. The data show that hospital A's reporting of higher level E/M codes has drastically increased since 2000. This increase coincides with the implementation of HOPPS (August 2000). A medical record audit should be performed to verify that medical record documentation supports the assignment of these CPT codes.

Check Your Understanding 2.2

1. The new coding assistant at the Glen Ellyn Medical Group office coded and submitted a claim to Blue Cross for an initial evaluation and management office visit when in fact the patient was established with the practice and was seen strictly for a follow-up medical check. The resulting error was an example of _____.

2. All of the following are efforts to fight healthcare fraud and abuse **except:**
   a. Operation Restore Trust
   b. Medicare Integrity Program
   c. Tax Equity and Fiscal Responsibility Act of 1982 (TEFRA)
   d. Medicare and Medicaid Patient and Program Protection Act of 1987

Figure 2.11.   E/M code distribution—2003

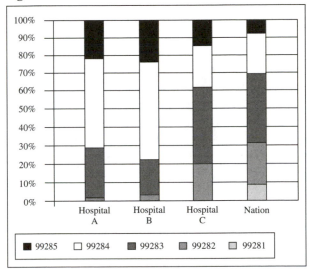

Figure 2.12.   Hospital A E/M distribution trend— 2000–2003

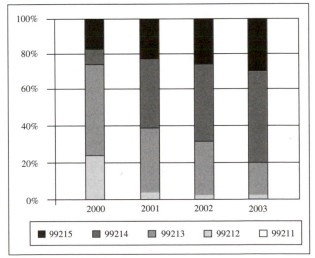

3. What are the core areas of the coding compliance plan?

4. Audit data has demonstrated that when coding managers conduct internal audits of coding quality, they do not require external audits to build effective coding compliance plans. True or false?

5. In DRG relationships reporting, DRG pairs are examined for _____.

Summary

Compliance is directly related to hospital reimbursement. The rules and regulations of public and private third party payers must be strictly followed to ensure that facilities receive reimbursement for which they are entitled. Good compliance practices not only reduce payment errors but also establish coding and billing diligence that leads to more focused employees. Compliance awareness is heightened through education and fostering higher-skilled employees who perform their job functions accurately and efficiently.

Chapter 2 Review Quiz

Match each coding system on the left with its description of uses on the right.

1. ICD-9-CM   _____   a. Medical and
                                  surgical supplies

2. HCPCS Level II   _____   b. Physician inpatient
                                  or outpatient
                                  procedures

3. CPT   _____   c. Diagnoses
                                  and inpatient
                                  procedures

4. Common forms of fraud and abuse include all of the following **except:**
    a. Upcoding
    b. Unbundling
    c. Refiling claims after denials
    d. Billing for services not furnished to patients

5. Name and describe three of the seven OIG elements of an effective compliance plan.

6. Name the legislation that created Medicare Summary Notices and describe their use.

7. What is the focus of quality improvement organizations (QIOs), and how do they help to improve quality?

8. What are three target areas of the First-look Analysis Tool for Hospital Outlier Monitoring (FATHOM) software?

9. What version of the OIG Scope of Work is being used, and when will it expire?

10. What HHS tool is available for healthcare providers to use in developing coding, HIM, and corporate compliance plans?

11. For what can a manager use internal benchmarking (trending)?

12. What resource can managers use to discover current hot areas of compliance?

13. What is the primary use of a case mix index analysis?

14. How do QIOs use site-of-service reviews?

15. What payment approach has created new compliance challenges related to E/M coding of emergency department services?

17. The International Classification of Diseases (ICD) is maintained by the American Medical Association. True or false?

18. CPT Category I codes include sections for Radiology and Medicine. True or false?

19. HCPCS Level II temporary codes may be replaced with permanent codes. True or false?

20. When the 8th SOW was implemented in August 2005, the Hospital Payment Monitoring Program ended. True or false?

References and Bibliography

American Hospital Association. 2004. AHA Central Office. www.hospitalconnect.com.

American Medical Association. 2005. *Current Procedural Terminology 2005*. Chicago: American Medical Association.

American Medical Association. 2004. AMA Web page. www.ama-assn.org.

American Medical Association. 1989 to 2005. *CPT Assistant*. Chicago: American Medical Association.

Beebe, M., 2003. CPT Category III codes cover new, emerging technologies: New codes developed to address issues in light of HIPAA. *Journal of American Health Information Management Association* 74(9): 84–85.

Centers for Medicare and Medicaid Services. 2004a. Healthcare Common Procedure Coding System (HCCPS). www.cms.hhs.gov/medicare/hcpcs.

Centers for Medicare and Medicaid Services. 2004b. Fighting fraud and abuse. www.cms.hhs.gov/providers/fraud.

Centers for Medicare and Medicaid Services. 2005 (April 7). Medicare takes major step toward improving quality of care. www.cms.hhs.gov/media/press/release.asp.

Department of Health and Human Services. 2005 (January 31). OIG supplemental compliance program guidance for hospitals. *Federal Register* 70 (19): 4858–4876.

Estrella, Rento. 2003. What happened to PEPP? QIOs plan for hospital payment monitoring program. *Journal of American Health Information Management Association* 74(7):43–48.

First Coast Service Options, Inc.1999, *Medicare Fraud & Abuse: A Practical Guide of Proactive Measures to Avoid Becoming a Victim*. Health Care Financing Administration.

KePRO. 2004. www.ohiokepro.com/providers/casereview/hpmp.asp.

KePRO. 2005. *A User Guide to PEPPER*. Available online from www.ohiokepro.com/providers/hospital/telemats/PepperFINAL.pdf.

KePRO. 2005. PEPPER: The Program for Evaluating Payment Patterns Electronic Report. Available online from www.ohiokepro.com/providers/hospital/events.asp#.

LaTour, K., and S. Eichenwald, eds. 2002. *Health Information Management: Concepts, Principles, and Practice*. Chicago: American Health Information Management Association.

Office of the Inspector General. 1991. www.oig.hhs.gov/fraud/complianceguidance.

Schraffenberger, L. A., ed. 2005. *Effective Management of Coding Services*. Chicago: American Health Information Management Association.

Chapter Appendix
Standards for Ethical Coding

In this era of payment based on diagnostic and procedural coding, the professional ethics of health information coding professionals continue to be challenged. A conscientious goal for coding and maintaining a quality database is accurate clinical and statistical data. The following standards of ethical coding, developed by AHIMA's Coding Policy and Strategy Committee and approved by AHIMA's Board of Directors, are offered to guide coding professionals in this process.

1. Coding professionals are expected to support the importance of accurate, complete, and consistent coding practices for the production of quality healthcare data.

2. Coding professionals in all healthcare settings should adhere to the ICD-9-CM (International Classification of Diseases, 9th revision, Clinical Modification) coding conventions, official coding guidelines approved by the Cooperating Parties,* the CPT (Current Procedural Terminology) rules established by the American Medical Association, and any other official coding rules and guidelines established for use with mandated standard code sets. Selection and sequencing of diagnoses and procedures must meet the definitions of required data sets for applicable healthcare settings.

3. Coding professionals should use their skills, their knowledge of currently mandated coding and classification systems, and official resources to select the appropriate diagnostic and procedural codes.

4. Coding professionals should only assign and report codes that are clearly and consistently supported by physician documentation in the health record.

5. Coding professionals should consult physicians for clarification and additional documentation prior to code assignment when there is conflicting or ambiguous data in the health record.

6. Coding professionals should not change codes or the narratives of codes on the billing abstract so that meanings are misrepresented. Diagnoses or procedures should not be inappropriately included or excluded because payment or insurance policy coverage requirements will be affected. When individual payer policies conflict with official coding rules and guidelines, these policies should be obtained in writing whenever possible. Reasonable efforts should be made to educate the payer on proper coding practices in order to influence a change in the payer's policy.

---

*The Cooperating Parties are the American Health Information Management Association, American Hospital Association, Health Care Financing Administration, and National Center for Health Statistics. All rights reserved. Reprint and quote only with proper reference to AHIMA's authorship.

7. Coding professionals, as members of the healthcare team, should assist and educate physicians and other clinicians by advocating proper documentation practices, further specificity, and resequencing or inclusion of diagnoses or procedures when needed to more accurately reflect the acuity, severity, and the occurrence of events.

8. Coding professionals should participate in the development of institutional coding policies and should ensure that coding policies complement, not conflict with, official coding rules and guidelines.

9. Coding professionals should maintain and continually enhance their coding skills, as they have a professional responsibility to stay abreast of changes in codes, coding guidelines, and regulations.

10. Coding professionals should strive for optimal payment to which the facility is legally entitled, remembering that it is unethical and illegal to maximize payment by means that contradict regulatory guidelines.

Revised 12/99

Article citation:

American Health Information Management Association. "Standards of Ethical Coding." *Journal of AHIMA* 71, no. 3 (2000): insert after p. 8.

Chapter 3
Voluntary Healthcare Insurance Plans

Objectives

- To differentiate major types of voluntary healthcare insurance plans

- To define basic language associated with reimbursement by commercial healthcare insurance plans and by Blue Cross and Blue Shield plans

- To explain common models and policies of payment for commercial healthcare insurance plans and for Blue Cross and Blue Shield plans

Key Terms

Actual charge
Allowable charge
Benefit cap
Benefits
Catastrophic expense limit
Certificate holders
Claim
Coinsurance
Coordination of benefits
Copayments
Cost-sharing
Covered conditions
Covered services
Creditable coverage
Credited coverage
Deductibles
Dependents
Endorsements
Evidence of insurability
Exclusions
Explanation of benefits (EOB)
Formulary
Guarantor

Indemnity health insurance
Insureds
Late enrollees
Limitations
Maximum out-of-pocket cost
Medical emergency
Medical necessity
Member
Out-of-pocket
Policy
Policyholders
Precertification
Preexisting condition
Premiums
Primary insurer (payer)
Prior approval
Rider
Risk pool
Secondary insurer (payer)
Stop-loss benefits
Subscribers
Usual, customary, and reasonable
Waiting period

Voluntary Healthcare Insurance

Voluntary health insurance (VHI) is the umbrella term that includes private or commercial healthcare insurance plans and Blue Cross and Blue Shield plans. Voluntary health insurance is private and denotes employment (Koch 2002, 96). VHI is differentiated from social health insurance and public welfare. Social health insurance comprises government programs based on current or past employment. Public welfare is assistance to categories of low-income people or other defined subpopulations.

Payments from voluntary health insurance plans account for approximately 33 percent of healthcare expenditures in the United States (Koch 2002, 94). Therefore, understanding this form of healthcare insurance is integral to understanding healthcare reimbursement.

Types of Voluntary Healthcare Insurance

This chapter investigates two major categories of voluntary health insurance—private or commercial healthcare insurance plans and Blue Cross and Blue Shield plans—organized in three classifications as illustrated in figure 3.1.

Private/Commercial Healthcare Insurance Plans

The first major category is private or commercial healthcare insurance, which contains two classifications: (1) private healthcare insurance plans and (2) employer-based healthcare insurance plans. Differentiating these two classifications is the size of the **risk pool.** A risk pool is the group of people

Figure 3.1.   Three classifications of voluntary healthcare insurance

Commercial (Private*) Individual (Private*) Healthcare Insurance Plan
Commercial (Private*) Employer-Based Healthcare Insurance Plan
Blue Cross and Blue Shield Plans

*Private is used two ways in the healthcare insurance industry: (1) as a synonym for commercial healthcare insurance and (2) meaning purchased by an individual rather than by an employer for a group.

covered by the healthcare insurance plan. Private or individual plans have a pool of the one **member** and his or her family. Employer-based healthcare insurance plans are also termed "group plans" because the risk pools comprise groups of employees. Thus, for group plans the risk is distributed across a much larger pool.

Blue Cross and Blue Shield Plans

The second major category and the third classification in itself are the Blue Cross and Blue Shield plans. Historically, for-profit status differentiated private or commercial healthcare insurance from Blue Cross and Blue Shield plans. Private or commercial healthcare insurance companies were for-profit and Blue Cross and Blue Shield plans were not-for-profit. However, although commercial healthcare insurance companies continue to be for-profit, some Blue Cross and Blue Shield plans also converted to for-profit status from not-for-profit between 1993 and 2002 (Hall and Conover 2003, 510). These conversions blurred the distinction between commercial healthcare insurance companies and Blue Cross and Blue Shield plans.

Confusing Terminology

In this discussion, there are three potential areas of confusion arising because members of the healthcare industry give the same word different meanings in different contexts:

- The word *private* is used two ways in the healthcare insurance industry. First, the term is sometimes used as a synonym for commercial healthcare insurance. Second, the term is sometimes used to denote healthcare insurance purchased by an individual versus healthcare insurance purchased by an employer for a group of employees.

- Commercial healthcare insurance plans and Blue Cross and Blue Shield plans often have multiple divisions that offer options both to private individuals and to employers. For example, both Aetna and Blue Cross and Blue Shield of Florida have healthcare insurance plans for individuals and families and for groups of employees. Consequently, the classifications overlap through these diversified offerings.

- The word *individual* is used to mean "nongroup" and also to mean "no **dependents.**"

Healthcare insurance companies sell healthcare plans to both individuals and groups of people. Individual (nongroup) plans are more expensive than are group plans. Also, healthcare insurance companies allow people to purchase healthcare coverage for their spouses and other family members (known as *dependent* or *family coverage*) for additional **premiums.** Persons who do not purchase the family coverage have individual (single) coverage or an individual plan.

Healthcare professionals must be careful to differentiate how these words are used and in what context. Finally, and most importantly, classification of a healthcare insurance plan depends upon the provisions of the healthcare insurance plan and how the plan functions, rather than its name.

Provisions and Functioning of Healthcare Insurance Plans

Prior to the 1970s, almost all voluntary health insurance was **indemnity health insurance.** Indemnity healthcare insurance plans are also called *retrospective fee-for-service,* as described in Chapter 1. In indemnity health insurance plans, the health insurance company pays a predetermined percentage of the cost of healthcare services and the **guarantor** pays the remaining percentage. For example, an individual (guarantor) might pay 20 percent for services and the health insurance company pays 80

percent. The providers define the fees for services, and those fees vary from physician to physician. Indemnity health plans offer individuals the freedom to choose their healthcare professionals.

Healthcare insurance companies assume the financial risk of the costs of individuals' and groups' healthcare. Healthcare insurance companies assume this risk because individuals or groups purchase the insurance companies' healthcare plans. The purchasers of healthcare plans are **policyholders** or **insureds.** If an employer or association purchases the healthcare insurance, the entity is the *group policyholder* and the employees or association members receive certificates of insurance coverage and, thus, are **certificate holders** or **subscribers.** Spouses and other family members of the policyholders are known as dependents. Policyholders pay higher premiums for dependent coverage than for single coverage. In addition to premiums, policyholders also pay **deductibles, coinsurance,** and **copayments** as provided in the **policy.**

Contracts formalize the relationship between the healthcare insurance companies and the individuals or groups for whom the companies are assuming the risk. These contracts are healthcare insurance policies. In the policies, the healthcare insurance companies promise to pay for the healthcare expenses of the policyholders and dependents. Healthcare insurance companies issue policies to individuals or groups who purchase the healthcare plan. The policies stipulate all aspects of healthcare for which the healthcare plan will pay (**covered conditions**). Healthcare services related to covered conditions are **covered services** for which the plan will pay.

Although the term *healthcare services* is used throughout this text, some sectors of the healthcare industry are more specific in their usage of terms. *Medical services (care)* include diagnostic and therapeutic measures provided to persons who are sick, injured, or concerned about their health status. Healthcare services expand medical services to include *preventive care* (Rowell 2000, 22).

Sections of a Healthcare Insurance Policy

Healthcare insurance policies are divided into sections. Typically, these sections include definitions (commonly used terms), eligibility and enrollment, **benefits, limitations, exclusions,** procedures, and appeals processes. The sections build upon one another and one aspect of healthcare may be addressed in multiple sections. Because the sections interlock, reviewing multiple sections is often necessary to determine whether the healthcare insurance company will pay for (cover) a specific diagnostic procedure, treatment, or healthcare expense.

Definitions

Definitions are often in a separate section, but they may also be incorporated into the benefits section.

Example:

Definitions are important. The healthcare plan of the state of North Carolina defines **medical necessity** as follows:

> A service or supply provided for the diagnosis, treatment, cure, or relief of a health condition, illness, injury, or disease. The service or supply must not be experimental, investigational, or cosmetic in purpose. It must be necessary for and appropriate to the diagnosis, treatment, cure, or relief of a health condition, illness, injury, disease, or its symptoms. It must be within generally accepted standards of medical care in the community. It must not be solely for the convenience of the insured, the insured's family, or the provider (State Health Plan for North Carolina 2005, 7).

Thus, by definition, cosmetic services are not considered medically necessary and, therefore, would not be paid for by the healthcare insurance company.

Definitions sometimes are specific to the healthcare plan and may be more restrictive than ones in everyday usage or dictionaries. For example, a dictionary definition of *emergency* is "an unexpected situation or sudden occurrence of a serious and urgent nature that demands immediate attention"

(Pickett et al. 2000). The healthcare insurance plan may define *emergency* as life-threatening, a concept that is more extreme and less likely than demanding immediate attention. Terms often listed in definitions include the following:

- Accidental injury
- **Medical emergency**
- Medical necessity
- **Prior approval**
- **Preexisting condition**
- **Usual, customary, and reasonable**

Eligibility and Enrollment

Eligibility and enrollment sections specify the persons eligible for healthcare insurance and the procedures for obtaining coverage. Eligibility often involves the percentage of the appointment or position or duration of employment. A common provision is that persons must be employed at least 50 percent or half-time (0.5 full-time equivalent). Enrollment is the process of becoming a policyholder or certificate holder. A common step of the procedure is the application for healthcare insurance. There are specific times when applications are received and processed. Common requirements for enrollment include application within 30 days of hire to obtain initial coverage and during certain months, such as October or November, to change healthcare plans or coverage. During enrollment periods, new insureds specify whether the coverage will be single or family.

Benefits

Benefits are the healthcare services for which the healthcare insurance company will pay (will cover). Benefits include the following services:

- Healthcare services provided by physicians, allied health practitioners, and visiting nurses

- Confinement in an acute care hospital, long-term care hospital, partial day center, specialty hospital, and nursing home, including necessary services, supplies, and medications

- Inpatient and outpatient surgeries and associated anesthesia services

- Emergency room, physician office visits, home healthcare, mental health and chemical dependency care, vision and dental care, laboratory tests, x-rays, and other radiologic procedures and treatments

- Rental or purchase of durable medical equipment (DME), prosthetic and orthotic appliances, prescriptions, medical supplies, and blood transfusions and administration

- Emergency transport services

- **Stop-loss benefits**

For example, a stop-loss benefit is designed to provide coverage in the event of a catastrophic illness or injury. A stop-loss benefit is a specific amount, in a certain time frame, such as one year, beyond which all covered healthcare services for that policyholder or dependent are paid at 100 percent by the healthcare insurance plan. This benefit is also known as the **maximum out-of-pocket cost** and the **catastrophic expense limit.** The total is the maximum amount that the policyholder will pay **out-of-pocket** for covered healthcare services in the specified period. Included in the total may be deductibles, coinsurance, and copayments that the policyholder is responsible to pay out-of-pocket. Specific total amounts per year may vary, by category, such as $1,500 maximum in coinsurance and $2,500 maximum in prescription copayments per year.

Often the insureds may purchase differing levels of these benefits in policies. The levels vary widely in the range of services they cover. Premiums, deductibles, coinsurances, and copayments range accordingly, as can be seen in the following examples:

- *Hospital confinement indemnity* policies pay a per diem for each day in the hospital. This policy is typically supplemental.

- *Hospital and surgical* policies cover major expenses in the hospital and expenses related to surgeries, including outpatient surgery. Healthcare insurance payments may be percentages or specific dollar amounts. Hospitalization policies typically have high deductibles and high coverage limits.

- *Major medical (catastrophic)* policies are designed to reduce risk associated with catastrophic illness or injury. A fixed amount is available during the lifetime of the policyholder or dependent. Major medical policies typically have high deductibles and high coverage limits.

- *Comprehensive* policies provide coverage for most healthcare services, including hospitalization, surgery, emergency room, physician services, clinic visits, diagnostic and therapeutic x-rays, laboratory tests, preventive services, and prescriptions. The deductible must be met before the healthcare insurance company will pay for any covered expenses. Coinsurance for all covered expenses must be paid until the maximum out-of-pocket cost is reached. Additional covered expenses are paid in full.

- *Long-term (extended) care* policies provide benefits for nursing home care and services.

- *Disability income protection* policies provide weekly or monthly payments during a lengthy illness or recovery from an injury. Disability income protection policies only begin to pay after a period established in the contract (30 days to 6 months). Contracts usually contain maximum payment limits that are based on a percentage of the policyholder's salary, such as 60 percent.

- *Accidental death and dismemberment (loss)* policies cover expenses due to an accident that causes a loss, such as death, amputation of a limb, or blindness. Benefits vary greatly dependent upon the specific policy.

- *Specific disease or accident* policies provide coverage for diseases or accidents listed in the policy. An example is a cancer policy.

- *Medicare supplement (Medigap)* policies are designed to coordinate payments with those by Medicare. These policies may pay Medicare deductibles and coinsurance. Benefits vary by policy.

Limitations

Limitations are qualifications or other specifications that limit the extent of the benefits. Limitations can be placed on total dollar amount, time frame, duration, and number. For example, purchases of durable medical equipment exceeding $500 require prior approval. Some healthcare insurance plans limit the number of well-visit checks to three per year for children ages one through two.

Cost-Sharing Provisions

Other common limitations are **cost-sharing** provisions of policies. Cost-sharing provisions require policyholders to bear some of the costs of healthcare that they consume. Making policyholders bear some of the financial burden of healthcare is a mechanism to control healthcare costs. Examples of cost-sharing provisions include the following:

- Coinsurance is a preestablished percentage of eligible expenses after the deductible has been met. The percentage may vary by type or site of service.

- Copayment is a fixed dollar amount (flat fee). The fixed amount may vary by type of service, such as a visit or a prescription. For example, the healthcare plan may require that the policyholder pay $15 per outpatient clinic visit and $50 per outpatient surgery visit.

Use of Formulary

The use of a **formulary** is another limitation. A formulary is a list of preferred drugs. Formularies often contain both brand-name and generic drugs approved by the Food and Drug Administration. Although a policy's prescription benefit may cover drugs not in the formulary, the policyholder's cost-sharing for nonformulary products may be higher. Policies may also require higher cost-sharing contributions for nongeneric drugs (table 3.1).

Benefit Cap

A **benefit cap** is an overarching limitation. A benefit cap is also known as a *maximum dollar plan limit*. A benefit cap is the total dollar amount that a healthcare insurance company will pay for a policyholder and each covered dependent for covered healthcare services during a specified period, such as a year or lifetime. Benefit caps vary by the levels

Table 3.1. Example of limitations in prescription drug benefit

Prescription Drug	Copayment per Prescription for 34-Day Supply
Tier 1: Generic	$10
Tier 2: Formulary without Generic	$25
Tier 3: Formulary with Generic	$35
Tier 4: Non-Formulary	$40

of benefits that are purchased. Inexpensive health-care insurance policies tend to have low caps, such as $250,000 per individual. Two common lifetime benefit caps, depending upon the specific policy, are $1 million per individual or $5 million per individual.

Exclusions

Exclusions are situations, instances, conditions, injuries, or treatments that the healthcare plan states will not be covered and for which the healthcare plan will pay no benefits. A synonym for exclusion is impairment **rider.** Specific and unique definitions may serve as exclusions. Typical exclusions include:

- Experimental or investigational diagnostic and therapeutic procedures

- Medically unnecessary diagnostic or therapeutic procedures

- Procedures related to preexisting conditions (states), self-inflicted injury, sexually transmitted diseases, war-related injuries, and cosmetic procedures.

For example, a healthcare plan may deny coverage for a prescription to remove wrinkles (tretinoin) because the purpose is cosmetic. Contraceptives are also sometimes excluded. In another circumstance, should the healthcare expenses be related to an injury suffered in an automobile accident, the healthcare insurance may deny coverage because the automobile accident insurance is responsible for these expenses.

Because of their prevalence, exclusions related to preexisting conditions (states) require detailed discussion. A preexisting condition is a health condition, status, or injury that has been diagnosed prior to the application for healthcare insurance. Healthcare insurance plans deny coverage for costs related to a preexisting condition for a preestablished period of time. This preestablished period of time is known as the **waiting period.** Under the

Health Insurance Portability and Accountability Act (HIPAA), an employer-based group healthcare insurance plan can impose a waiting period for a preexisting condition only if the employee or dependent was diagnosed, received care or treatment, or had care or treatment recommended in the six months before the enrollment date. For group healthcare insurance, the maximum duration of the waiting period cannot exceed twelve months (eighteen months for **late enrollees** who applied after the earliest date on which coverage was available). However, any preexisting condition waiting period must be reduced by a preceding period of coverage under another group health plan or health maintenance organization (HMO), Indian Health Service, Medicare, military healthcare (TRICARE), or other governmental public healthcare plans **(creditable coverage).** This reduction is known as **credited coverage.** Moreover, a preexisting condition will be covered without a waiting period if an employee joins a new group plan if the employee had been insured for the previous 12 months under a group plan without a lapse in coverage exceeding 63 days. No preexisting condition clause may be imposed for pregnancy or childbirth, or a newborn or adopted child (under age 18). (See table 3.2 for examples of creditable coverage in various scenarios.)

The provisions of HIPAA regarding creditable coverage do not apply to the purchase of individual healthcare insurance. Purchasers of individual healthcare insurance are required to meet specified time requirements (up to 24 months) prior to benefits being paid for preexisting conditions.

Riders and Endorsements

Riders and **endorsements** are similar to limitations and exclusions. They provide additional details about coverage or noncoverage for special situations that are not usually included in standard policies. A rider is an additional document and an endorsement is language or statements within the policy itself.

Table 3.2. Examples of calculations of creditable coverage

	Scenario 1	Scenario 2	Scenario 3
Duration of Coverage under Group Healthcare Insurance	2 Years	7 Months	3 Years
Duration of No Coverage between Periods of Employment	45 Days	10 Days	6 Months
Credited Coverage	2 Years	7 Months	0
Maximum Duration of Waiting Period for Preexisting Condition	0 Days	5 Months	12 Months
Rationale	Lapse in Coverage <63 Days Duration of Previous Coverage >12 Months	Lapse in Coverage <63 Days Duration of Previous Coverage <12 Months	Lapse in Coverage >63 Days

Procedures

Procedures explain how policyholders obtain the healthcare benefit or qualify to receive the healthcare benefit. Healthcare plans may deny benefits because procedures are not followed. Moreover, the procedures can function as limitation and exclusions, even though they may be stated in the positive. For example, "all mental health and chemical dependency services must be rendered by an eligible provider." Therefore, if services were provided by an ineligible provider, they would not be covered (paid for).

Prior Approval

A common procedure is obtaining prior approval. During this approval process, the healthcare plan determines medical necessity. Types of services often requiring prior approval include:

- Outpatient surgeries
- Diagnostic, interventional, and therapeutic outpatient procedures
- Physical, occupational, and speech therapies
- Mental health and chemical dependency care
- Inpatient care including surgery, home health, private nurses, and nursing homes
- Organ transplants

If a policy requires prior approval for physical therapy services and the policyholder does not obtain the prior approval, the expenses related to the physical therapy services may be denied.

Coordination of Benefits

Another common procedure is **coordination of benefits.** Coordination of benefits becomes necessary when people have multiple healthcare insurance carriers that are providing coverage. Multiple carriers can occur in instances when both spouses or parents work and both employers provide healthcare insurance, or when automobile insurance company is paying for the treatment of injuries incurred in an automobile accident. The primary insurer (payer) is the healthcare insurance responsible for the greatest proportion or majority of the healthcare expenses. The secondary insurer (payer) is responsible for the remainder of the healthcare expenses.

Determination of primary or secondary insurer can be complicated. Some common rules are:

- Patient's healthcare insurance is primary over the spouse's healthcare insurance.
- Dependent child's primary insurer is the insurance of the parent whose birthday

comes first in the calendar year ("birthday rule").

- A legal decree, such as divorce agreement, dictates determination.
- The circumstances of the case, such as automobile accident insurance for injuries from an automobile accident, dictate determination.

In many instances, when policyholders enroll in a healthcare insurance plan, they are required to list all other healthcare insurance policies they may have. Often, clauses within the healthcare insurance policy state that the primary insurance will pay for the majority of the healthcare expenses and the secondary insurance will pay for the remaining costs. Thus, the payments from all healthcare insurance companies do not exceed 100 percent of the covered healthcare expenses. This integration of payments is known as coordination of benefits (Jones 2001, 495).

Appeals Processes

An appeal is a request for reconsideration of denial of coverage for healthcare services or rejection of a **claim.** A claim is a bill for healthcare services submitted by a hospital, physician's office, or other healthcare provider facility. Claims are submitted for reimbursement to the healthcare insurance plan by either the policy or certificate holder or the provider. The appeals section of a policy describes the steps that policyholders must take to appeal a decision about coverage or payment of a claim. Typically, the appeal must be in writing and within a specific time frame of the healthcare insurance company's decision concerning the issue.

Check Your Understanding 3.1

1. Who is included in a healthcare insurance policy offering dependent healthcare coverage?

2. Which type of policy offers the widest ranging coverage but requires the insured to pay

coinsurance until the maximum out-of-pocket costs are met?

3. Which of the following is **not** a type of healthcare policy limitation?
   a. Benefit cap
   b. Cost-sharing provision
   c. Geographic plan
   d. Use of formulary

4. Under HIPAA, any preexisting condition waiting period in a group healthcare plan must be reduced by _____.

5. Describe the types of procedures and services that typically require prior approval.

Determination of Covered Services

Healthcare insurance policies must be studied in their entirety to determine covered services. All the sections of the policy operate together to delineate covered services and noncovered services. An example from a mental health and chemical dependency benefit illustrates the linkage of policy sections (figure 3.2). The benefit is inpatient care for a mental health condition or chemical dependency. In the definitions section of a policy, both **precertification** and prior approval are defined. These definitions detail how to properly complete the procedures of obtaining precertification and prior approval. The limitations section notes that there is $100 copayment in addition to applicable deductibles and coinsurance. Moreover, the limitations for mental health facilities specify that patients must be in beds licensed as psychiatric or chemical dependency and that the eligible attending physician must have specialized credentials. Finally, the exclusions section specifies that care preceding precertification, delivered by a noneligible provider, or obtained at a noncontracting facility will be denied. This illustration demonstrates how intricately the sections of the policy integrate to define coverage.

Figure 3.2.   Illustration of linkage of policy sections for a mental health or chemical dependency benefit

Policy Section	Language Demonstrating Linkage
Definitions	Precertification for Mental Health and Chemical Dependency: Process of calling the mental health claim management representative prior to receiving services and obtaining approval for all continuing care. (This requirement is different from prior approval and is not a guarantee of payment.)
	Prior Approval: Review of request for coverage of services prior to services being rendered that ensures certain covered services are deemed medically necessary and appropriate in order to treat the patient's condition.
Benefits	Inpatient care
Limitations	$100 copayment in addition to deductible and coinsurance
	Inpatient mental health or psychiatric treatment must be in licensed psychiatric bed and have attending physician who is a psychiatrist
	Inpatient chemical dependency treatment must be in a licensed chemical dependency bed and have attending physician who is a psychiatrist or addictionologist
	Delivered by eligible provider listed on pages 61 through 62 of the benefits manual
Exclusions	Treatment preceding precertification
	Treatment provided by ineligible provider
	Treatment at a noncontracting facility
Procedures	Obtain prior approval
	Obtain precertification

Private (Individual) Healthcare Plans

Individuals and self-employed business persons purchase healthcare insurance for themselves and their families. Private healthcare plans are sometimes termed *individual plans* because individuals purchase them. For some persons, the private healthcare plan is their only plan for themselves and their families. However, some persons purchase private healthcare plans to supplement their employer-based group insurance or their Medicare.

In general, individual healthcare insurance plans provide fewer covered services at a higher cost than group healthcare insurance plans.

Purchasers of individual healthcare plans usually must provide **evidence of insurability.** This evidence includes completing a survey about current and past health status and undergoing a physical examination. Based on the evidence, the healthcare insurance company may reject the applicant or may specify exclusionary clauses in the policy. Reasons for rejection include health habits, past medical history, age, income and other factors that affect risk of illness or accident.

Typically, private healthcare plans have higher premiums and deductibles, lower maximum plan dollar limits, and more restrictions on coverage for preexisting conditions than group healthcare insurance plans have. Policyholders of private healthcare insurance pay higher premiums to obtain and to maintain their healthcare insurance. Also higher are the deductibles that the policyholder must pay before the healthcare insurance will assume its share of liability for the remaining costs. Maximum plan dollar limits may be lower than for group healthcare plans.

Employer-Based (Group) Healthcare Plans

Employer-based healthcare plans are group plans for groups of employees or members. Employer-based healthcare plan is a misnomer because the type includes all plans that cover groups. Individuals may form groups through professional associations and other entities. An example of an "other entity" is the Mississippi Comprehensive Health Insurance Risk Pool Association (MCHIRPA). The MCHIRPA is a nonprofit legal entity created to make the advantages of group healthcare insurance available to Mississippi's citizens who cannot secure other healthcare insurance because of their health conditions.

Employer-based healthcare plans have lower premiums and deductibles and greater benefits than private healthcare plans. Persons with pre-existing conditions and who cannot obtain private healthcare insurance can obtain coverage (after a period of time) under an employer-based health-care plan.

Blue Cross and Blue Shield Plans

Blue Cross and Blue Shield plans began in Dallas, Texas, in 1929, when Justin Ford Kimball established a health insurance plan for schoolteachers. In the plan, schoolteachers prepaid $6 per year for twenty-one days of hospitalization (Blue Cross 2005). Similar plans were also formed in Michigan and New Jersey (Koch 2002, 98). In 1934, the American Hospital Association (AHA) united the plans under its auspices (Koch 2002, 98). In 1939, the AHA adopted the symbol of the blue cross to indicate the health insurance plans that met specific criteria for covering hospital care. Also, in 1939, Blue Shield was founded in California to cover physician services (Blue Cross 2005). In 1972, the AHA's sponsorship of Blue Cross ended. Blue Cross and Blue Shield merged in 1982 to form the Blue Cross and Blue Shield Association (Blue Cross 2005).

Today Blue Cross and Blue Shield is a federation of forty independent, locally operated plans united through membership in the Blue Cross and Blue Shield Association (BCBSA). Plans can operate at the state level, such as Blue Cross of Alabama or at the substate level, such as Blue Cross and Blue Shield of Western New York being one of six Blue plans in the state. The plans contract with hospitals, physicians, and other health care providers to offer services to their subscribers (policyholders). BCBSA is one of the most influential groups in healthcare (Hall and Conover 2003, 509).

The Blue Companies insure nearly one in three Americans (Grossman and Strunk 2004, 1). In June 2003, 88.3 million Americans were enrolled in the Blue Companies, a 28-year high (Grossman and Strunk 2004, 1). The Blue Companies offer their subscribers a wide range of options such as health maintenance organizations, point-of-service plans, preferred provider organizations, and indemnity plans.

Profit Versus Nonprofit Status

The Blue Companies had operated traditionally as nonprofit. However, in 1994, BCBSA decided to allow local plans to convert to for-profit status (Grossman and Strunk 2004, 1). Between 1993 and 2003, Blue Cross and Blue Shield plans in 15 states, including Blue Cross of California and Empire Blue Cross of eastern New York converted to for-profit status (Hall and Conover 2003, 510). The result is more than one in four Blue Cross subscribers belong to a for-profit plan (Hall and Conover 2003, 510).

Types of Blue Cross and Blue Shield Accounts

Blue Cross and Blue Shield have two types of accounts: geographic plans at the state or substate level and the federal employee program (FEP). Geographic plans cover subscribers (members) in a specific state or region. The FEP covers all enrolled federal government employees across the nation and the globe.

Geographic Plans

Geographic plans cover specific geographic areas, such as Blue Cross and Blue Shield of Missouri or Regence Blue Cross and Blue Shield of Utah. The geographic plans are locally administered and have long-standing relationships with their local hospitals and medical communities (Hall and Conover 2003, 509). The subscribers carry cards with the name of the plan, their subscribers' names, and contract and group numbers.

Federal Employee Program

The government-wide federal employee program (FEP) has 4.4 million members. The FEP is also known as the Service Benefit Plan. The following notation on the insured's cards—Government-Wide Service Benefit Plan and FEP—identify the federal program.

Explanation of Benefits

An **explanation of benefits (EOB)** is a report from Blue Cross and Blue Shield that is sent from a healthcare insurer to the policyholder and to the provider. The report lists the following data elements:

- Healthcare service with provider and date

- Cost or **actual charge** of the healthcare service

- **Allowable charge** which is the amount the healthcare insurer will cover

- Applicable cost-sharing, such as coinsurance and copayment

- The remainder of the costs, which is the policyholder's responsibility

Figure 3.3 is a sample explanation of benefits illustrating how a Blue plan provides specific benefits for a subscriber (member).

Figure 3.3. Explanation of benefits

Blue Cross of Some State					
Member's Name: Jane Green **ID Number:** 123-45-6789 **Date** June 15, 200*					
Patient's Name: Jane Green (Member)					
Service	**Amount of Bill**	**Amount You Do Not Owe**	**Amount Paid by Plan**	**Your Balance**	**Explanation of Your Balance**
Surgicenter of Smith County 05-10-200* Ambulatory Surge	536.01	181.34	To Provider 150.00	204.67	**Your $150 wellness benefit maximum has been met.** 50.00 Outpatient services copay. 154.67 Applied to Plan year deductible.
City Physicians Group 05-10-200* Surgery	271.00	163.46	0.00	107.54	**Your $150 wellness benefit maximum has been met.** 107.54 Applied to Plan year deductible.
Smith County Hospital 05-16-200* X-Ray Services	450.63	72.10	To Provider 232.59	145.94	**Your $150 wellness benefit maximum has been met.** 58.15 Your 20% coinsurance. 87.79 Applied to Plan year deductible.
TOTAL			382.59	458.15	
350 of 350 Deductible met for 07-01-200* to 06-30-200*		58.15 of 1500.00 Coinsurance met for 07-01-200* to 06-30-200*			

Summary

Voluntary health insurance includes private or commercial healthcare insurance plans and Blue Cross and Blue Shield plans. This sector of the healthcare industry is very important as approximately 33 percent of healthcare expenditures in the U.S. are payments from voluntary health insurance plans. Healthcare insurance policies are comprised of sections, such as definitions, eligibility and enrollment, benefits, limitations, exclusions, procedures, and appeals processes. The sections operate together to clearly delineate healthcare services for which the healthcare insurance company will pay.

Types of healthcare insurance include private or commercial healthcare insurance, which can be purchased by individuals or employers and other entities. Employer-based group plans tend to be more flexible and provide greater benefits at less cost than individual policies. Blue Cross and Blue Shield is a federation of 40 independent, locally-operated plans that collectively form one of the most influential private groups in the healthcare industry.

Chapter 3 Review Quiz

1. What is the relation between covered conditions and covered services in private or commercial insurance plans?

2. Name at least two of the three benefit terms that mean the amount beyond which all covered healthcare services for an insured or dependent are paid 100 percent by the insurance plan.

3. What type of insurance policy provides benefits to (a) a resident requiring nursing home care and services, (b) an insured who becomes blind, and (c) a homeowner who requires an eight-month recuperation after a fall down her basement stairs?

4. Why can use of a formulary be considered a policy limitation?

5. List at least three typical exclusions found in insurance plan riders.

6. Describe the health insurance plan that covers federal government employees.

7. How does Blue Cross and Blue Shield notify insureds about the extent of payments made on a claim? What data elements does that notification include?

8. Voluntary health insurance plan payments account for about one-fourth of U.S. healthcare expenditures. True or false?

9. Copayments are cost-sharing provisions of policies that require insureds to pay a flat fee to healthcare service providers and suppliers. True or false?

10. Individuals having preexisting conditions are financially better off using private healthcare plans than either employer group plans or managed care alternatives. True or false?

References and Bibliography

Blue Cross. 2005. Available online from www.brainy encyclopedia.com/encyclopedia/b/bl/blue_cross.html.

Grossman, J. M., and B. C. Strunk. 2004. For profit conversions and merger trends among Blue Cross Blue Shield health plans. *Issue Brief/Center for Studying Health System Change* 76 (January): 1–6.

Hall, M. A., and C. J. Conover. 2003. The impact of Blue Cross conversions on accessibility, affordability, and the public interest. *The Milbank Quarterly* 81 (December) (4): 509–542.

Jones, L. M., ed. 2001. Glossary. In *Reimbursement Methodologies for Healthcare Services* [CD-ROM]. Chicago: American Health Information Management Association.

Koch, A. L. 2002. Financing health services. In *Introduction to Health Services.* 6th ed., edited by S. J. Williams and P. R. Torrens. Albany, N.Y.: Delmar.

Pickett, J. P. et al., eds. 2000. *American Heritage Dictionary of the English Language.* 4th ed. Boston: Houghton Mifflin Company.

Rowell, J. C. 2000. *Understanding Health Insurance: A Guide to Professional Billing,* 5th ed. Albany, N.Y.: Delmar.

State Health Plan for North Carolina. 2005. Available online from www.statehealthplan.state.nc.us.

Chapter 4
Government-Sponsored Healthcare Programs

Objectives

- To differentiate among and to identify the various government-sponsored healthcare programs

- To understand the history of the Medicare and Medicaid programs in America

- To recognize the impact that government-sponsored healthcare programs have on the American healthcare system

Key Terms

Beneficiary

Centers for Medicare and Medicaid Services (CMS)

Civilian Health and Medical Program: Veterans Administration (CHAMPVA)

Federal Employees' Compensation Act of 1916 (FECA)

Indian Health Service

Medicaid

Medicare

Medicare Advantage

Medicare Modernization Act of 2003 (MMA)

Medicare Part A

Medicare Part B

Medicare Part C

Medicare Part D

Medigap

Programs of All-Inclusive Care for Elderly (PACE)

Social Security Act

State Children's Health Insurance Program (SCHIP)

Temporary Assistance for Needy Families Program (TANF)

TRICARE

Workers' Compensation

Introduction

The various levels of government administer several health plans for various populations as mandated by laws and regulations. Perhaps the most well-known is **Medicare** for persons who qualify for social security benefits and are 65 years of age or older. This chapter discusses Medicare and several other federal and state sponsored programs.

Medicare

The **Social Security Act** was amended in 1965 to create the Medicare program (Title XVIII). Medicare is a national health insurance program that provides health services to elderly and other qualifying persons. Medicare benefits are available for persons:

- Sixty-five years or older who are eligible for Social Security or Railroad Retirement benefits

- Individuals entitled to Social Security or Railroad Retirement disability benefits for at least twenty-four months

- Government employees with Medicare coverage who have been disabled for more than twenty-nine months

- Insured workers (and their spouses) with end-stage renal disease

- Children with end-stage renal disease

The most significant recent legislative change to Medicare was the **Medicare Modernization Act of 2003 (MMA).** MMA created an outpatient prescription drug benefit, provided beneficiaries with expanded coverage choices, and improved benefits.

Medicare is divided into four parts: Part A, Part B, Part C, and Part D.

Medicare Part A for Inpatients

Medicare Part A, inpatient hospital insurance, is provided with no premiums to most beneficiaries. Most services covered under this benefit require an annual deductible and copayment to be paid by the **beneficiary.** Services included in this benefit are:

- Inpatient hospitalization

- Long-term care hospitalization

- Skilled nursing facility services

- Home health services

- Hospice care

Each site of service has specific limitations with regard to cost-sharing provisions per benefit period (see table 4.1).

Medicare Part B

Medicare Part B, supplemental medical insurance, is an optional insurance package that beneficiaries may purchase. For 2006, the monthly premium is $88.50 (CMS 2005a). Part B insurance covers physician services, medical services, and medical supplies not covered by Part A. Most of these services are provided on an outpatient basis. In addition to the monthly premium, beneficiaries are responsible for an annual deductible and service copayments. Table 4.2 provides a summary of the services and cost-sharing provisions.

Medicare Part C

Several services are excluded from Part A and Part B Medicare coverage. Beneficiaries can purchase additional coverage or choose **Medicare Part C** coverage, a managed care option known as **Medicare Advantage,** to gain insurance for these services. The Part A and Part B excluded services which are provided under Part C are:

- Long-term nursing care

- Custodial care

- Dental services

- Vision services

Table 4.1.   Part A services

Site of Service	Benefit Period	Patient Responsibility
Hospital Inpatient and Long-Term Care Hospital	First 60 days	$952 annual
	Days 61–90	$238 per day
	Days 91–150 (lifetime reserve days*)	$476 per day
	Beyond 150 (lifetime reserve days*)	All costs
Skilled nursing facility	First 20 days	Nothing
	Days 21–100	$114 per day
	Beyond 100 days	All costs
Home health	No time limit—based on medical necessity criteria	Nothing for services, 20% for durable medical equipment (DME)
Hospice	No time limit—based on physician certification	Limited costs for outpatient drugs and inpatient respite care

*Nonrenewable lifetime reserve of up to 60 additional days of inpatient hospital care.

Table 4.2.   Part B services

Site of Service	Benefit	Patient Responsibility
Medical services	Physician services, medical and surgical services and supplies, DME	$124 annual deductible, plus 20% of approved amount (excludes hospital outpatient, see below)
	Mental health care	50% of most care
	Occupational, physical, and speech therapy	20% of approved amount
Clinical laboratory services	Blood tests, urinalysis, and more	Nothing
Home health	Intermittent skilled care, home health aide service, DME and supplies, and other services	Nothing for services, 20% for durable medical equipment (DME)
Outpatient hospital services	Services for diagnosis and/or treatment of an illness or injury	$124 deductible, plus established copayment amount per covered service
		100% charges for noncovered services

- Routine examinations, except initial preventive medicine examination added by MMA

- Health and wellness education

- Acupuncture

- Hearing aids

Medicare Part C, Medicare Advantage, is available for beneficiaries participating in Part A, B, and D (drug benefit) coverage. In addition to the Part B premium, members of an approved Medicare Advantage program pay an additional premium for the full scope of services offered by the program that are not typically covered by Medicare.

Example:

Routine physical examinations and vision services are excluded from Medicare Parts A and B. However, these services are provided by Medicare Advantage programs.

MMA revised several components of the Medicare Advantage program including a new process for determining beneficiary premiums. Monthly premiums range from $50 to $350 depending on the scope of service the beneficiary elects to purchase.

Medicare Part D

Medicare Part D, Medicare drug benefit, was created by the MMA of 2003. The benefit was scheduled to be fully implemented on January 1, 2006. The program offers outpatient drug coverage provided by private prescription drug plans and Medicare Advantage. Beneficiaries pay monthly premiums of $35, have an annual deductible of $250, and make copayments of 25 percent. Low-income beneficiary provisions are built into the program for seniors who cannot afford the standard copayment amounts. MMA also established improved access to pharmacies, an up-to-date formulary, and emergency access for Medicare beneficiaries.

Medigap

Medicare beneficiaries may elect to purchase private insurance policies to supplement their Medicare Part A and/or Part B coverage. This supplemental insurance, known as **Medigap,** covers most cost-sharing expenses as shown in tables 4.1 and 4.2. Medigap policies must meet federal standards and are offered by various private insurance companies.

Medicaid

Originally known as the Medical Assistance Program, **Medicaid** (Title XIX) was added to the Social Security Act in 1965. Medicaid is a joint program between the federal and state governments to provide healthcare benefits to low-income persons and families. This program is designed to allow each individual state to develop and maintain a Medicaid program unique to its state. Each state determines specific eligibility requirements and services to be offered. Therefore, coverage varies greatly from state to state. A person qualifying for services in one state may not qualify in any other state. Further, coverage determination for services is state-specific. Federal funds allocated to each state are based on the average income per person for that state. However, for a state to qualify to receive Medicaid federal funds, the state's program must provide coverage to at least the following groups:

- Low-income families with children including those who meet eligibility for Temporary Assistance for Needy Families (TANF)

- Supplemental Security Income recipients (or others who meet criteria in more restrictive states)

- Infants born to Medicaid-eligible pregnant women

- Children under the age of six whose family income is at or below 133 percent of the federal poverty level

- Recipients of adoption assistance and foster care (Title IV-E of the Act)

- Certain Medicare beneficiaries

- Special protected groups

Additionally, the state program must offer a designated set of services to members in order to receive federal matching funds (see figure 4.1). Eligibility and services may be expanded by individual states based on that state's laws and regulations. For example, states may elect to provide members with optometry services and eyeglasses, or dental services. States are also afforded the flexibility to determine cost-sharing (in terms of deductible and copayments) terms for their programs for certain services and members. For example, family planning services are exempt from cost-sharing as well as services to pregnant women and children under the age of eighteen. State programs may also offer managed care options. In 2004, 60.68 percent of all Medicaid enrollees chose the managed care option; that is up from 32.1 percent in 1995 (CMS 2005b; 2005c).

Check Your Understanding 4.1

1. Match each Medicare part with the type of benefits it provides:

    a. Part A   _____ Medicare drug benefit
    b. Part B   _____ Supplemental medical insurance
    c. Part C   _____ Inpatient hospital services
    d. Part D   _____ Medicare Advantage

2. What types of costs do Medigap policies cover?

3. Why is Medicaid coverage not identical in New Jersey, California, and Idaho?

Other Government-Sponsored Healthcare Programs

Other government-sponsored healthcare programs include the following:

- The Temporary Assistance for Needy Families (TANF) program

Figure 4.1.   Medicaid-required services

Inpatient hospital services	Rural health clinic services
Outpatient hospital services	Laboratory and x-ray services
Physician services	Pediatric and family nurse practitioner services
Medical and surgical dental services	Federally-qualified health center services
Nursing facility services for individuals aged 21 or older	Nurse-midwife services
Home health care for persons eligible for nursing facility services	Early and periodic screening, diagnosis, and treatment services for individuals under age 21
Family planning services and supplies	

- Programs of All-Inclusive Care for the Elderly (PACE)

- The State Children's Health Insurance Program (SCHIP)

- TRICARE Programs

- Civilian Health and Medical Program: Veterans Administration (CHAMPVA)

- Indian Health Services (IHS)

- Worker's Compensation

Each of these programs serves a specific target group and has specific eligibility requirements, plan requirements, and participant benefits.

The Temporary Assistance for Needy Families Program

The Personal Responsibility and Work Opportunity Reconciliation Act of 1996 (also known as *welfare reform*) brought about many changes to Medicaid eligibility. For example, welfare reform repealed the Aid to Families with Dependent Children (AFDC) program. AFDC was replaced with the TANF program which provides states with grant money designated to provide low-income families with case assistance. However, because welfare reform made significant changes to eligibility, individuals may not realize that they are eligible for Medicaid benefits under this program (CMS 2005d).

Programs of All-Inclusive Care for the Elderly

The Balanced Budget Act of 1997 (BBA) authorized the creation of Programs of All-Inclusive Care for the Elderly (PACE). PACE is a joint Medicare–Medicaid venture that offers states the option of creating and administering this managed care option for the frail elderly population (DHHS 1999). PACE was designed to enhance the quality of life for the frail elderly population by enabling them to live in their own homes and communities, and to preserve and support their family units.

States electing to administer PACE must be approved and provide designated services (see figure 4.2). States must provide services in at least one facility in a geographical service area. The facilities must be accessible and offer adequate services to meet the needs of all participants in the programs. Additional facilities must be staffed and supply a full range of services when warranted by the growth of the PACE population in a service area. Participants may frequent the facility as determined by the multidisciplinary team and the patient's needs. Each facility must have in place a multidis-

ciplinary team consisting of at least the following members (DHHS 1999):

- Primary care physician
- Registered nurse
- Social worker
- Physical therapist
- Occupational therapist
- Recreation therapist or activity coordinator
- Dietician
- PACE center coordinator
- Home care coordinator
- Personal care attendants or representatives
- Drivers or representatives

Beneficiaries of PACE, frail elderly persons, must meet the following eligibility requirements:

- Minimum age of fifty-five
- Resident in the PACE service area
- Assessed by the PACE multidisciplinary team
- Certified by the State Medicaid Agency as eligible for nursing home level of care

PACE programs are not offered in all states or even all service areas within states.

State Children's Health Insurance Program

The State Children's Health Insurance Program (SCHIP) or Title XXI of the Social Security Act, was created in 1997 by the Balanced Budget Act (BBA). SCHIP is a state/federal partnership that

Figure 4.2. PACE-required services

Multidisciplinary assessment and treatment plan	Medical specialty services
Primary care services	Laboratory and x-ray services
Social work services	Drugs and biologicals
Physical, occupational, and speech therapies	Prosthetics and DME
Personal care and supportive services	Acute inpatient care
Nutritional counseling	Nursing facility care
Recreational therapy	All Medicaid covered services
Transportation	
Meals	

*Services in this column must be provided at each PACE facility.

targets the growing number of children not covered by health insurance. It is designed to provide health insurance to children of families whose income level is too high to qualify for Medicaid, but too low to afford private healthcare insurance. Specifically, to qualify for the program, the child must reside with a family whose income is below 200 percent of the federal poverty level or whose family has an income no more than 50 percent higher than the state's Medicaid eligibility threshold.

SCHIP varies from state to state. Each state may determine how it would like to deliver the healthcare benefit to qualifying persons. The state may elect to expand Medicaid eligibility to children who would qualify for SCHIP. The state may design a separate program to provide the benefit. Or the state may combine the Medicaid expansion and separate program concepts. Regardless of the individual program design, state plans and revisions must be approved by the **Centers for Medicare and Medicaid Services (CMS).** By September 30, 1999, each state and territory had an approved SCHIP plan in place (CMS 2005e). States must provide the following services to SCHIP beneficiaries:

- Inpatient hospital services

- Outpatient hospital services

- Physicians' medical and surgical services

- Laboratory and radiology services

- Well-baby/child care services, including immunizations

States may impose cost-sharing provisions on individuals who are enrolled in the program. The cost-sharing cannot exceed 5 percent of a family's gross or net income. States cannot impose cost-sharing for preventive or immunization services. Further, American Indian/Alaskan native children who are members of a federally recognized Tribe may not be charged any cost-sharing fees.

TRICARE

The Department of Defense provides a healthcare program for active duty and retired members of one of the seven uniformed services of the United States: Air Force, Army, Coast Guard, Marine Corps, Navy, National Oceanic and Atmospheric Administration (NOAA) Commissioned Corps, and Public Health Service Commissioned Corps. Additionally, coverage is provided for their families and survivors. The healthcare program is now titled TRICARE replacing Civilian Health and Medical Program of the Uniformed Services (CHAMPUS) that was enacted in 1966 by amendments to the Dependents Medical Care Act. There is only one program option for active duty members, but several for active duty family members, retirees, and their family members and survivors.

TRICARE Prime and TRICARE Prime Remote

TRICARE Prime and TRICARE Prime Remote are the program's managed care options. All active duty service members (ADSMs) are automatically covered by one of these programs, although the individual must complete an enrollment form and submit it to the regional contractor. TRICARE Prime is required when ADSMs live and work within fifty miles or an hour's drive of a military treatment facility.

TRICARE Prime Remote is required when ADSMs live and work in remote areas. In this option, the member may access primary care from a nonnetwork provider if network providers are unavailable in the area. There are no enrollment fees, deductibles, or copayments for authorized medical services and prescriptions with either TRICARE option.

Active duty family members (ADFMs) may also enroll in TRICARE Prime or TRICARE Prime Remote. This is the most economical program available for military families because there are no enrollment, deductible, or copayment fees for covered services. In order to participate in the managed care option, ADFMs must enroll during an open enrollment period.

TRICARE Standard and TRICARE Extra

If ADFMs do not want to enroll in the managed care options, they can participate in TRICARE Standard or TRICARE Extra. TRICARE Standard requires members to pay an annual deductible as well as a 25 percent cost-share of allowed charges. Participants in this program may receive care from any TRICARE authorized provider. TRICARE Extra also requires an annual deductible, but only requires a 20 percent copayment for negotiated codes. Care must be provided by a TRICARE network provider. With this option, there are no claims to file by the beneficiary. The ADFM does not need to enroll in either of these programs. Rather, each family member enrolls in the Defense Enrollment Eligibility Reporting System (DEERS), which outlines eligibility dates. Service members are responsible for maintaining up-to-date information in DEERS.

Military retirees under age sixty-five and their families may enroll in TRICARE Prime or participate in TRICARE Standard or TRICARE Extra. TRICARE Standard and TRICARE Extra require deductibles and copayments for covered services. TRICARE Prime for retirees and their families requires an annual enrollment fee ($230 per individual or $460 per family) and a $12 per visit copayment for in-network providers. There is no copayment for covered services at a military treatment facility.

In addition to health services, TRICARE provides dental services for ADFMs and members of the Individual Ready and Selected Reserve and their families. There are single and family plans that consist of monthly premiums and copayments for covered services. Additionally, TRICARE provides a dental program for retirees and their families. Single, two-party, and family plans are available with monthly premiums, deductibles, and copayments for covered services.

The National Defense Authorization Act for federal fiscal year 2005 expanded TRICARE coverage to be available for Reserve Component (RC) members and their dependents when the RC member is called to active duty (on orders) for more than thirty consecutive days. RC dependents become eligible for TRICARE Standard or TRICARE Extra on the first day of the RC member's orders if the orders are for more than thirty days. RC dependents may choose to enroll in TRICARE Prime or TRICARE Prime Remote any time during the first month of the RC member's activation.

TRICARE for Life

TRICARE for Life (TFL) is TRICARE's secondary coverage for beneficiaries who become entitled to Medicare Part A. TRICARE becomes the secondary payer to Medicare. Members are required to participate in Medicare Part B and pay Medicare Part B premiums.

CHAMPVA

The Department of Veterans Affairs provides covered healthcare services and supplies to eligible beneficiaries through the Civilian Health and Medical Program of the Department of Veterans Affairs (CHAMPVA). This benefits program is available for the spouse or widow(er) and for the children of a veteran who meets one of the following criteria:

- Is permanently and totally disabled due to a service-connected disability
- Was permanently and totally disabled due to a service-connected condition at the time of death
- Died of a service-connected disability
- Died on active duty

Persons eligible for TRICARE benefits cannot participate in CHAMPVA. This program covers most healthcare services and supplies that are medically and psychologically necessary. CHAMPVA becomes a secondary payer when another health insurance benefit is available. For example, when a beneficiary reaches the age of 65, Medicare is the primary payer and CHAMPVA becomes the secondary payer.

The Indian Health Service

The Indian Health Service (IHS) was created to uphold the federal government's obligation to promote healthy American Indian and Alaskan native people, communities, and cultures (IHS 2005). A government-to-government relationship between the United States and Indian tribes was established in 1787 based on Article I, Section 8, of the U.S. Constitution. From this relationship came the provision of health services for members of federally recognized tribes. Principal legislation for authorizing federal funds for Indian Health Services is the Snyder Act of 1921. The IHS is an agency within the Department of Health and Human Services.

Following are the functions of the IHS:

- Assists Indian tribes in the development of their own health programs

- Facilitates and assists Indian tribes in coordinating health planning

- Promotes using health resources available through federal, state, and local programs

- Provides comprehensive healthcare services

Healthcare services offered by the IHS include inpatient and outpatient care, preventive and rehabilitative services, and development of community sanitation facilities. The federal IHS healthcare delivery system consists of hospitals, health centers, health stations, and residential treatment centers.

Workers' Compensation

The workers' compensation benefit is provided to most employees to cover healthcare costs and lost income that results from a work-related injury or illness. Federal government employees are covered under the **Federal Employees' Compensation Act (FECA).** Other employees are covered under state workers' compensation insurance funds if that program is established in the state in which the employees work.

FECA was established in 1916 and ensures that civilian employees of the federal government are provided medical, death, and income benefits for work-related injuries and illnesses. FECA is administered by the Office of Workers' Compensation Programs (OWCP), a division of the Department of Labor. OWCP also administered the Longshore and Harbor Workers' Compensation Act of 1927 and the Black Lung Benefits Reform Act of 1977.

State workers' compensation insurance funds are established by each state. Benefits may include burial, death, income, and medical. Rather than contracting individually with insurance companies for coverage, employers pay premiums into the nonprofit workers' compensation fund for their state. This allows the workers' compensation premiums to remain low and affordable for small business owners.

In states where no fund is mandated for workers' compensation, employers must purchase insurance from private carriers or provide self-insurance coverage. (LaTour and Eichenwald, 296–297).

Check Your Understanding 4.2

1. Match each TRICARE program on the left with its description on the right:

   a. ADFMs with deductible   ____ TRICARE for
      and 20% copay   Life (TFL)
   b. ADFMs with deductible   ____ TRICARE
      and 25% cost-share   Prime
   c. Managed care   ____ TRICARE
      for ADSMs   Extra
   d. Secondary coverage for   ____ TRICARE
      Medicare beneficiaries   Standard

2. When a CHAMPVA beneficiary reaches the age of 65, Medicare is the primary payer and CHAMPVA becomes the secondary payer. True or false?

3. Services offered by the IHS to Indian tribes include all of the following except:
   a. Rehabilitative services
   b. Death benefits
   c. Outpatient care
   d. Development of sanitation facilities

Summary

Government-sponsored healthcare plans such as Medicare, Medicaid, TANF, PACE, the TRICARE programs, CHAMPVA, the IHS, and workers' compensation make affordable healthcare options available to many people who would otherwise go without coverage and the quality healthcare services they need. The market for government-sponsored healthcare plans is large and growing, with federally sponsored programs now covering more than 60 million beneficiaries. Such programs, due to their size, have a unique and pervasive influence on private insurance plans and other public-sector plans in terms of coverage, quality of care, and cost-effectiveness, as well as the processes employed in healthcare reimbursement.

Chapter 4 Review Quiz

1. Which program replaced the Aid to Families with Dependent Children (AFDC)?

2. What recent legislation made a substantive change to Medicare benefits, and how did they change?

3. List at least three types of Medicaid recipients required for states to qualify for federal matching funds.

4. How was the PACE venture designed to enhance the quality of life for the frail elderly population?

5. What is the target population of the State Children's Health Insurance Program (SCHIP) (Title XXI)?

6. Which TRICARE program is the most economical program for military families, and why is it less expensive than the other options?

7. What program covers healthcare costs and lost income from work-related injuries or illness of federal government employees?

8. Individuals eligible for Railroad Retirement disability or retirement benefits are ineligible for Medicare. True or false?

9. Individuals who are eligible may choose between TRICARE benefits and CHAMPVA. True or false?

10. In states having no mandated workers' compensation fund, employers must purchase insurance from private carriers or provide self-insurance coverage. True or false?

References and Bibliography

Centers for Medicare and Medicaid Services. 2005a. Available online from www.cms.hhs.gov/providerupdate/regs/cms8027N.pdf.

Centers for Medicare and Medicaid Services. 2005b. Available online from www.cms.hhs.gov/medicaid/managedcare/pctoftot.pdf.

Centers for Medicare and Medicaid Services. 2005c. Available online from www.cms.hhs.gov/medicaid/managedcare/trends04.pdf.

Centers for Medicare and Medicaid Services. 2005d. State requirements and options under Federal Medicaid law. Available online from www.cms.hhs.gov/medicaid/welfareref/welfare.asp#ch1State.

Centers for Medicare and Medicaid Services. 2005e. State Children's Health Insurance Program (SCHIP). Available online from www.cms.hhs.gov/schip/about-SCHIP.asp.

Department of Health and Human Services. 1999. *Federal Register*. Medicare and Medicaid programs: Programs of all-inclusive care. 64 (226): 66233–66304.

Indian Health Service. 2005. www.ihs.gov.

LaTour, K., and S. Eichenwald, eds. 2002. *Health Information Management: Concepts, Principles, and Practice*. Chicago: American Health Information Management Association.

Chapter 5
Managed Care Plans

Objectives

- To describe origins of managed care

- To trace evolution of managed care

- To describe types of managed care plans

Key Terms

Capitation
Case management
Community rating
Disease management
Episode-of-care reimbursement
Evidence-based clinical practice guidelines
Exclusive provider organization (EPO)
Fee-for-service reimbursement
Gatekeeper
Global payment
Group practice model
Health maintenance organizations (HMOs)
Independent practice association (IPA)
Integrated delivery system
Managed care
Managed care organizations (MCOs)
Medical foundation
Network

Out-of-pocket
Per member per month (PMPM)
Point-of-service (POS) healthcare insurance plan
Preadmission review
Preadmission certification
Preauthorization
Preauthorization (precertification) number
Precertification
Preferred provider organizations (PPOs)
Prescription management
Primary care provider
Prior approval (authorization)
Second opinion
Staff model
Third opinion
Utilization review
Withhold
Withhold pool

Introduction to Managed Care

The purpose of **managed care** is to provide affordable, high-quality healthcare. Managed care systematically merges clinical, financial, and administrative processes to manage access, cost, and quality of healthcare.

Managed care traces its origins to the early 1900s. As early as 1910, Western Clinic in Tacoma, Washington, offered its members medical services for $0.50 per month (American College of Managed Care Medicine 2005). The first Blue Cross plan, established in Dallas, Texas, was a form of managed care. In 1929, schoolteachers in this plan prepaid $6 per year for twenty-one days of hospitalization (Blue Cross 2005). In the 1930s, Kaiser Construction Company established a plan for its workers (American College of Managed Care Medicine 2005).

In the United States between 1966 and the early 1970s, the costs of healthcare escalated quickly (Foster 2000). To control costs and provide affordable quality healthcare, federal legislation encouraged the growth of **health maintenance organizations (HMOs).** The Health Maintenance Organization (HMO) Act of 1973 provided federal grants and loans for new HMOs.

Through the 1980s and 1990s, additional economic constraints encouraged the growth of HMOs and other types of managed care as employers sought to reduce their healthcare costs. Contributing to the growth of hybrid types were the consumers' desires for freedom of choice and access to specialists. The result is that there are numerous types of managed care.

Managed Care Organizations

Managed care organizations (MCOs) are healthcare plans that attempt to manage care. In the Balanced Budget Act of 1997, these plans are termed *coordinated care plans.* MCOs implement provisions to manage both the costs and outcomes of healthcare. Managed care plans integrate the financing and delivery of specified healthcare services.

Benefits and Services of MCOs

MCOs offer differing levels of benefits, depending on the cost of their premiums and copayments. Typical covered services include:

- Physician services (inpatient and outpatient)
- Inpatient care
- Preventive care and wellness, such as immunizations, well-child examinations, adult periodic health maintenance examinations, and pap smears
- Prenatal care
- Emergency services
- Diagnostic and laboratory tests
- Certain home health services

Access to mental and behavioral health and specialty care is through referral from the **primary care provider.**

Characteristics of MCOs

Managed care organizations share characteristics associated with providing quality care and cost-effective care (table 5.1 and table 5.2). The lines between quality care and cost-effective care blur considerably. Moreover, these characteristics are not unique to MCOs; other payers also implement them. However, these characteristics are often associated with MCOs because of the characteristics' prevalence and extent of use in MCOs. MCOs coordinate and control healthcare services to improve quality and to contain expenditures.

Quality Patient Care

Managed care organizations focus on providing quality patient care. They achieve this goal through careful selection of providers, an emphasis on the health of their populations of members, use of care management tools, and maintenance of accreditation or participation in quality improvement programs.

Table 5.1. Managed care characteristics associated with quality care

Characteristic	Description
Selection Criteria for Providers	Criteria Include Quality, Scope of Services, Cost, and Location Credentialing and Periodic Re-credentialing Procedural Selection Process at Senior Clinical Staff Level
Population	Responsible for Delivery of Healthcare Services on Continuum of Care (Prevention, Wellness, Acute, and Chronic) Population Receives Recommended Preventive Care and Appropriate Care for Chronic Conditions Health and Wellness Management
Care Management Tools	Coordination of Care by Primary Care Provider Evidence-Based Clinical Practice Guidelines Disease Management
Quality Assessment and Improvement	Entities Accredited and Engage in Performance Improvement Joint Commission on Accreditation of Healthcare Organizations (JCAHO) National Committee for Quality Assurance (NCQA) URAC (formerly Utilization Review Accreditation Commission) CAHPS®* HEDIS®** Member Satisfaction

*CAHPS® is a registered trademark of the Agency for Healthcare Research and Quality (AHRQ) and private research organizations.
**HEDIS® is a registered trademark of the National Committee for Quality Assurance (NCQA).

Selection of Providers

MCOs stress the use of criteria in their selection of providers. Senior clinicians in the upper echelons of the MCO select providers using preestablished procedures and standards. These criteria are based on quality, scope of services, cost, and location. Timelines for credentialing and recredentialing are followed. This emphasis ensures their members' access to superior and eminent providers throughout a geographic area.

Services Across the Continuum of Care

Managed care organizations emphasize the health of their entire populations of members. These organizations are responsible for the delivery of healthcare services across the continuum of care in terms of setting and type. Examples of settings include the physicians' offices, home health agencies, and hospitals. Examples of types of care are preventive, wellness-oriented, acute, and chronic. The MCO is clinically responsible for the health outcomes of its population.

For preventive care, members receive appropriate testing for preventive care, such as timely mammograms and pap smears. Moreover, members with chronic conditions receive appropriate assessment and therapeutic procedures, as recommended by **evidence-based clinical practice guidelines.** In addition, managed care organizations often support their members' participation in health and wellness management. Wellness programs are one component of health and wellness management. These programs stress the habits of healthy lifestyles, such as exercise and proper nutrition. Other aspects of health and wellness management include smoking cessation, alcohol moderation, and harm reduction.

Table 5.2.   Managed care characteristics associated with cost-effective care

Characteristic	Description
Service Management Tools	Medical Necessity Review
	Utilization Management
	Case Management
	Prescription Management
Episode-of-Care Reimbursement	Capitated Reimbursement
	Global Payment
Financial Incentives	Providers to Meet Fiscal Targets
	Members to Use Providers Associated with the Plan

Care Management Tools

Care management tools include coordination of care, **disease management,** and the application of evidence-based clinical practice guidelines. Together, these tools foster continuity of healthcare services and accessibility and reduce fragmentation and misuse of resources and facilities.

Coordination of care is achieved through the use of primary care providers (PCPs). In many managed care organizations, one PCP provides, supervises, or arranges for a patient or client's healthcare and makes necessary and appropriate referrals. Primary care providers may be physicians, nurse practitioners, or physician assistants (Felt-Lisk 1996, 97–98). Primary care physicians are often family practitioners, general practitioners, internists, pediatricians, and obstetricians/gynecologists.

Disease management focuses on preventing exacerbations of chronic diseases and promoting healthier lifestyles for patients and clients with chronic diseases. In disease management, patients are monitored to promote adherence to treatment plans and to detect early signs and symptoms of exacerbations. Disease management programs often focus on diabetes, congestive heart failure, coronary heart disease, chronic obstructive pulmonary disease, and asthma. Often the management of chronic diseases requires treatment plans and

complex medication regimens involving multiple healthcare providers. Therefore, disease management is closely aligned with coordination of care because the efforts of multiple providers must be synchronized.

Evidence-based clinical practice guidelines are the foundation of members' care for specific clinical conditions. Evidence-based clinical practice guidelines are explicit statements that guide clinical decision making. They outline the

- Key diagnostic indicators

- Timelines

- Alternatives in interventions and treatments

- Potential outcomes

They have been systematically developed from scientific evidence and clinical expertise to answer clinical questions. Other terms for these guidelines are evidence-based guidelines, clinical practice guidelines, clinical guidelines, clinical pathways, clinical criteria, and medical protocols. Sources of these guidelines are the Agency for Healthcare Research and Quality (AHRQ), the Centers for Disease Control and Prevention, the National Guideline Clearinghouse, and specialty organizations, such as the American College of Cardiology, the American Academy of Family Physicians, the American Academy of Ophthalmology, and the American College of Obstetricians and Gynecologists. These guidelines are benchmarks of best practices in the care and treatment of patients and clients.

These guidelines are used to manage the wellness of members and to direct the care of acute illnesses and chronic conditions. The guidelines typically address:

- Entire plan of care across multiple delivery sites

- Appropriate diagnostic and therapeutic procedures for given diseases and conditions

- Reasons for referrals to specialists

- Clinical decision factors and decision points

Therefore, evidence-based clinical practice guidelines serve as a means to standardize optimum care for all patients and to deliver comprehensive, coordinated care across multiple providers.

Accreditation Processes and Performance Improvement Initiatives

Managed care organizations also participate in rigorous accreditation processes and in performance improvement initiatives. Organizations with accreditation standards for managed care include the Joint Commission on Accreditation of Healthcare Organizations (JCAHO), the National Committee for Quality Assurance (NCQA), and the URAC (formerly the Utilization Review Accreditation Commission). Plans also participate in performance improvement initiatives, such as the AHRQ's CAHPS® (formerly Consumer Assessment of Health Plans) project and the NCQA's Health Plan Employer Data and Information Set (HEDIS®). Often as a part of HEDIS, managed care organizations also survey their members to assess members' feedback on such issues as:

- Satisfaction with administrative, clinical services, and customer services

- Perceptions of the plan's strengths and weaknesses

- Suggestions for improvements

- Intentions regarding reenrollment

In addition to surveying members, MCOs conduct satisfaction surveys of patients, physicians, providers, customers, employers, and disenrolled members. Commitment to accreditation and performance improvement demonstrates MCOs' dedica-

tion to their members and to the delivery of quality healthcare.

Cost Controls

Managed care plans implement various forms of cost controls. These cost controls include service management tools, the method of reimbursement, and financial incentives. Examples of service management tools are review of medical necessity, utilization management, and case and prescription management. The method of reimbursement is **episode-of-care reimbursement** with its inherent features of cost reduction. Financial incentives include those for both providers and members. The MCO is fiscally accountable for the health outcomes of its population.

Medical Necessity and Utilization

Several cost controls are related to medical necessity and utilization. These cost controls contain and monitor use of healthcare services by evaluating the need for and intensity of the service prior to it being provided. As stated in chapter 3, *medical necessity* can be defined as:

> A service or supply provided for the diagnosis, treatment, cure, or relief of a health condition, illness, injury, or disease. The service or supply must not be experimental, investigational, or cosmetic in purpose. It must be necessary for and appropriate to the diagnosis, treatment, cure, or relief of a health condition, illness, injury, disease, or its symptoms. It must be within generally accepted standards of medical care in the community. It must not be solely for the convenience of the insured, the insured's family, or the provider (State health plan 2005, 7).

Utilization review assesses the appropriateness of the setting for the healthcare service in the continuum of care and the level of service. Also factored in are patients' severity of illness and other medical conditions and illnesses. Review of medical necessity and utilization are often performed concomitantly.

MCOs and other insurers review medical necessity and utilization in a three-step process: initial clinical review, peer clinical review, and appeals consideration (Table 5.3). Steps two and three are only implemented if the previous step results in a negative decision. If a step results in a positive decision, the process stops at that step.

Medical necessity and utilization are reviewed using objective, clinical criteria. Multiple sets of criteria exist:

- Intensity of Service, Severity of Illness, and Discharge Screens (ISD)

- Appropriateness Evaluation Protocol (AEP)

- Managed Care Appropriateness Protocol (MCAP) (Kalant et al. 2000, 1809)

- Milliman and Robertson (M&R) guidelines (Rutledge 1998, 579)

- Solucient (formerly HCIA-Sachs) length of stay guidelines

- American Society of Addiction Medicine's Patient Placement Criteria, Second Edition-Revised (ASAM PPC-2R)

- Federal and state-specific guidelines

Medical necessity and utilization are often reviewed for the following services:

Table 5.3.   Review of medical necessity and utilization

Step	Responsible Party	Activity or Resource
Clinical Review	Licensed Health Professional	Review against Established Criteria
Peer Clinical Review	Peer Clinician	Clinician Qualified to Render Clinical Opinion Performs Clinical Review
Appeals Consideration	Qualified, Expert Clinician in Same Specialty	Clinician Not Involved in Initial Decision and Qualified to Render Clinical Opinion Performs Clinical Review

- Confinement in acute care hospital, long-term acute care facility, long-term care facility psychiatric hospital, partial-day hospital, hospice, and rehabilitation services

- Surgical procedures

- Emergency room services

- Emergent care received from out-of-**network** (out-of-plan) providers

- High-cost or high-risk diagnostic, interventional, or therapeutic outpatient procedures

- Physical, occupational, speech and other rehabilitative therapies

- Mental health and chemical dependency care

- Home health services, private duty nurses, and referrals to medical specialists

- Durable medical equipment, prosthetic and orthotic appliances, medical supplies, blood transfusions and administration, and medical transport

Gatekeeper Role of Primary Care Provider

The **gatekeeper** role of the primary care provider is a cost control. As the coordinator of all the healthcare a member may access, the primary care provider determines whether referrals are warranted. These referrals may be to (a) medical specialists, (b) other healthcare sites for diagnostic or therapeutic procedures, or (c) hospitals or other healthcare facilities. Gatekeepers determine the appropriateness of the healthcare service, the level of healthcare personnel, and the setting in the continuum of care.

Prior Approval

Prior approval (authorization) is also a cost control. Prior approval is the formal administrative process of obtaining prior approval for healthcare services. Alternate terms for this process are

preauthorization and **precertification.** Terms for prior approval specific to inpatient services are **preadmission review** and **preadmission certification.** Inpatient admissions, surgeries, visits to medical specialists, elective procedures, and expensive or sophisticated diagnostic tests are all types of services requiring prior approval. Occasionally, for healthcare services such as mental or behavioral health, providers must submit entire treatment plans for prior approval. A **preauthorization** or **precertification number** is issued when the healthcare service is approved. Managed care organizations may deny coverage and third party payers may deny payment for healthcare services for which required prior approval was not obtained. Policies identify the healthcare services for which prior approval must be obtained.

Second/Third Opinions

Second and **third opinions** are cost containment measures to prevent unnecessary tests, treatments, medical devices, or surgical procedures. Second or third opinions are obtained from medical experts within the healthcare plan. They are particularly sought when the:

- Test, treatment, medical device or surgical procedure is high risk or high cost

- Diagnostic evidence is contradictory or equivocal

- Experts' opinions are mixed about efficacy

Utilization Review

Utilization review is also a means of cost control that evaluates both effectiveness and efficiency. Utilization review answers the following two questions:

- Should this healthcare service occur?

- If yes, then what setting is the most efficient in terms of delivery and cost?

Utilization review determines the medical necessity of a procedure and the appropriate setting (inpatient or outpatient), given the severity of a patient's illness. For example, utilization review assesses whether the services could be provided more efficiently and economically in an ambulatory setting rather than in the inpatient hospital. Generally, then, utilization review saves money through its prevention of overutilization. Overutilization is the unnecessary consumption of healthcare services or the consumption of unnecessarily expensive or sophisticated healthcare services.

Case Management

Case management coordinates an individual's care, especially in complex and high-cost cases. Individuals are assigned case managers who are typically nurses or physicians. With patients or clients and their families, case managers coordinate the efforts of multiple healthcare providers at multiple sites over time. Consultants, specialists, primary care providers, ancillary services, ambulatory care, inpatient services, and long-term care may all be involved. Case managers are often assigned to patients or clients with catastrophic illnesses or injuries, such as severe head injury. Workers' compensation cases may involve a case manager. Goals of case management include continuity of care, cost-effectiveness, quality, and appropriate utilization.

Prescription Management

Prescription management is also a cost control measure. Prescription management expands the use of a **formulary** (chapter 3) to a comprehensive approach to medications and their administration. This approach includes patient education; electronic screening, alert, and decision-support tools; expert and referent systems, especially related to drug-drug interactions, food-drug interactions, and cross-sensitivities; and criteria for drug utilization. Some electronic prescription management systems include point-of-service order entry, electronic transmission of the prescription to the pharmacy, and patient-specific medication profiles. As discussed in chapter 3, generic, less-expensive drugs are preferred to brand-name, expensive drugs. However, the comprehensive approach also enhances quality patient care. Considering the cost of medications, prescription management is a powerful tool of cost containment.

Episode-of-Care Reimbursement Method

Managed care organizations utilize the episode-of-care reimbursement method. The purpose of the episode-of-care reimbursement method is to reduce the inflation of costs in a **fee-for-service reimbursement** environment. Episode-of-care reimbursement pays providers one pre-determined amount for all the care a patient or client may receive during a period. The MCO does not increase payments for the complexity or extent of healthcare services. Therefore, the incentive to provide higher volumes of services to generate higher reimbursements is eliminated.

Episode-of-care reimbursement is based upon averages. On average, the majority of enrolled members will rarely or never use healthcare services within a period. These low or nonusers offset the acutely or chronically ill members. In the aggregate, the low or nonusers balance out the heavy users. Managed care organizations most commonly use two of the episode-of-care payment methods: **capitation** and **global payment.**

Capitation

In capitation, providers are reimbursed a pre-determined, fixed amount per member per period. The common phrase is **"per member per month"** (PMPM). The volume of services and their expense does not affect the reimbursement. Typically, capitation involves a group of physicians or an individual physician.

Global Payment

Global payment extends the scale of capitation. In global payment, providers in an **integrated delivery system** or other type of network receive one fixed amount for members of the MCO. These providers include physicians, hospitals, and other care providers. The single payment is divided among all the providers. Therefore, in global payment, the scale of capitation is increased from the single group to an entire delivery system.

Financial Incentives

Financial incentives exist for both providers and members. These incentives prevent the waste of financial resources through the provision of excessive or unnecessarily expensive healthcare services.

For providers, these incentives involve the provision of cost-efficient care. Incentives involve meeting targets for cost-efficiency. The following types of healthcare services were the focus of incentives (Grumbach et al. 1998, 1517):

- Referrals to specialists

- Use of laboratory or other ancillary services

- Inpatient admissions or days

- Settings of care, such as office preferred to emergency room

- Productivity, in terms of number of visits per day

- Pharmaceuticals

For example, primary care providers in MCOs may order less expensive generic drugs rather than the more expensive brand-name drugs. Medicaid managed care organizations also set targets, such as "the number of emergency room visits for mental health or substance abuse treatment shall not exceed 8.5 visits per 1000 enrollee months" (Carlson 2000, 13–14).

Incentives can be both positive and negative. As a positive incentive, providers may receive bonuses for meeting cost-containment targets. Conversely, a penalty may be assessed as a negative incentive (disincentive). Examples of penalties include percentage reduction of the PCP's salary if the provider does not meet the target or the loss of withholds (also known as physician contingency reserve [PCR]). A **withhold** is a part of the provider's capitated payment that the MCO deducts and holds to pay for excessive expenditures for expensive healthcare services, such as referrals to specialists. Withholds transfer risk to the providers. For a group practice, the withholds from individual providers are combined to form a **withhold pool.** At the end of period, surplus withheld funds are dispersed for meeting efficiency (utilization) or performance targets. Providers who do not meet targets do not receive their withholds at the end of the period.

It should be noted that, effective January 1, 1997, a federal rule governs financial incentives in managed care Medicaid and Medicare plans (Gallagher, Alpers, and Lo 1998, 409). This rule is Medicare and Medicaid Programs: Requirements for Physician Incentive Plans in Prepaid Health Care Organizations. The rule prohibits incentives that limit medically necessary referrals and requires MCOs to report information about financial incentives regarding referrals to the CMS and state Medicaid offices. Moreover, the rule mandates that MCOs disclose summaries about financial incentives to Medicare and Medicaid members who ask.

As financial incentives to members, MCOs set varying rates of **cost-sharing.** For example, MCOs require higher **out-of-pocket** payments when members use out-of-plan providers than in-plan providers. Other MCOs offer members levels of prescription drug benefits. The drug benefit with the most restrictive formulary is the least expensive while the member's cost-sharing increases with the liberality of the formulary. Incentives influence members' behavior without eliminating freedom of choice.

Contract Management

Contract management is critical in the episode-of-care reimbursement method. Providers and plans must be able to accurately project their expenditures in order to negotiate contracts that cover the costs of treating members. If a provider or plan underestimates the costs to treat plan members, the provider or plan loses money. Moreover, once the contract is established, entities must monitor and evaluate utilization and costs to assess whether projections align with reality. If variances are detected, the plan or provider must implement corrective interventions on a timely basis.

Types of MCOs

As managed care has evolved, lines have blurred among the types of MCOs. The blurring across types makes a continuum a better conceptualization of managed care than individual, separate categories. The different types of MCOs can be placed on a continuum of control. On this continuum, the HMOs represent the most controlled and the **preferred provider organizations (PPOs),** represent the least controlled. This chapter discusses several managed care plans across the continuum of control.

Health Maintenance Organization

Health maintenance organizations (HMOs) combine the provision of healthcare insurance and the delivery of healthcare services. The HMO Act of 1973 was an initiative to control healthcare costs. Subsequent amendments were enacted in 1976, 1978, and 1981 implementing regulations (42 CFR Part 417). Included in the act were conditions for becoming a federally qualified health HMO. The conditions were a minimum benefits package, open enrollment, and **community rating.** In community rating, the rates for healthcare premiums are determined by geographic area (community) rather than by age, health status, or company size.

The act recognized three basic types of HMOs. These basic types are the **staff model,** the **group practice model,** and the **independent practice association (IPA).** Since the 1970s, the **network model** HMO has developed. In some types of HMOs, the HMO hires the healthcare providers and owns the hospitals and other facilities. In other types of HMOs, the plans contract with providers, such as physicians, hospitals, and other healthcare professionals, to provide service. The negotiated payment rates in the contract are discounted. Providers accept the discounted rate because of the increased certainty of referrals and income. The different types of HMOs reflect these differing means of compensation.

HMOs share the following characteristics:

- Organized system of healthcare delivery to a geographic area

- Established set of basic and supplemental health maintenance and treatment services

- Voluntarily enrolled members

- Predetermined, fixed, and periodic prepayments for enrollees

HMOs emphasize preventive care in the belief that, in the long term, preventive care saves money by preventing acute illness and chronic conditions. HMOs are the most restrictive form of managed care because they allow patients and clients the least freedom in choosing a provider. Offsetting this loss of freedom is the reduced out-of-pocket expenses and wide range of benefits.

Staff Model
The staff model HMO provides hospitalization and physicians' services through its own staff. It owns its facility. Its physicians are employees of the HMO and paid on salary or on a capitated basis. Both the staff model and the group model are sometimes called **"closed panel."**

The staff model is the most controlled of the HMOs. Primary care physicians strictly control referrals to specialists within the HMO. Members who seek healthcare services outside the HMO receive no compensation for their healthcare costs.

Group Practice Model
In the group practice model, the HMO contracts with a medical group. The health professionals in this medical group provide services on a fee-for-service or capitation basis. The medical group bears the risk.

Network Model
A network model is the same as a group model HMO except that a network model contracts with two or more independent group practices.

Independent Practice Model
The independent (individual) practice association (IPA) (or organization, IPO) is a type of MCO in which participating physicians maintain their private practices. In the independent practice model, the HMO contracts with the IPA. The IPA, in turn, contracts with individual health providers. The HMO reimburses the IPA on a capitated basis. However, the IPA may reimburse the physicians on a capitated basis or a on a fee-for-service basis. The participating physicians have patients and clients who are members of the HMO as well as patients and clients who are not members. Existing facilities of the independent health professionals are used rather than a free-standing facility. Local, county, or state medical societies may sponsor this type of HMO.

Preferred Provider Organization

A preferred provider organization (PPO) is an entity that contracts with employers and insurers to render healthcare services to a group of members. Its common characteristics are as follows:

- Virtual rather than physical entity

- Decentralized

- Flexibility of choice for members

- Negotiated fees (may include discounts)

- Financial incentives to induce members to choose preferred option

- No prepaid capitation (retains aspects of fee-for-service)

- Not subject to regulatory requirements of HMOs

- Limited financial risk for providers

The PPO also contracts with providers for healthcare services at fixed or discounted rates. The providers are a network of physicians, hospitals, and other healthcare providers. Members can choose to use the healthcare services of any physician, hospital, or other healthcare provider. However, the PPO influences members to use the healthcare services of in-network (in-plan) providers. Members' out-of-pocket expenses are lower if they use in-network providers; members' out-of-pocket expenses are higher if they use the services of out-of-network (out-of-plan) providers. A PPO may be a separate legal entity or it may be a functional unit of another MCO, such as an HMO. A PPO may also be a functional unit of a larger indemnity insurer. The PPO may be sponsored by the network of physicians, hospitals, and other healthcare providers. PPOs offer greater freedom of choice for patients and clients than HMOs. Because there is greater uncertainty about the number of referrals, PPOs typically reimburse providers at a higher rate than HMOs.

Point-of-Service Plan

A **point-of-service (POS) healthcare insurance plan** is one in which members choose how to receive services at the time they need the services. For example, members can choose "at the point of service" whether they want an HMO, a PPO, or a fee-for-service plan. They do not need to make this decision during an open enrollment period. These healthcare insurance plans are also known as open-ended HMOs. Patients' out-of-pocket costs are increased if they receive services outside a referral network (out-of-network or out-of-plan).

Similar to a point-of-service plan is the *provider-sponsored organization (PSO)*. The PSO differs from the point-of-service plan in that the physicians that practice in a regional or community hospital organize the plan. Various levels of benefits are offered, including aggressiveness of gatekeeping, cost-sharing for out-of-network healthcare services, and prescription drug benefits.

Exclusive Provider Organization

An **exclusive provider organization (EPO)** is an MCO that is sponsored by self-insured (self-funded) employers or associations. The EPO is very much a hybrid. Along a continuum of freedom of choice, EPOs feature characteristics of both HMOs and PPOs. Similar to operations of HMOs, a small network of primary care physicians frequently act as gatekeepers. Similar to the system of PPOs, many EPOs reimburse providers on a discounted fee schedule. A few EPOs, however, do reimburse providers through capitation. Members are influenced to seek healthcare services from in-network providers. Patients or clients who choose to receive care outside the network receive lower—and in some cases, no—recompense. Contracts are created between the EPO and providers. Because they offer greater choice, EPOs ensure cost efficiency by aggressively reviewing medical necessity and utilization.

Medicare Advantage

Medicare Advantage, or Medicare Part C (formerly Medicare+Choice), is a form of MCO for Medicare beneficiaries. Medicare beneficiaries who are entitled to Part A and enrolled in Part B have the option to switch to a Medicare Advantage plan, if a plan exists in their area. Types of plans available include HMOs, POSs, PPOs, and PSOs.

Deductibles and copayments are lower in Medicare Advantage. Other benefits may include:

- Preventive care

- Prescription drug plan

- Eyeglasses and hearing aids

- Day care, respite care, assisted care, and long-term care insurance

- Health transport

- Education and health promotion programs

Because the elderly often present complex medical conditions, Medicare Advantage plans may incorporate case management and disease management.

Check Your Understanding 5.1

1. How does a member of an MCO plan obtain coverage for an oncologist?

2. List three types of care delivered by MCOs.

3. _____ supported by MCOs stress the habits of healthy lifestyles, such as exercise and proper nutrition.

Integrated Delivery Systems

Stephen Shortell, a leader in health services management, defines an integrated delivery system (IDS) as "various components that work together in an integrated fashion to provide a continuum of healthcare to a defined patient population" (Manus 1995, 24). *Integrated delivery system* is a generic term referring to the collaborative integration of healthcare providers. Financial agreements, contracts, or both underpin the legal entity. The goal of the IDS is the seamless delivery of care along the continuum of care. Other terms for IDS are health delivery network, horizontally integrated system, integrated services network (ISN), and vertically integrated system.

Shortell states that there are four types of integrated delivery systems, differentiated by who organizes or leads them (Manus 1995, 24), as follows:

- Hospital-led IDS. This type of IDS is the most common. In addition to hospitals and physicians, this system may include group practices; home health agencies; hospices; nursing homes; ambulatory surgery, outpatient care centers, and urgicenters; and ancillary providers, such as podiatrists, psychologists, and others.

- Physician-led IDS. An example of a physician-led IDS is the Mayo Clinic in Rochester, Minnesota (Manus 1995, 24).

- Physician-hospital organization (PHO). In this hybrid of the hospital-led and physician-led IDSs, hospitals and physicians share leadership.

- Insurance-led IDS. The fourth type is led by a healthcare insurance company.

Shortell states that integrated delivery systems are evolving and various "permutations" of these generic types exist (Manus 1995, 25). The permutations are based on specifics of accountability and organization. Examples of these various permutations include:

- Network or horizontal integration

- Vertical integration

- With-or-without healthcare plan

The existence of the healthcare plan alters the regulations under which the entity operates. If the IDS includes a healthcare plan, the IDS is governed by applicable state and federal regulations for healthcare plans, insurance, or HMOs, as relevant. If the IDS does not include a healthcare plan, the IDS is governed by the regulations for each type of organization in the entity. Hospital regulations govern hospitals; clinic regulations govern clinics.

The variance in the degree of integration adds more complexity to this sector of the healthcare industry. Scanlan describes four degrees of integration: affiliation, acquisition, consolidation, and merger (Scanlan 1995, 33–34). The least binding is affiliation. In affiliation, the components influence one another. In acquisition, one component purchases part or all the assets of the other component. *Consolidation* is a catch-all term in which operations are legally combined. In a merger, two similar components permanently combine to form one unit. Finally, *partnership* is a term that can refer to all four of the degrees of integration and any other integrative effort (Scanlan 1995, 34).

This section describes the following models of integration including the integrated provider organization, the group practice without walls, the physician-hospital organization, the management service organization, and the medical foundation.

Integrated Provider Organization

An integrated provider organization (IPO) is an entity that includes one or more hospitals, a large physician group practice, other healthcare organizations, or various configurations of these businesses. An IPO is the corporate umbrella for the management of an IDS.

Group Practice Without Walls

A group practice without walls (PWW) or clinic without walls (CWW) is a group practice in which the physicians have maintained their separate practices and offices in a geographic area. The individual practices share administrative systems to form the group practice. The PWW is similar to an independent practice association. The purpose of the PWW is to gain bargaining power in the negotiation of managed care contracts. Economies of scale also accrue from the centralization of administrative systems.

Physician-Hospital Organization

A physician-hospital organization (PHO) is a legal entity formed by a hospital and a group of physicians. The single corporate umbrella gives the PHO bargaining power when the provider organization negotiates contracts with managed care organizations. The PHO also fosters the delivery of seamless healthcare to its patients and clients.

Management Service Organization

A management service organization or medical service organization (MSO) is a specialized entity that provides management services and administrative and information systems to one or more physician group practices or small hospitals. An MSO may be owned by a hospital, physician group, PHO, IDS, or investors. The MSOs' services and systems are infrastructure for the smaller healthcare organizations. Patient billing and claims management are examples of services that an MSO provides.

Medical Foundations

A **medical foundation** is a nonprofit service organization. Members include physicians and other healthcare providers. Medical foundations are typically geographically based, such as a local organization or county organization. Medical foundations have many purposes other than serving as a managed care organization. For example, medical foundations may be involved with offering continuing medical education for their members. Medical foundations have, though, also involved themselves in some aspects of managed care. Medical foundations have established PPOs, EPOs, and MSOs. As physician-led organizations, the common characteristics are freedom of choice and preservation of the physician–patient relationship.

Future Trends

Consumer-directed (driven) healthcare plans (CDHPs) are a trend of the future. In consumer-directed healthcare, patients and clients are more involved in the design of their packages of health benefits. CDHPs provide patients and clients with information about packages' costs and with incentives to select the more cost-efficient package. With decision-support tools and information, the patients and clients determine the level of cost-sharing appropriate for their health and their economic situation. Three models of CDHPs exist: health reimbursement accounts (HRAs), premium-tiered, and point-of-service tiered (Rosenthal and Milstein 2004, 1055).

The model of health reimbursement accounts (personal care account, personal medical fund) combines an employer-funded account with a high deductible. For example, a member may have a

$500 HRA and a $1500 deductible. After the member has used the $500 HRA, the member must pay $1000 out-of-pocket before insurance becomes effective (Rosenthal and Milstein 2004, 1059).

The tiered models are focused on influencing healthcare behaviors by linking freedom of choice and either premiums or cost-sharing. Premium-tiered models link freedom of choice and premiums. Less restrictive packages have higher premiums; more restrictive packages allow greater freedom of choice. Point-of-service tiered models link freedom of choice and cost-sharing. Copayments are higher when members select providers outside the preferred network (Rosenthal and Milstein 2004, 1059).

In these plans, patients and clients (consumers) are made more aware of and responsible for the costs of their healthcare than in fee-for-service or other types of reimbursement. Experts believe that awareness and responsibility will influence patients and clients to choose the lower-priced package. For employers, CDHPs are a means to control the costs of their employees' health benefits. For consumers, CDHPs give them flexibility in choosing how they spend their healthcare benefit dollars.

Check Your Understanding 5.2

1. Which type of integrated delivery system is most common, and what types of providers may be included?

2. List the four types of integration models.

3. Name two ways that practices having integrated structures lower their overhead costs.

Summary

Managed care is the provision of cost-effective, quality healthcare through the integration of administrative, financial, and clinical systems. Managed care organizations (MCOs) implement the concepts and techniques of managed care to both deliver and finance healthcare. Managed care organizations share characteristics associated with providing quality care, such as an emphasis on coordination of care, techniques of disease management, application of evidence-based clinical practice guidelines, and maintenance of accreditation. MCOs also share characteristics associated with cost efficiency, such as review of medical necessity and utilization and financial incentives. Also associated with cost savings is capitation, a reimbursement method common to MCOs in which the providers share risk. Multiple types of MCOs exist on a continuum of control with health maintenance organizations representing the most controlled and preferred provider organizations, the least controlled. An integrated delivery system is a separate legal entity that healthcare providers have formed to offer a comprehensive set of healthcare services to a population. Consumer-directed healthcare plans are a trend of the future in which patients and clients assume more responsibility and accountability for the costs of their healthcare.

Review Quiz

1. Describe at least three ways in which MCOs work toward their goal of quality patient care.

2. From where do evidence-based clinical guidelines originate?

3. List at least two reasons that MCOs survey their members for feedback.

4. Name the three steps in medical necessity and utilization review.

5. Describe three types of cost controls used by MCOs.

6. Which type of HMO offers patients the least selection in referrals to specialists?

7. Describe the major advantage of consumer-driven healthcare plans (CDHPs) for employer-sponsors and healthcare consumers.

8. Disease management is closely associated with coordination of care tools of MCOs because efforts of multiple providers must be synchronized in disease management. True or false?

9. Integrated delivery systems typically have horizontal rather than vertical integration of services. True or false?

10. The least binding degree of healthcare service integration is affiliation, and the highest degree of integration is the merger. True or false?

References and Bibliography

American College of Managed Care Medicine. 2005. A history of managed care. Available online from www.managingmanagedcare.com/Resources/HxMgdCare.htm.

Blue Cross. 2005. www.brainyencyclopedia.com/encyclopedia/b/bl/blue_cross.html.

Carlson, B. 2000. Many state Medicaid agencies use financial incentives to boost quality. *Managed Care* 9 (4): 13–14.

Felt-Lisk, S. 1996. How HMOs structure primary care delivery. *Managed Care Quarterly* 4 (4): 96–105.

Foster, R. S. 2000. Trends in Medicare expenditures and financial status, 1966–2000. *Health Care Financing Review* 22 (1): 35–49.

Gallagher, T., A. Alpers, and B. Lo. 1998. Health Care Financing Administration's new regulations for financial incentives in Medicaid and Medicare managed care: One step forward? *American Journal of Medicine* 105 (5): 409–415.

Grumbach, K., et al. 1998. Primary care physicians' experience of financial incentives in managed-care systems. *New England Journal of Medicine* 339 (21): 1516–1521.

Kalant, N., M. Berlinguet, J. Diodati, L. Dragatakis, and F. Marcotte. 2000. How valid are utilization review tools in assessing appropriate use of acute care beds? *Canadian Medical Association Journal* 162 (13): 1809–1813.

Manus, P. and S. Shortell. 1995. The future of integrated systems. *Healthcare Financial Management* 49 (1): 24–30.

Rosenthal, M. and A. Milstein. 2004. Awakening consumer stewardship of health benefits: Prevalence and differentiation of new health plan models. *Health Services Research* 39 (4) Part II: 1055–1070.

Rutledge, R.. 1998. An analysis of 25 Milliman & Robertson Guidelines for surgery: Data-driven versus consensus-derived clinical practice guidelines. *Annals of Surgery* 228 (4): 579–587.

Scanlan, L. 1995. Building consensus for integration. *Healthcare Financial Management* 49 (1): 32–43.

State health plan for North Carolina. 2005. Available online from statehealthplan.state.nc.us/yourbenefits/benefits.pdf.

Chapter 6
Medicare-Medicaid Prospective Payment Systems for Inpatients

Objectives

- To differentiate major types of Medicare and Medicaid prospective payment systems for inpatients

- To define basic language associated with reimbursement under Medicare and Medicaid prospective payment systems

- To explain common models and policies of payment for inpatient Medicare and Medicaid prospective payment systems

Key Terms

Add-ons
Arithmetic mean length of stay (AMLOS)
Average length of stay (ALOS)
Base payment rate
Case mix
Case mix group (CMG)
Case mix index (CMI)
Clean claim
Code range
Complication or comorbidity (CC)
Cost reports
Cost-of-living adjustment (COLA)
Diagnosis related groups (DRGs)
Encounter
Etiologic diagnosis
Fiscal intermediaries
Fiscal year (FY)
Functional independence assessment tool
Functional status
Geometric mean length of stay (GMLOS)
Grouper (pricer)
High-cost outliers
Impairment group code (IGC)
Indirect medical education (IME) adjustment
Inpatient Rehabilitation Validation and Entry (IRVEN)

Interrupted stays
Labor-related share
Long-term care diagnosis related groups (LTC-DRGs)
Long-term care hospital (LTCH)
Major diagnostic categories (MDCs)
Market basket
Market basket index
Minimum data set (MDS)
New technology
Nonlabor share
Outliers
Prospective payment systems (PPSs)
Qualifying OR procedure
Quintiles
Rehabilitation impairment category (RIC)
Relative weight (RW)
Resource utilization groups (RUGs)
Short-stay outliers
Sole-community
Standard federal rate
Standardized payment
Teaching hospitals
Title
Transfer
Trim points

Introduction to Inpatient Prospective Payment Systems (PPSs)

Federal legislators are demanding that healthcare costs be controlled. These demands have led to federal healthcare reimbursement reform. Reform in the federal method of reimbursing providers for healthcare services resulted from three trends:

- Rising healthcare payments using the funds in the Medicare Trust at a rate faster than U.S. workers were contributing dollars

- Fraud and abuse in the system, which wasted funding

- Payment rules that were not uniformly applied across the nation

Federal analysts noted that the inpatient **prospective payment system (PPS),** implemented in 1983, had successfully curbed payments for inpatient charges. In the first three years of the prospective payment system, the rate of growth of Medicare Part A payments decreased from 7.3 percent in the five years prior to its implementation to 4 percent (Lave 1989, 152). Reporting on longer time periods, the staff of the Office of the Inspector General wrote that Medicare hospital payments increased by 88 percent between 1970 and 1980 (Gottlober 2001, 3) and the payment rates decreased by 52 percent between 1985 and 1990; and by 37 percent between1990 and 1995.

This success of the inpatient prospective system prompted Congress to authorize the Department of Health and Human Services (DHHS) to develop and implement prospective payment systems across the continuum of care. Today, the original acute care PPS has been augmented by prospective payment systems for all types of inpatients through the skilled nursing facility prospective payment system, long-term care hospital prospective payment system, inpatient rehabilitation prospective payment system, and inpatient psychiatric facility prospective payment system. Also, Chapter 7 describes reimbursement systems for ambulatory encounters and physicians.

Acute Care Prospective Payment System

The inpatient prospective payment system (IPPS) is the Medicare reimbursement system for inpatient services provided in an acute care setting. The system provides payment to facilities but does not include payment for professional services.

Conversion from Cost-Based Payment to Prospective Payment

From the implementation of the Medicare Program in 1966 until 1983, Medicare hospital inpatient claims were reimbursed based on the cost of services, reasonable cost, and/or per-diem costs (LaTour and Eichenwald, 303). This meant a hospital was reimbursed for approximately 80 percent of their costs for treating Medicare beneficiaries. From the hospital's perspective, there was no incentive to reduce costs—if its costs associated with patient care increased, so did its payments. By the late 1970s, healthcare costs, hand in hand with Medicare reimbursement payments, were sharply on the rise. The steep increase in healthcare costs had a dramatic impact on the Medicare Program, as illustrated by the following facts (Averill 2001, 105):

- Medicare payments to hospitals grew on average by 19 percent annually (three times the average overall rate of inflation).

- The Medicare hospital deductible expanded, creating a burden for Medicare beneficiaries.

- The solvency of the Medicare Trust Fund was endangered due to the increase of hospital costs.

- The increase in Medicare expenditures for hospital inpatient care jeopardized the ability of Medicare to fund other needed health programs.

- Under the variable cost-based payment system, Medicare paid up to sixfold differences across hospitals for comparable services.

- The reporting requirements of the cost-based system were some of the most burdensome in the federal government.

In response to the rising healthcare costs, Medicare administrators began to search for a different payment mechanism in the early 1970s to help control the rising healthcare costs.

Concept of Prospective Payment

The system that they began to investigate was based on the concept of prospective payment. In 1972, Congress authorized CMS (then HCFA) to begin prospective payment demonstration projects (Averill 2001, 83). The demonstration projects had to follow four guiding principles of prospectivity in their study:

- Payment rates are to be established in advance and fixed for the fiscal period to which they apply.

- Payment rates are not automatically determined by the hospital's past or current actual cost.

- Prospective payment rates are considered to be payment in full.

- The hospital retains the profit or suffers a loss resulting from the difference between the payment rate and the hospital's cost, thus creating an incentive for cost control (Averill 2001, 106).

Demonstration Projects

Between 1972 and 1983, Connecticut, Maryland, Massachusetts, New Jersey, New York, Rhode Island, Washington, and Wisconsin implemented prospec-

tive payment systems (PPSs) by participating in the demonstration projects (Averill 2001, 106). Based on these demonstration projects, CMS concluded:

- Prospectivity itself was effective in reducing the rate of increase in hospital costs.

- All state systems required consideration of hospital case mix.

- Failure to adequately address the case mix issue results in an active appeals process.

- Small rural hospitals frequently required special exceptions unless case mix was explicitly recognized in the payment system.

- Prospective payment rates were established through use of actual hospital costs for a base year.

- Successful systems had a firm legal basis with strict enforcement and could not be manipulated by the hospitals.

- Individual hospitals' budget review systems were often managed by exceptions and were complex to administer.

- All prospective payment systems had some inherent undesirable incentives that required the insertion of countermeasures.

The projects proved that hospital costs could be controlled under a prospective payment system and still allow for adequate reimbursement of hospital services rendered to Medicare beneficiaries.

New Jersey Model

Medicare chose the New Jersey model, which was based on **diagnosis related groups (DRGs)** as the prospective payment system to use. The DRG system was created at Yale University in the late 1960s through early 1970s. The initial charge for the DRG developers was to create a classification system that would monitor quality of care and use of services in a hospital setting. Although DRGs can be used to monitor quality and utilization, they are best known for their use as the foundation for the Medicare Inpatient Prospective Payment System implemented in 1983.

Prospective Payment Legislation

The Tax Equity and Fiscal Responsibility Act of 1982 (TEFRA) mandated extensive changes to the Medicare program. Many of the changes focused on controlling the rising costs of healthcare. TEFRA called for the implementation of a prospective payment system for hospital inpatients (Johns 2002, 256). In 1983, Public Law 98–21 amended Sections 1886(d) and 1886(g) of the Social Security Act (the Act) and mandated DRGs as the prospective payment system for the operating and capital-related costs of acute care hospital inpatient stays under Medicare Part A (DHHS 2004e, 48920).

Diagnosis Related Group Classification System

The diagnosis related group (DRG) system takes into consideration the role that a hospital case mix plays in influencing costs (Averill 2001, 83). Each DRG is assigned a relative weight that is intended to represent the resource intensity of the clinical group. It is also used to determine the payment level for the group. **Case mix index (CMI)** is an average of the sum of the relative weights of all patients treated during a specified time period. It should be noted that **case mix** is defined in many different ways, based on one's healthcare perspective. From a clinician's or physician's perspective, case mix complexity or description of the patient population can refer to the severity of illness, risk of mortality, prognosis, treatment difficulty, or need for intervention. This viewpoint uses sickness as a proxy for resource consumption.

However, from the DRG perspective, the case mix complexity is a direct measure of the resource consumption and, therefore, the cost of providing care. A high case mix in the DRG system means patients are consuming more resources, and, therefore, the cost of care is higher. However, it is a weak measure of the severity of illness, risk of mortality, prognosis, treatment difficulty, or need for intervention for the patient population (Averill 2001, 84). Therefore, this case mix complexity viewpoint allows DRGs to be an adequate system for hospital reimbursement because it measures the resources consumed for clinically like patients.

Classification System Development

The hospital inpatient business is vast, with great variation in the types of diseases treated and procedures performed. Consequently, the task of creating a classification system to encompass the industry was understandably daunting. After statistical analysis and physician consultation, four guidelines were established as guiding principles for the DRG system's formation:

- The patient characteristics used in the definition of the DRGs should be limited to information routinely collected on the hospital billing form.

- There should be a manageable number of DRGs, which encompass all patients seen on an inpatient basis.

- Each DRG should contain patients with a similar pattern of resource intensity.

- Each DRG should contain patients who are similar from a clinical perspective (that is, each class should be clinically coherent) (Averill 2001, 85).

Medicare has been successful at implementing the DRG system because it strictly adheres to these guiding principles. All hospitals are able to compute a DRG because they routinely collect all data needed to calculate the DRG assignment. Version 22.0 (effective dates October 1, 2004–September 30, 2005) of the DRG system included 520 DRGs, which is a reasonable number of groupings for hospitals to evaluate and manage. Linking like-patients with like resource consumption allows hospitals to perform cost management by DRG or DRG groupings. In addition, because DRGs were developed to monitor quality of care and resource use, hospitals can benchmark by DRG and continually improve upon their quality and resource indicators.

Only one DRG can be assigned and reimbursed for a single **encounter.** All hospital services performed during an encounter are packaged into this single DRG payment. The payment provided for the DRG is intended to cover the costs of all hospital services performed during the patient stay. Therefore, individual tests, services, pharmaceuticals, and supply items are not paid separately from the DRG payment. One component of a prospective payment system is that the predetermined payment for the clinical group is considered payment in full. Therefore, hospitals accept profit or loss based on their cost of providing services. The fully packaged concept drives facilities to practice cost management for inpatient services. Physician services are separately reimbursed under RBRVS and are not included in the DRG reimbursement to the hospital.

Structure of the DRG System

The DRG system is hierarchal in design. (See figure 6.1.) The highest level in the hierarchy is **major diagnostic categories (MDCs),** which represent the body systems treated by medicine. At the system's inception, there were twenty-three MDCs, plus a group for DRGs associated with all MDCs and the pre-MDC. However, in Version 8.0 (October 1, 1990–September 30, 1991) two new MDCs were added to represent the Human Immunodeficiency Virus Infections and Multiple Significant Trauma categories (see table 6.1). The next level in the hierarchy divides each MDC group into surgical and

Figure 6.1.   Hierarchical DRG system

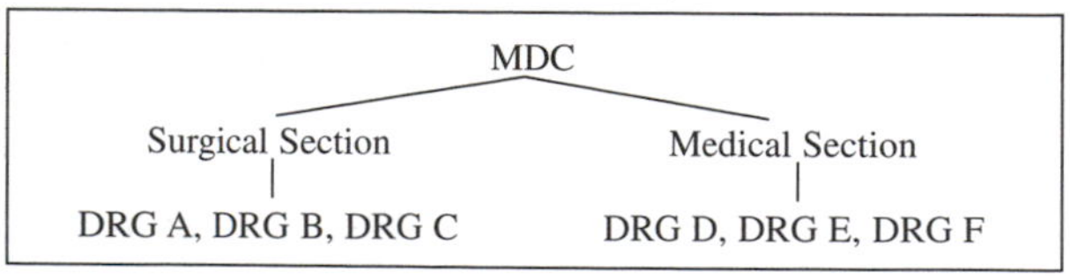

```
                         MDC
              _____
              |                      |
        Surgical Section        Medical Section
              |                      |
      DRG A, DRG B, DRG C      DRG D, DRG E, DRG F
```

Table 6.1.   Major diagnostic categories

MDC	Title
	DRGs associated with all MDCs and the Pre-MDC
1	Diseases and disorders of the nervous system
2	Diseases and disorders of the eye
3	Diseases and disorders of the ear, nose, mouth, and throat
4	Diseases and disorders of the respiratory system
5	Diseases and disorders of the circulatory system
6	Diseases and disorders of the digestive system
7	Diseases and disorders of the hepatobiliary system and pancreas
8	Diseases and disorders of the musculoskeletal system and connective tissue
9	Diseases and disorders of the skin, subcutaneous tissue and breast
10	Endocrine, nutritional and metabolic diseases and disorders
11	Diseases and disorders of the kidney and urinary tract
12	Diseases and disorders of the male reproductive system
13	Diseases and disorders of the female reproductive system
14	Pregnancy, childbirth and the puerperium
15	Newborns and other neonates with conditions originating in the perinatal period
16	Diseases and disorders of the blood and blood-forming organs and immunological disorders
17	Myeloproliferative diseases and disorders and poorly differentiated neoplasms
18	Infectious and parasitic diseases
19	Mental diseases and disorders
20	Alcohol/drug use and alcohol/drug-induced organic mental disorders
21	Injury, poisoning and toxic effects of drugs
22	Burns
23	Factors influencing health status and other contacts with health services
24	Multiple significant trauma
25	Human immunodeficiency virus infections

medical sections. The third and final level in the hierarchy divides the DRGs into the surgical or medical sections amongst the twenty-five MDC groups. Table 6.2 presents the ten DRGs reported to Medicare most frequently in fiscal year 2004.

Each version of the DRG system defines the same components: **title, geometric mean length of stay (GMLOS), arithmetic mean length of stay (AMLOS), relative weight (RW),** and ICD-9-CM **code range** that drives the DRG assignment. (See figure 6.2.) The code range may consist of the principal diagnosis, operating room (OR) procedure, or a diagnosis/procedure combination.

Assigning DRGs

Computer programs that assign patients to case mix groups are generically called **groupers or pricers.** Groupers have internal logic, or an algorithm, that determines the patients' groups. Although groupers are available and widely used for DRG assignment, a good understanding of the assignment process is necessary to help coding and reimbursement professionals ensure proper payment for services communicated. A four-step process is used to assign DRGs for hospital inpatient encounters. (See figure 6.3.)

Step One: Pre-MDC Assignment

The pre-MDC assignment step was added during the version 8 revision of DRGs. A set of procedures was identified that crossed all MDCs. The principal diagnosis is not considered for DRG assignment; rather, the principal ICD-9-CM procedure is used to assign the DRG. These procedures, transplants, and tracheostomies, can be performed for diagnoses from multiple MDCs. Once the encounter has been determined to qualify for preMDC assignment, the DRG assignment is made and the process is complete. No other steps are taken to assign the payment group. The nine DRGs that qualify for preMDC assignment are displayed in table 6.3. If the DRG assignment is made during step one, all other steps are ignored.

Step One Example:

A pancreas transplant can be performed for a variety of clinical conditions including diabetes with renal, ophthalmic, neurological, or peripheral circulatory manifestations (MDC 10), hypertensive renal disease (MDC 05), chronic pancreatitis (MDC 06), chronic renal failure (MDC 11), and complications of

Table 6.2. Medicare top 10 DRGs for FY 2004

DRG	Description	Relative Weight (FY 2005)	Volume (FY 2004)
127	Heart failure and shock	1.0390	669,664
089	Simple pneumonia and pleurisy, age greater than 17 with CC	1.0479	532,893
209	Major joint and limb reattachment procedures of lower extremity	2.0332	450,627
088	Chronic obstructive pulmonary disease	0.9089	399,409
430	Psychoses	0.6608	327,413
462	Rehabilitation	0.8865	303,482
182	Esophagitis, gastroenteritis and miscellaneous digestive disorders, age greater than 17 with CC	0.8255	281,991
174	GI hemorrhage with CC	1.0109	259,323
296	Nutritional and miscellaneous metabolic disorders, age greater than 17 with CC	0.8420	246,799
143	Chest pain	0.5643	237,926

Figure 6.2.   DRG components

DRG 127	
Title:	Heart Failure and Shock
Geometric Mean Length of Stay (GMLOS):	4.1
Arithmetic Mean Length of Stay (AMLOS):	5.2
Relative Weight:	1.0390

Principal Diagnosis

398.91	Failure, heart, congestive, rheumatic
402.01	Hypertensive heart disease, malignant, with heart failure
402.11	Hypertensive heart disease, benign, with heart failure
402.91	Hypertensive heart disease, unspecified, with heart failure
404.01	Hypertensive heart and renal disease, malignant, with failure, heart
404.03	Hypertensive heart and renal disease, malignant, with failure, heart and renal
404.11	Hypertensive heart and renal disease, benign, with failure, heart
404.13	Hypertensive heart and renal disease, benign, with failure, heart and renal
404.91	Hypertensive heart and renal disease, unspecified, with failure, heart
404.93	Hypertensive heart and renal disease, unspecified, with failure, heart and renal
*428	Failure, heart
785.50	Shock, unspecified, without mention of trauma
785.51	Shock, cardiogenic

*Entire code range is included.

transplanted organs (MDC 21). The diagnoses that warrant a pancreas transplant can be found in multiple MDCs. In order to maintain a manageable number of DRGs and to adhere to the concept of like-resource consumption groupings, there is only one DRG for all pancreas transplants regardless of the principal diagnosis. Therefore, the patient who received a pancreas transplant would be assigned to DRG 513 regardless of the principal diagnosis.

Step Two: MDC Determination

The principal diagnosis assigned to an encounter is the reason "established after study to be chiefly responsible for occasioning the admission of the patient to the hospital for care" (Schraffenberger 2005, 49). The principal diagnosis is used to place the encounter into one of the 25 MDCs. (See table 6.1.) Once the MDC is established for the encounter, step two is completed and the case moves on to step three.

Step Two Example:

Patient A presents and is treated for pneumonia due to Streptococcus, Group A. The ICD-9-CM code for Group A Streptococcus pneumonia is 482.31 and is assigned to MDC 04, Diseases and Disorders of the Respiratory System.

Step Three: Medical/Surgical Determination

The next step is to determine if an OR procedure was performed. If a **qualifying OR procedure** was performed, the case is assigned a surgical status. Many ICD-9-CM Code Books provide a flag or indicator for procedure codes that qualify as a valid OR procedure. Minor procedures and testing are not qualifying procedures. If a qualifying OR procedure was not performed, the case is assigned a medical status.

Step Three Example:

Patient A presents and is treated for an acute myocardial infarction of the anterolateral wall, initial episode (heart attack). The ICD-9-CM code for this diagnosis is 410.01 and is assigned to MDC 05, Diseases and Disorders of the Circulatory System (step two). During the hospital stay a percutaneous transluminal coronary angioplasty (PTCA) is performed on the right coronary artery. The ICD-9-CM code for this procedure is 36.01 and is a valid OR procedure. Therefore, this case is a surgical case in MDC 05.

Patient B is also evaluated for an acute myocardial infarction of the anterolateral wall, initial episode (heart attack). The ICD-9-CM code for this diagnosis is 410.01 and is assigned to MDC 05, Diseases and Disorders of the Circulatory System (step two). However, no procedures were performed for this patient during the hospital stay. This case is a medical case in MDC 05.

Once the medical/surgical status is assigned, step three is complete, and the case proceeds to step four.

Figure 6.3. DRG decision tree for medical MDC ##

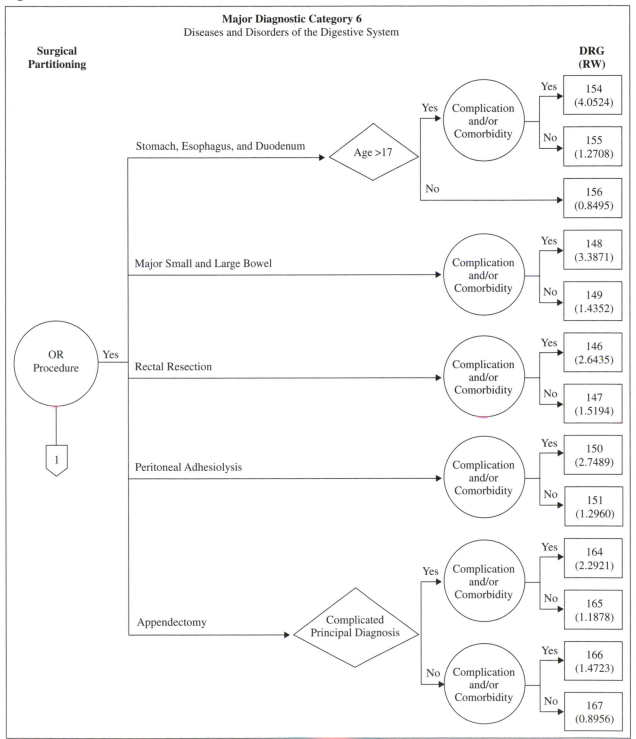

Table 6.3.   Pre-MDC assignment DRGs

DRG	Title
103	Heart transplant or implant of heart assist system
480	Liver transplant
481	Bone marrow transplant
482	Tracheostomy for face, mouth and neck diagnosis
495	Lung transplant
512	Simultaneous pancreas/kidney transplant
513	Pancreas transplant
541	Tracheostomy with mechanical ventilation 96+ hours or principal diagnosis except face, mouth, and neck diagnoses with major OR procedures
542	Tracheostomy with mechanical ventilation 96+ hours or principal diagnosis except face, mouth, and neck diagnoses without major OR procedures

Step Four: Refinement

Step four uses various refinement questions to isolate the correct DRG assignment. This refinement process allows for the DRG system to group together like patients from the clinical perspective with like resource consumption. The refinement questions get to the heart of grouping patients by like resource consumption. The refinement questions are:

- Is a **complication or comorbidity (CC)** present?

- Is the principal diagnosis complicated?

- Is a major complication or complex diagnosis present?

- Is the patient's age greater or less than seventeen years?

- What is the patient's sex?

- What is the patient's discharge disposition (alive, expired, or against medical advice)?

- For neonates, what is the birth weight of the baby?

Step Four Surgical Example:

Patient A is sixty-seven years old and is admitted for a duodenum fistula closure procedure. The patient also has type 1 diabetes, not stated as uncontrolled. The ICD-9-CM diagnosis codes are 537.4 (Duodenum fistula) and 250.01 (Diabetes mellitus, type 1, not specified as uncontrolled), and the ICD-9-CM procedure code is 46.72. Code 537.4 is assigned to MDC 06, Diseases and Disorders of the Digestive System (step two). Code 46.72 is a valid OR procedure (step three). Therefore, the case is a surgical MDC 06 case.

There are two applicable pathway questions for this encounter. First, is the patient's age greater than seventeen years? The answer is yes, the patient is sixty-seven years old. Second, is there a complication or comorbidity present? Type 1 diabetes is a comorbidity; therefore, the answer is yes. Now that all the refinement questions have been answered, the DRG assignment can be made. The DRG assignment for this case is DRG 154, Stomach, Esophageal, and Duodenal Procedures, Age Greater than 17 with CC.

Step Four Medical Example:

Patient B is sixty-eight years old and is admitted for cellulitis of the right ankle. Nonexcisional debridement is performed on the right ankle. The patient also has chronic obstructive pulmonary disease (COPD). The ICD-9-CM diagnosis codes are 682.6 (Cellulitis of leg, except foot) and 496 (COPD) and the ICD-9-CM procedure code is 86.28. Code 682.6 is assigned to MDC 09, Diseases and Disorders of the Skin, Subcutaneous Tissue and Breast (step two). Code 86.28 is not a valid OR procedure (step three). Therefore, the case is a medical MDC 09 case.

There are two applicable pathway questions for this encounter. First, is the patient's age greater than seventeen years of age? The answer is yes, the patient is sixty-eight years old. Second, is there a complication or comorbidity present? COPD is a comorbidity; therefore, the answer is yes. Now that all the refinement questions have been answered, the DRG assignment can be made. The DRG assignment for this case is DRG 277, Cellulitis, Age Greater than 17 with CC.

Invalid Coding and Data Abstraction

Accurate diagnosis/procedure coding and health-care information abstracting are vital to DRG assignment. When invalid codes or data are submitted on the patient claim form, one of two DRGs is assigned. DRG 469, Principal Diagnosis Invalid as Discharge Diagnosis, is assigned when the principal diagnosis reported is not specific enough for DRG assignment. DRG 470, Ungroupable, is assigned when an invalid diagnosis code, age, sex, or discharge status code is reported. Payment for each of these DRG is $0. The claim is returned to the provider and should be corrected, then resubmitted to Medicare.

Provisions of the DRG System

The DRG system uses provisions to provide additional payments for specialized programs and unusual admissions that historically have added significant cost to patient care. Without the additional payments associated with these provisions, it may not be feasible for acute care facilities to provide all services to Medicare beneficiaries.

Disproportionate Share Hospital

Effective for discharges occurring on or after May 1, 1986, Disproportionate Share Hospital (DSH) status was enacted for facilities with a high percentage of low-income patients (CMS n.d). Additional payment is provided for these hospitals because they experience a financial hardship by providing treatment for patients who are unable to pay for the services rendered. There are two methods of qualification for this provision. First, a hospital may qualify by exceeding 15 percent on the statutory formula. The statutory formula takes into consideration Medicare inpatient days for patients eligible for Medicare Part A and Supplemental Security Income (SSI), and total inpatient days for patients eligible for Medicaid but not Medicare Part A.

The second method for DSH qualification applies to large urban hospitals. If large urban hospitals are able to demonstrate that more than 30 percent of their total net inpatient care revenues

come from state and local governments for indigent care (excluding Medicare and Medicaid) then they can be granted DSH status (CMS 2005). The DSH payment adjustment is hospital-specific and is based on a formula that incorporates the hospital bed size and hospital type (rural, **sole-community,** urban). The SSI/Medicare Part A Disproportionate Share Percentage File is updated once a year for the IPPS Final Rule and can be found on the Medicare Web site at www.cms.hhs.gov.

Indirect Medical Education

Approved **teaching hospitals** are provided an **indirect medical education (IME) adjustment.** The hospitals must have residents in an approved graduate medical education (GME) program. Teaching hospitals experience an increased patient care cost in comparison to nonteaching hospitals. Therefore, Medicare provides IME hospitals with additional reimbursement to help offset the costs of providing education to new physicians. The IME payment adjustment is hospital-specific. The adjustment factor is based on the hospital's ratio of residents to beds and a multiplier established by Congress. This formula is traditionally described as "a certain percentage increase in payment for every 10 percent increase in the resident-to-bed ratio."

Several acts of Congress have decreased the percentage increase during the past nine years. The most recent, Benefits Improvement and Protection Act (BIPA) of 2000, established the transition to a 5.5 percent increase to take effect in 2003. The percent increase of 5.5 percent in IME payment for every 10 percent increase in the resident-to-bed ratio is effective for the 2005 fiscal year.

High-Cost Outlier Cases

Because the Medicare payment for inpatient services is prospective, hospitals will experience profit or loss for individual cases whose reimbursements exceed or fall short of the cost incurred for a particular case. The payment provided to facilities is an average amount, meaning that some cases will result in a profit and some, a loss. For the most part, costs are covered if reasonable cost management is performed. However, there are extreme cases, **outliers,** for which the costs are very high when compared to the average costs for cases in the same DRG. The outlier payment provision provides some financial relief for those cases.

For an encounter to qualify for an outlier payment, the hospital's Medicare-approved charges reported on the claim are converted to costs, using the cost-to-charge ratio (CCR), and compared to the threshold limit established for that **fiscal year (FY).** If the threshold is exceeded, additional payment is made. The payment is 80 percent of the difference between the hospital's entire cost for the stay and the threshold amount (CMS 2005). Outlier payments for the Burn DRGs (DRGs 504-511) are 90 percent rather then 80 percent.

New Medical Services and New Technologies

New medical services, new technologies, and innovative methods for treating patients are often very costly. A **new technology** is an advance in medical technology that substantially improves, relative to technologies previously available, the diagnosis or treatment of Medicare beneficiaries (CMS 2005). Applicants for the status of new technology must submit a formal request, including a full description of the clinical applications of the technology and the results of any clinical evaluations demonstrating that the new technology represents a substantial clinical improvement, along with data to demonstrate the technology meets the high-cost threshold.

Providing these innovative services in a prospective system could, in many cases, lead to inadequate payments. These financial losses may prohibit a facility from offering new and innovative services to patients because they are simply not affordable. Therefore, in order to ensure that new and innovative services and technologies are provided to Medicare beneficiaries, the IPPS allows additional payments to be made for new medical services and new technologies. This payment provision allows for the full DRG payment plus 50 percent of the cost for the new technology or service.

Payment

Medicare provides a six-step methodology for calculating total DRG payment (CMS 2005). **Fiscal intermediaries** use grouper (pricer) software to calculate the DRG and payment for each hospital encounter.

Step One: DRG Assignment

Hospitals must submit a claim to Medicare for payment using an electronic claim to its designated Medicare fiscal intermediary. The fiscal intermediary performs electronic auditing of the claim to ensure that the claim contains correct information (also referred to as **clean claim**) based on edits found in the Medicare Code Editor (MCE). Once the claim is deemed clean, the grouper software assigns a DRG based on the demographic and coded data submitted.

Step Two: Establishment of Initial Payment Rate

A **base payment rate** is established for each Medicare-participating hospital for each fiscal year (FY). The base payment rate is a per encounter rate that is based on historic claims data. The standardized amounts are derived from 1981 hospital costs per Medicare discharge figures. The 1981 costs established the base year amount that was adjusted to explain differences among facilities for case mix, wage rates, DSH status, IME status, and certain hospital costs. The base-year amount has been updated each year since 1981 by an update factor that is established by Congress and is intended to account for inflation.

Each year, the standardized amount is divided into a labor-related portion and a nonlabor portion. The **labor-related share** is adjusted by the wage index for the hospital's geographic location based on core based statistical areas (CBSA). The **nonlabor share** is modified by a **cost-of-living adjustment (COLA)** if the hospital is located in Alaska or Hawaii. These adjustments establish the base payment rate for the effective fiscal year. A listing of the wage index and COLA values can be found in the IPPS Final Rule released each year via the

Federal Register. Past and current *Federal Register* publications can be located via the government printing office at www.gpoaccess.gov. Current prospective payment system rules are also posted on the Medicare website at www.cms.hhs.gov.

The base payment rate is multiplied by the relative weight for the DRG that was assigned in step one.

Example:

Patient A was seen for congestive heart failure (428.0) and no OR procedures were performed. DRG 127 is assigned for the encounter. The relative weight for DRG 127 is 1.0390. The hospital base rate is $7,325. In order to calculate the initial payment rate, the relative weight is multiplied by the hospital base rate. The initial payment rate for this case is $7,610.68 (1.0390 × $7,325).

Step Three: Add-on for Disproportionate Share Hospital

If the hospital has DSH status, the established percentage for that year for that facility is added on to the initial payment rate.

Step Four: Add-on for Indirect Medical Education

If the hospital qualifies for IME payments, then the established percentage for that year for that facility is added on.

Step Five: Add-on for High Cost Outlier

The costs incurred for providing services for the encounter are calculated and examined to determine whether the case qualifies for an outlier payment. If an outlier payment is warranted, the additional payment is added on during this step.

Step Six: Add-on for New Medical Service and Technology

The encounter is reviewed to determine whether any qualifying new services or technology were used during the course of patient treatment. If a new service or technology was used, the costs are calculated for the service or supply. Fifty percent of the calculated costs are added onto the payment.

Pricer Software

The pricer software is used to completes steps two through six. When the six steps are completed, payment is made to the facility and the data from the encounter is included in the National Claims History File. The Medicare Provider Analysis Review (MedPAR) file, an extract from the National Claims History File, is used for statistical analysis and research.

Transfer Cases

There are two types of **transfer** cases under the IPPS. The first category is a patient transfer between two IPPS hospitals. A type 1 transfer is when a patient is discharged from an acute IPPS hospital and is admitted to another acute IPPS hospital on the same day. If a patient leaves an acute IPPS hospital against medical advice (AMA) and is admitted to another acute IPPS hospital on the same day, this situation is treated the same as a transfer between two IPPS hospitals.

Payment is altered for the transferring hospital and is based on a per-diem rate methodology. The DRG is established for the case and the full payment rate is calculated. This payment rate is divided by the GMLOS established for the DRG, thus creating a per-diem rate. The transferring facility receives double the per-diem rate for the first day plus the per-diem rate for each day thereafter for the patient LOS. DHS, IME, and outlier add-ons are applied after the per-diem rate is established. The receiving facility receives full PPS payment for the case. The one exception to this rule is DRG 385, Neonates Died or Transferred to Another Acute Care Facility. The payment and GMLOS established for DRG 385 are based on historical data; no reduction is necessary because it is a transfer-related DRG.

A transfer that occurs from an IPPS hospital to a hospital or unit excluded from IPPS is known as a type 2 transfer. For this type of transfer case, the full PPS payment is made to the transferring hospital and the receiving hospital or unit is paid on a reasonable cost basis or under prospective payment, whichever is applicable for that setting (CMS 2004, 1). However, there are exceptions to the payment policy, known as the post-acute care transfer policy, for type 2 transfer cases. One hundred and eighty two DRGs (see table 6.4.) qualify for the post-acute care transfer policy and for these DRGs, a discharge from an acute IPPS hospital to an excluded IPPS hospital or unit is considered a type 1 transfer rather than a discharge. The facilities that are excluded from IPPS are:

- Inpatient rehabilitation facilities or units

- Long-term care hospitals

- Psychiatric hospitals and units

- Children's hospitals

- Cancer hospitals

Additionally, the case is considered a transfer instead of a discharge when a patient is discharged from an acute IPPS hospital and is admitted to a skilled nursing facility (SNF) or is sent home with a written plan of care for home health services that will begin within three days after discharge from the IPPS hospital. In these three situations, the same transfer payment provision used for IPPS-to-IPPS transfer cases (type 1 transfer cases) is enacted and followed for the 169 of the 182 qualifying DRGs. For the remaining thirteen DRGs, there is a special payment policy which allows for 50 percent of the full DRG payment plus the per diem amount to be made for the first day of stay, and then 50 percent of the per diem amount each day thereafter. These thirteen DRGs have significantly higher costs upon admission. Creating this special payment policy better reimburses facilities in the post-acute care transfer situation for these thirteen DRGs.

The post-acute care transfer policy ensures that an incentive is not created for hospitals to discharge patients early in order to reduce costs while still receiving full DRG payment. Additionally, this concept allows for proper reimbursement levels when the full course of treatment is divided across two healthcare settings.

Maintenance of the DRG System

CMS is responsible for updating the DRG system. Each payment rate for each DRG is intended to reimburse the costs for average resources required to care for encounters grouping to that DRG. Therefore, adjustments are made to the DRG system to account for changes in treatment patterns, technology, and other elements that influence resource cost. Section 1886(d)(4)(C) of the Act requires that DRG classifications and relative weights are adjusted at least annually (DHHS 2004e, 48925). Claims from the MedPAR file are used to evaluate possible changes to the system. Non-MedPAR issues are also considered. Interested parties (such as hospitals, supply companies, and national associations representing healthcare groups) can submit change requests to Medicare. Non-MedPAR issues should be submitted to CMS no later than December for consideration for the next federal fiscal year (FY), which begins annually on October 1. The group adjustments and recalibration of group weights are published in the *Federal Register* at least forty-five days prior to the start of the new federal FY.

Summary

The IPPS for hospital inpatient services provided to Medicare beneficiaries was successfully implemented in 1983. The concept of prospective payment has spread to other third party payers, and many have implemented payment systems using DRGs or a modified version of DRGs. In response, hospitals have adopted cost analysis and containment practices in order to remain profitable under prospective systems. IPPS was the first prospective payment system and has paved the way for the implementation of many other systems in other healthcare settings, such as skilled nursing, rehabilitation, and for a variety of outpatient services, as described in Chapter 7.

Table 6.4.   Postacute-care transfer DRGs for FY 2006

DRG	Title	GMLOS	Relative Weight
001	Craniotomy age >17 with CC	7.6	3.4347
002	Craniotomy age >17 without CC	3.5	1.9587
007*	Peripheral and cranial nerve & other nervous system procedures with CC	6.7	2.6978
008*	Peripheral and cranial nerve & other nervous system procedures without CC	2.0	1.5635
010	Nervous system neoplasms with CC	4.6	1.2222
011	Nervous system neoplasms without CC	2.9	0.8736
012	Degenerative nervous system disorders	4.3	0.8998
013	Multiple sclerosis & cerebellar ataxia	4.0	0.8575
014	Intracranial hemorrhage or cerebral infarction	4.5	1.2456
015	Nonspecific CVA & precerebral occlusion without infarct	3.7	0.9421
016	Nonspecific cerebrovascular disorders with CC	5.0	1.3351
017	Nonspecific cerebrovascular disorders without CC	2.5	0.7229
018	Cranial & peripheral nerve disorders with CC	4.1	0.9903
019	Cranial & peripheral nerve disorders without CC	2.7	0.7077
020	Nervous system infection except viral meningitis	8.0	2.7865
024	Seizure and headache, age >17 with CC	3.6	0.9970
025	Seizure and headache, age >17 without CC	2.5	0.6180
028	Traumatic stupor & coma, coma <1 hour, age >17 with CC	4.4	1.3353
029	Traumatic stupor & coma, coma <1 hour, age >17 without CC	2.6	0.7212
034	Other disorders of nervous system with CC	3.7	1.0062
035	Other disorders of nervous system without CC	2.4	0.6241
073	Other ear nose, mouth & throat diagnoses age >17	3.3	0.8527
075	Major chest procedures	7.6	3.0732
076	Other respiratory system OR procedures with CC	8.4	2.8830
077	Other respiratory system OR procedures without CC	3.3	1.1857
078	Pulmonary embolism	5.4	1.2427
079	Respiratory infections & inflammations age >17 with CC	6.7	1.6238
080	Respiratory infections & inflammations age >17 without CC	4.4	0.8947
082	Respiratory neoplasms	5.1	1.3936

(Continued on next page)

Table 6.4.   (Continued)

DRG	Title	GMLOS	Relative Weight
083	Major chest trauma with CC	4.2	0.9828
084	Major chest trauma without CC	2.6	0.5799
085	Pleural effusion with CC	4.8	1.2405
086	Pleural effusion without CC	2.8	0.6974
089	Simple pneumonia & pleurisy, age >17 with CC	4.7	1.0320
090	Simple pneumonia & pleurisy, age >17 without CC	3.2	0.6104
092	Interstitial lung disease with CC	4.8	1.1853
093	Interstitial lung disease without CC	3.1	0.7150
101	Other respiratory system diagnoses with CC	3.3	0.8733
102	Other respiratory system diagnoses without CC	2.0	0.5402
104	Cardiac valve & other major cardiothoracic procedures with cardiac cath	12.7	8.2201
105	Cardiac valve & other major cardiothoracic procedures without cardiac cath	8.4	6.0192
108	Other cardiothoracic procedures	8.6	5.8789
113	Amputation for circulatory system disorders except upper limb and toe	10.8	3.1682
114	Upper limb and toe amputation for circulatory system disorders	6.7	1.7354
120	Other circulatory system OR procedures	5.9	2.3853
121	Circulatory disorders with acute myocardial infarction and major complications, discharged alive	5.3	1.6136
126	Acute & subacute endocarditis	9.4	2.7440
127	Heart failure and shock	4.1	1.0345
130	Peripheral vascular disorders with CC	4.4	0.9425
131	Peripheral vascular disorders without CC	3.2	0.5566
144	Other circulatory diagnoses with CC	4.1	1.2761
145	Other circulatory diagnoses without CC	2.1	0.5835
146	Rectal resection with CC	8.6	2.6621
147	Rectal resection without CC	5.2	1.4781
148	Major small & large bowel procedures with CC	10.0	3.4479
149	Major small & large bowel procedures without CC	5.4	1.4324
150	Peritoneal adhesiolysis with CC	8.9	2.8061

Table 6.4.   (Continued)

DRG	Title	GMLOS	Relative Weight
151	Peritoneal adhesiolysis without CC	4.0	1.2641
154	Stomach, esophageal & duodenal procedures age >17 with CC	9.9	4.0399
155	Stomach, esophageal & duodenal procedures age >17 without CC	3.1	1.2889
157	Anal & stomal procedures with CC	4.1	1.3356
158	Anal & stomal procedures without CC	2.1	0.6657
170	Other digestive system OR procedures with CC	7.8	2.9612
171	Other digestive system OR procedures without CC	3.1	1.1905
172	Digestive malignancy with CC	5.1	1.4125
173	Digestive malignancy without CC	2.7	0.7443
176	Complicated peptic ulcer	4.1	1.1246
180	GI obstruction with CC	4.2	0.9784
181	GI obstruction without CC	2.8	0.5614
188	Other digestive system diagnoses age >17 with CC	4.2	1.1290
189	Other digestive system diagnoses age >17 without CC	2.4	0.6064
191	Pancreas, liver & shunt procedures with CC	9.0	3.9680
192	Pancreas, liver & shunt procedures without CC	4.3	1.6793
197	Cholecystectomy except by laparoscope without common duct exploration with CC	7.5	2.5425
198	Cholecystectomy except by laparoscope without common duct exploration without CC	3.7	1.1604
205	Disorders of liver except malignancy, cirrhosis, alcoholic hepatitis with CC	4.4	1.2059
206	Disorders of liver except malignancy, cirrhosis, alcoholic hepatitis without CC	3.0	0.7292
210*	Hip & femur procedures except major joint age >17 with CC	6.1	1.9059
211*	Hip & femur procedures except major joint age >17 without CC	4.4	1.2690
213	Amputation for musculoskeletal system & connective tissue disorders	7.2	2.0428
216	Biopsies of musculoskeletal system & connective tissue	3.3	1.9131
217	Wound debridement & skin graft except hand, for musculoskeletal & connective tissue disorders	9.3	3.0596
218	Lower extremity & humerous procedures except hip, foot, femur age >17 with CC	4.4	1.6648
219	Lower extremity & humerous procedures except hip, foot, femur age >17 without CC	2.6	1.0443
225	Foot procedures	3.7	1.2251

(Continued on next page)

Table 6.4.   (Continued)

DRG	Title	GMLOS	Relative Weight
226	Soft tissue procedures with CC	4.5	1.5884
227	Soft tissue procedures without CC	2.1	0.8311
233*	Other musculoskeletal system & connective tissue OR procedures with CC	4.6	1.9184
234*	Other musculoskeletal system & connective tissue OR procedures without CC	2.0	1.2219
235	Fractures of femur	3.8	0.7768
236	Fractures of hip & pelvis	3.8	0.7407
238	Osteomyelitis	6.7	1.4401
239	Pathological fractures & musculoskeletal & connective tissue malignancy	5.0	1.0767
240	Connective tissue disorders with CC	5.0	1.4051
241	Connective tissue disorders without CC	3.0	0.6629
244	Bone diseases & specific arthropathies with CC	3.6	0.7200
245	Bone diseases & specific arthropathies without CC	2.5	0.4583
250	Fracture, sprain, strain & dislocation of forearm, hand, foot age >17 with CC	3.2	0.6974
251	Fracture, sprain, strain & dislocation of forearm, hand, foot age >17 without CC	2.3	0.4749
253	Fracture, sprain, strain & dislocation of upper arm, lower leg, except foot age >17 with CC	3.8	0.7747
254	Fracture, sprain, strain & dislocation of upper arm, lower leg, except foot age >17 without CC	2.6	0.4588
256	Other musculoskeletal system & connective tissue diagnoses	3.9	0.8509
263	Skin graft &/or debridement for skin ulcer or cellulitis with CC	8.6	2.1130
264	Skin graft &/or debridement for skin ulcer or cellulitis without CC	5.0	1.0635
265	Skin graft &/or debridement except for skin ulcer or cellulitis with CC	4.4	1.6593
266	Skin graft &/or debridement except for skin ulcer or cellulitis without CC	2.3	0.8637
269	Other skin, subcutaneous tissue & breast procedures with CC	6.2	1.8352
270	Other skin, subcutaneous tissue & breast procedures without CC	2.7	0.8313
271	Skin ulcers	5.6	1.0195
272	Major skin disorders with CC	4.5	0.9860
273	Major skin disorders without CC	2.9	0.5539
277	Cellulitis, age >17 with CC	4.6	0.8676
278	Cellulitis, age >17 without CC	3.4	0.5391

Table 6.4.   (Continued)

DRG	Title	GMLOS	Relative Weight
280	Trauma to the skin, subcutaneous tissue & breast age >17 with CC	3.2	0.7313
281	Trauma to the skin, subcutaneous tissue & breast age >17 without CC	2.3	0.4913
283	Minor skin disorders with CC	3.5	0.7423
284	Minor skin disorders without CC	2.4	0.4563
285	Amputation of lower limb for endocrine, nutritional & metabolic disorders	8.2	2.1831
287	Skin grafts & wound debridement for endocrine, nutritional & metabolic disorders	7.8	1.9470
292	Other endocrine, nutritional & metabolic O.R. procedures with CC	7.3	2.6395
293	Other endocrine, nutritional & metabolic O.R. procedures without CC	3.2	1.3472
294	Diabetes, age >35	3.3	0.7652
296	Nutritional & miscellaneous metabolic disorders, age >17 with CC	3.7	0.8187
297	Nutritional & miscellaneous metabolic disorders, age >17 without CC	2.5	0.4879
300	Endocrine disorders with CC	4.6	1.0922
301	Endocrine disorders without CC	2.7	0.6118
304	Kidney, ureter & major bladder procedures for non-neoplasm with CC	6.1	2.3761
305	Kidney, ureter & major bladder procedures for non-neoplasm without CC	2.6	1.1595
316	Renal failure	4.9	1.2692
320	Kidney & urinary tract infections, age >17 with CC	4.2	0.8658
321	Kidney & urinary tract infections, age >17 without CC	3.0	0.5652
331	Other kidney & urinary tract diagnoses age >17 with CC	4.1	1.0619
332	Other kidney & urinary tract diagnoses age >17 without CC	2.4	0.6160
395	Red blood cell disorders, age >17	3.2	0.8328
401	Lymphoma & non-acute leukemia with other OR procedure with CC	8.0	2.9678
402	Lymphoma & non-acute leukemia with other OR procedure without CC	2.8	1.1810
403	Lymphoma & non-acute leukemia with CC	5.8	1.8432
404	Lymphoma & non-acute leukemia without CC	3.0	0.9265
415	OR procedure for infectious & parasitic diseases	11.0	3.9890
416	Septicemia age >17	5.6	1.6774
418	Postoperative & post-traumatic infections	4.8	1.0716
423	Other infectious & parasitic diseases diagnoses	6.0	1.9196

(Continued on next page)

Table 6.4.   (Continued)

DRG	Title	GMLOS	Relative Weight
429	Organic disturbances & mental retardation	4.3	0.7919
430	Psychoses	5.8	0.6483
440	Wound debridements for injuries	5.9	1.9457
442	Other OR procedures for injuries with CC	6.0	2.5660
443	Other OR procedures for injuries without CC	2.6	0.9943
444	Traumatic injury age >17 with CC	3.2	0.7556
445	Traumatic injury age >17 without CC	2.2	0.5033
462	Rehabilitation	8.9	0.8700
463	Signs & symptoms with CC	3.1	0.6960
464	Signs & symptoms without CC	2.4	0.5055
468	Extensive OR procedure unrelated to the principal diagnosis	9.7	4.0031
471*	Bilateral or multiple major joint procedures of lower extremity	4.5	3.1391
475	Respiratory system diagnosis with ventilator support	8.1	3.6091
477	Non-extensive OR procedure unrelated to principal diagnosis	5.8	2.0607
482	Tracheostomy for face, mouth & neck diagnosis	9.6	3.3387
485	Limb reattachment, hip and femur procedure for multiple significant trauma	8.4	3.4952
487	Other multiple significant trauma	5.3	1.9459
497*	Spinal fusion except cervical with CC	5.0	3.6224
498*	Spinal fusion except cervical without CC	3.4	2.7791
501	Knee procedures with principal diagnosis of infection with CC	8.5	2.6462
502	Knee procedures with principal diagnosis of infection without CC	4.9	1.4462
521	Alcohol/drug abuse or dependence with CC	4.2	0.6939
522	Alcohol/drug abuse or dependence with rehabilitation therapy without CC	7.7	0.4794
529	Ventricular shunt procedures with CC	5.3	2.3160
530	Ventricular shunt procedures without CC	2.4	1.2041
531	Spinal procedures with CC	6.5	3.1279
532	Spinal procedures without CC	2.8	1.4195
537	Local excision & removal of internal fixation device except hip & femur with CC	4.8	1.8360
538	Local excision & removal of internal fixation device except hip & femur without CC	2.1	0.9833

Table 6.4. (Continued)

DRG	Title	GMLOS	Relative Weight
541	ECMO or tracheostomy with mechanical ventilation 96+ hours or principal diagnosis except face, mouth, and neck diagnoses with major OR procedures	38.1	19.8038
542	Tracheostomy with mechanical ventilation 96+ hours or principal diagnosis except face, mouth, and neck diagnoses without major OR procedures	279.1	12.8719
543	Craniotomy with implant of chemotherapy agent or acute complex CNS principal diagnosis	8.5	4.4184
544*	Major joint replacement or reattachment of lower extremity	4.1	1.9643
545*	Revision of hip or knee replacement	4.5	2.4827
547	Coronary bypass with cardiac cath with major cardiovascular diagnosis	10.8	6.1948
548	Coronary bypass with cardiac cath without major cardiovascular diagnosis	8.2	4.7198
549*	Coronary bypass without cardiac cath with major cardiovascular diagnosis	8.7	5.0980
550*	Coronary bypass without cardiac cath without major cardiovascular diagnosis	6.2	3.6151
553	Other vascular procedures with CC with major cardiovascular diagnosis	6.6	3.0957
554	Other vascular procedures with CC without major cardiovascular diagnosis	4.0	2.0721

*Indicates one of thirteen special payment DRGs.

Skilled Nursing Facility Prospective Payment System

Section 4432 of the Balanced Budget Act of 1997 mandated a prospective payment system (PPS) and consolidated billing for skilled nursing facilities (SNFs). Under the PPS, SNFs are paid through per-diem prospective, case mix adjusted payment rates applicable to all covered SNF services. These payment rates cover all the costs of furnishing covered skilled nursing services. Included in the payment rates are routine care, ancillary services, and capital costs. Operational costs associated with defined, approved educational activities are excluded. The payment system was effective for cost reporting periods beginning on or after July 1, 1998.

Consolidated billing requires the SNF to pay for outpatient services that a resident may receive from outside vendors. Outside vendors will no longer bill Medicare for services provided to the SNF for a resident with Part A benefits. The laboratory, x-ray service, and pharmacy must bill the SNF and the SNF is responsible for paying for the services. Emergency services, inpatient services, and other extensive procedures (such as radiation therapy) are not consolidated.

Data Collection

Since the late 1980s, CMS has required SNFs to prepare the **Minimum Data Set (MDS).** The MDS is an extensive database of clinical data. These clinical data include comprehensive assessments and treatment plans and are reported within prescribed time frames. The PPS treatment plan is integral; thus, services outside the scope of the treatment plan may be excluded from payment. The PPS also requires SNFs to use HCPCS coding.

The MDS data determine the classification into one of forty-four **resource utilization groups (RUGs).** The resource utilization groups, version

III (RUG-III) form a schema that classifies nursing home residents into forty-four homogeneous groups. Residents within groups are similar in terms of their health characteristics and use of resources. The RUG-III schema is hierarchical with the first level being seven categories. The second hierarchical level is the forty-four groups. The groups are allocated among the seven categories:

- Rehabilitation (fourteen RUG-III groups)
- Extensive services (three RUG-III groups)
- Special care (three RUG-III groups)
- Clinically complex (six RUG-III groups)
- Impaired cognition (four RUG-III groups)
- Behavior function (four RUG-III groups)
- Physical function (ten RUG-III groups)

CMS analysts believe that MDS data that classify patients into one of the upper twenty-six RUGs (rehabilitation, extensive services, special care, and clinically complex) justify the patients' admissions to SNFs. These patients by definition require skilled care. The coverage of patients classified into the lower eighteen RUGs (impaired cognition, behavior function, and physical function) is determined on an individual basis.

Grouping and Payment

The PPS uses per-diem federal payment rates based on mean SNF costs that are updated for inflation. The payment rates were calculated using allowable costs from SNF **cost reports.** Cost reports are reports that providers are required to submit to Medicare. The base year of the cost reports was 1995. Separate payment rates were established for urban and rural areas. Annually, the rates are adjusted using the SNF **market basket index.** A **market basket** is a mix of goods and services. The market basket index is a relative measure that averages the costs of an appropriate mix of goods and services for the SNF PPS.

The per-diem rates are case-mix adjusted using the resident classification system, RUG III. The forty-four RUG-III groups are derived from data in the resident assessments of the MDS. Each of the forty-four groups has an associated rate (table 6.5). Therefore, federal payment is then based on the RUG. A forty-fifth default group also exists. This group represents patients for whom the SNF has made an error in assessment or has missed a deadline.

In addition, the rates are adjusted for geographic variations in wages. The total federal rate includes both the labor-related portion and the nonlabor-related portion (table 6.6), which vary from year to year.

Example:

In 1999, the labor and nonlabor portions for the RVC category were $245.23 and $57.20, respectively (DHHS 1999, 41686). In 2004, the corresponding rates were $274.56 and $85.65 (DHHS 2004d, 45784).

To adjust for local geographic variations in wages, the labor portion is multiplied by the local wage index that also varies from year to year. Finally, to calculate the payment, the wage-adjusted total federal rate is multiplied by the number of covered Medicare days. (See the sample calculation in table 6.7.)

Federal acts subsequent to the BBA of 1997 initiated additional, *temporary* payment adjustments. These acts are the:

- Medicare, Medicaid, and SCHIP Balanced Budget Refinement Act of 1999 (BBRA) (P.L. 106–113)
- Medicare, Medicaid, and SCHIP Benefits Improvement and Protection Act of 2000 (BIPA) (P.L. 106–554)
- Medicare Prescription Drug, Improvement, and Modernization Act of 2003 (MMA) (P.L. 108–173)

The adjustments authorized by these acts are termed **add-ons.**

Table 6.5.   Case-adjusted skilled nursing facility rates by resource utilization groups, version III (RUG-III)

Urban Case-Mix Adjusted Federal Rate (Effective October 1, 2004)		
No.	RUG III Category	Total Federal Rate ($)
1	RUC	467.21
2	RUB	420.56
3	RUA	397.90
4	RVC	360.21
5	RVB	348.21
6	RVA	317.55
7	RHC	330.36
8	RHB	303.70
9	RHA	278.37
10	RMC	325.28
11	RMB	290.63
12	RMA	273.30
13	RLB	259.15
14	RLA	217.83
15	SE3	307.84
16	SE2	266.52
17	SE1	237.20
18	SSC	231.87
19	SSB	221.20
20	SSA	215.87
21	CC2	230.53
22	CC1	213.21
23	CB2	202.54
24	CB1	193.21
25	CA2	191.88
26	CA1	181.22
27	IB2	173.22
28	IB1	170.55
29	IA2	157.23
30	IA1	151.89
31	BB2	171.89
32	BB1	167.89
33	BA2	155.89
34	BA1	145.23
35	PE2	186.55
36	PE1	183.88
37	PD2	177.22
38	PD1	174.55
39	PC2	167.89
40	PC1	166.56
41	PB2	149.23
42	PB1	147.90
43	PA2	146.56
44	PA1	142.56

Source: Department of Health and Human Services. 2004 (July 30). *Federal Register.* 69 (146): 45781–45782.

The BBRA authorized a temporary 20 percent increase in the payment rates of fifteen RUGs:

RHC	SE1	CC1
RMC	SSC	CB2
RMB	SSB	CB1
SE3	SSA	CA2
SE2	CC2	CA1

After the enactment of BIPA, the temporary 20 percent increase remained in effect for twelve RUGs:

SE3	SSB	CB2
SE2	SSA	CB1
SE1	CC2	CA2
SSC	CC1	CA1

The BIPA corrected an anomaly in the structure of the payment rates of the rehabilitation RUGs. In this anomaly, the payment rates for less intensive rehabilitation groups were higher than the payment rates of more intensive rehabilitation groups. The BIPA reduced the temporary rate increase from 20 percent to 6.7 percent for three RUGs (RHC, RMC, RMB). For eleven other rehabilitation RUGs, BIPA also temporarily authorized a 6.7 percent rate increase:

RUC	RVB	RMA
RUB	RVA	RLB
RUA	RHB	RLA
RVC	RHA	

The MMA provided a temporary increase of 128 percent for SNF residents with Acquired Immune Deficiency Syndrome (AIDS; diagnosis code 042). The act identifies no particular RUG. Applying the AIDS add-on (128 percent) excludes the application of other add-ons (DHHS 2004d, 45777). (See table 6.8.)

These temporary adjustments remain in effect until case mix refinements are made in the SNF PPS. A compilation of the RUGs affected by the temporary add-ons is shown in table 6.8. The impact of these temporary add-ons on the SNF payment calculation is demonstrated in table 6.9.

Table 6.6.   Resource utilization groups, version III (RUG-III) and labor adjustments

	Excerpt from Urban Case-Mix Adjusted Federal Rate Showing Labor and Nonlabor Portions (Effective October 1, 2004)			
No.	RUG III Category	Labor ($)	Nonlabor ($)	Total Federal Rate ($)
4	RVC	274.56	85.65	360.21
7	RHC	251.81	78.55	330.36
9	RHA	212.18	66.19	278.37
18	SSC	176.74	55.13	231.87
21	CC2	175.71	54.82	230.53
29	IA2	119.84	37.39	157.23
30	IA1	115.77	36.12	151.89
31	BB2	131.02	40.87	171.89
32	BB1	127.97	39.92	167.89

Source: Department of Health and Human Services. 2004 (July 30). *Federal Register.* 69 (146): 45784.

Table 6.7.   Generic calculation of skilled nursing facility payment

	Sample Calculation of Wage-Adjusted Federal Payment						
RUG III	Labor Portion ($)	Wage Index (Greenville, NC)*	Adj. Labor Portion ($)	Nonlabor Portion ($)	Adjusted Rate [Adj. Labor Portion + Nonlabor Portion] ($)	Medicare Days	Payment [Adj. Rate × Days] ($)
RVC	274.56	0.9183	252.13	85.65	337.78	50	16,889.00
RHC	251.81	0.9183	231.24	78.55	309.79	100	30,979.00
RHA	212.18	0.9183	194.84	66.19	261.03	16	4,176.48
SSC	176.74	0.9183	162.30	55.13	217.43	30	6,522.90
CC2	175.71	0.9183	161.35	54.82	216.17	10	2,161.70
IA2	119.84	0.9183	110.05	37.39	147.44	30	4,423.20

Adapted source: Department of Health and Human Services. 1999 (July 30). *Federal Register.* 64 (146): 41697; and 2004 (December 30). *Federal Register.* 69 (250): 78463, with information from 2004 (July 30). *Federal Register.* 69 (146): 45784.

*Greenville, NC is in the Metropolitan Statistical Area [MSA] 3150. Department of Health and Human Services. 2004 (December 30). *Federal Register.* 69 (250): 78452.

Table 6.8.   Temporary rate increases by resource utilization groups, version III (RUG-III)

No.	RUG III Category	Remaining BBRA Add-On (20%)	BIPA Add-On (6.7%)	Potential for AIDS MMA Add-On (042 Diagnosis Code Present; 128%)—Not Applicable in Conjunction with Other Add-On
1	RUC		√	√
2	RUB		√	√
3	RUA		√	√
4	RVC		√	√
5	RVB		√	√
6	RVA		√	√
7	RHC		√	√
8	RHB		√	√
9	RHA		√	√
10	RMC		√	√
11	RMB		√	√
12	RMA		√	√
13	RLB		√	√
14	RLA		√	√
15	SE3	√		√
16	SE2	√		√
17	SE1	√		√
18	SSC	√		√
19	SSB	√		√
20	SSA	√		√
21	CC2	√		√
22	CC1	√		√
23	CB2	√		√
24	CB1	√		√
25	CA2	√		√
26	CA1	√		√
27	IB2			√
28	IB1			√
29	IA2			√
30	IA1			√
31	BB2			√
32	BB1			√
33	BA2			√
34	BA1			√
35	PE2			√
36	PE1			√
37	PD2			√
38	PD1			√
39	PC2			√
40	PC1			√
41	PB2			√
42	PB1			√
43	PA2			√
44	PA1			√

Information source: Department of Health and Human Services. 2004 (July 30). *Federal Register.* 69 (146): 45775–45777.

Table 6.9.   Calculation of skilled nursing facility payment with temporary add-ons

Sample Calculation of Wage-Adjusted Federal Payment (2005)								
RUG III	**Labor Portion ($)**	**Wage Index (Greenville, NC)***	**Adj. Labor Portion ($)**	**Nonlabor Portion ($)**	**Adjusted Rate [Adj. Labor Portion + Nonlabor Portion] ($)**	**Temporarily Percentage Increased Adjusted Rate [% + Adj. Rate]**	**Medicare Days**	**Payment [Increased Adj. Rate × Days] ($)**
RVC	274.56	0.9183	252.13	85.65	337.78	**360.41	50	$18,020.50
RHC	251.81	0.9183	231.24	78.55	309.79	**330.54	100	$33,054.59
RHA	212.18	0.9183	194.84	66.19	261.03	**278.52	16	$4,456.32
SSC	176.74	0.9183	162.30	55.13	217.43	***260.92	30	$7,827.60
CC2	175.71	0.9183	161.35	54.82	216.17	****492.87	10	$4,928.70
IA2	119.84	0.9183	110.05	37.39	147.44	147.44	30	$4,423.20

Adapted source: Department of Health and Human Services. 2004 (December 30). *Federal Register.* 69 (250): 78463.

*Greenville, NC is in the Metropolitan Statistical Area [MSA] 3150 (p. 78452).

**6.7% BIPA add-on.

***20% BBRA add-on.

****128% MMA add-on effective only for 042 diagnosis code.

Other Applications

At the state level, Pennsylvania instituted a new case mix reimbursement system for its Medicaid recipients in nursing facilities in 1994. This prospective case mix reimbursement system replaced a retrospective cost-based methodology. Administrators in Pennsylvania hope that prospective payment will improve long-term care and payment for this care. The cost-based system reimbursed nursing facilities at an interim payment cost per day during the fiscal year. Using the prospective case mix reimbursement system, the Department of Public Welfare (DPW) determines a payment rate based on the facility resident population, adjusted to reflect resource usage of the Medical Assistance population, administrative costs, and other costs. This payment rate is determined quarterly based on the resident population information provided to the DPW via the Commonwealth of Pennsylvania Access to Social Services (COMPASS). Each facil-

ity knows in advance its payment rate under the Medical Assistance system.

The case mix system enhances incentives for facilities to admit residents who require a more skilled, intensive type care. This system eliminates any incentives for providers to admit and care for the least disabled residents. The payment system was established at 120 percent of the median cost for each facility peer group. The rate of 120 percent directs a higher amount of revenue to those activities most related to resident care. The case mix reimbursement system also reimburses facilities for capital costs based on the appraised value rather than depreciation and interest.

Check Your Understanding 6.1

1. When and where was the DRG system created?

2. In the four-step DRG assignment process, if a coder is able to assign the DRG in step one, the

pre-MDC assignment, all subsequent steps in the process are _____.

3. List two refinement questions that help coders group together patients with like resource consumption.

4. How are Medicare base payment rates increased to reflect inflation?

5. What tool does the SNF PPS use annually to adjust payment rates?

Long-Term Care Hospital Prospective Payment System

Prior to October 2002, Medicare reimbursed **long-term care hospitals (LTCHs)** under a cost-based (retrospective) payment system. LTCHs were exempt from the acute care hospital prospective payment system of diagnosis related groups (DRGs). On August 30, 2002, CMS published the final rule for PPS for LTCHs (DHHS 2002). Starting in October 2002, the LTCH PPS became effective as each LTCH began its new fiscal year. The PPS will be phased in incrementally (20 percent per year) until full implementation in 2006.

The Balanced Budget Refinement Act (BBRA) of 1999 (P.L. 106–113), as amended by the Benefits Improvement and Protection Act (BIPA) of 2000 (P.L. 106–554) mandated that a budget neutral, per discharge PPS for LTCHs based on diagnosis related groups (DRGs) be implemented for cost reporting periods beginning on or after October 1, 2002. This LTCH PPS was to replace the reasonable cost-based payment system mandated by the Tax Equity and Fiscal Responsibility Act (TEFRA) of 1982.

Covered Organizations

Long-term care hospitals treat groups of patients who have longer than average lengths of stay. Some patients have chronic diseases, such as tuberculosis and respiratory ailments. Other patients have acute diseases requiring long-term therapy, such as cancer and head trauma. LTCHs can provide both general acute care and specialized services, such as comprehensive rehabilitation and ventilator-dependent therapy.

A facility can meet the Centers for Medicare and Medicaid Services (CMS) definition of long-term care hospital (LTCH) in two ways (DHHS 2002, 55957):

- Its **average length of stay (ALOS)** is twenty-five days or more. The calculation is based only on the lengths of stay of Medicare patients and it includes both covered and noncovered days. In addition, the calculation must be based on data from the past six months.

- It was excluded from the diagnosis related group (DRG) PPS on or after August 5, 1997, and has an ALOS of twenty days or more for both Medicare and nonMedicare patients. In addition, 80 percent of the hospital's annual inpatient Medicare discharges in the fiscal year had principal diagnoses of neoplastic diseases, such as cancer.

Approximately 270 LTCHs meet these qualifying circumstances (Dougherty 2002, 72). Excluded from the LTCH PPS are Department of Veterans Affairs (VA) hospitals, hospitals reimbursed under state cost-control systems or authorized demonstration projects, and nonparticipating hospitals furnishing emergency services to Medicare beneficiaries.

Long-term care hospitalizations are covered under Part A Medicare. Beneficiaries have up to ninety days of hospital services within the benefit period. Admissions to both acute care hospitals and long-term care hospitals are counted in the benefit period. One inpatient deductible is required for each ninety-day benefit period. For the sixty-first through ninetieth days, a daily coinsurance payment is also required. The sixty lifetime reserve days may also be used after the ninetieth day (DHHS 2002, 55960–55961).

Long-Term Care Diagnosis Related Groups

The LTCH PPS is based on categorizing patients into classes with similar clinical characteristics. Generally, classes of patient discharges with similar clinical characteristics are called **case mix groups (CMGs).** For the LTCH PPS, these case mix groups are the **long-term care diagnosis related groups (LTC-DRGs).** The LTC-DRGs are exactly the same as the acute care DRGs. The number of LTC-DRGs varies from year to year just as the number of acute care DRGs varies. In 2003, there were 510 LTC-DRGs (DHHS 2002, 55979). In 2004, there were 518 LTC-DRGs (DHHS 2004b, 25679). Just like acute care DRGs, LTC-DRGs are based on:

- The principal diagnosis

- Up to eight additional diagnoses

- Up to six procedures

- Age

- Sex

- Discharge status

The difference between the acute care DRGs and the LTC-DRGs is the weight assigned to the groups. LTC-DRGs have higher weights to account for the increased complexity of the patients' conditions (DHHS 2004b, 25678). Another difference is the grouping of low-volume LTC-DRGs (less than 25 LTCH cases) in five **quintiles** based on average charge per discharge (DHHS 2004b, 25678). A third difference is the classification of **short-stay outliers.** A short-stay outlier is defined as an LTCH admission that is five-sixths of the geometric average length of stay (DHHS 2004b, 25678).

Grouping and Payment

A computer software program called a grouper classifies the patient discharges into LTC-DRGs. Groupers have internal logic or an algorithm that determines the patients' groups. The groupers use the principal diagnosis, additional diagnoses, procedures, age, sex, and discharge status to determine the LTC-DRG.

The principal diagnosis is the primary determinant of the LTC-DRG. Additional (secondary) diagnoses also affect the assignment of the LTC-DRG. Additional diagnoses represent comorbid conditions that were present at admission, conditions that occurred subsequent to admission, or both. These comorbid conditions or complications (CCs) group a patient's discharge to a higher weight LTC-DRG.

LTC-DRGs have assigned relative weights (table 6.10). These weights reflect the resources necessary to treat the medically complex LTCH patients. Patients who consume more resources are grouped to LTC-DRGs that have higher relative weights. The weights are adjusted annually because changes in the delivery of healthcare change the resource consumption. For example, the relative weight of LTC-DRG 148 decreased between 2002 and 2004 from 2.8488 to 2.0841. On the other hand, the relative weight of LTC-DRG 009 increased between 2002 and 2004 from 1.3118 to 1.5025.

Of the 518 LTC-DRGs, 516 have weights. Two of the LTC-DRGs are administrative and have no assigned weights (469, Principal Diagnosis is invalid and 470, Ungroupable). There are 161 low-volume LTC-DRGs. They are divided into quintiles and each quintile has a specific relative weight. No volume LTC-DRGs are crosswalked to one of the low-volume quintiles. Organ transplants should not occur at an LTCH. Therefore, CMS has assigned weights of 0.0000 to TC-DRGs for organ transplants: 103 (heart), 302 (kidney), 480 (liver), and 495 (lung).

The weights of the LTC-DRGs in the federal prospective payment include the following costs:

- Operating

- Capital-related

- Routine

- Ancillary

Excluded from the prospective payment are the following costs:

- Bad debts

- Approved educational activities

- Blood-clotting factors

- Anesthesia

- Photocopying costs for records sent to the quality improvement organization (QIO)

The LTCH can bill these costs separately to CMS. There are also adjustments for the following:

- Short stays

- Interrupted stays

- High cost outliers

- Area wage differences

The unit of payment is the discharge. A budget-neutral conversion factor (CF) converts the LTC-DRG

Table 6.10.   Selected long-term care diagnosis related groups (LTC-DRG) relative weights

Excerpts: LTC-DRG Relative Weights					
			2002**	2003***	2004****
LTC-DRG	Description		Relative Weight	Relative Weight	Relative Weight
001	Craniotomy age >17 with CC[5]		1.8783	1.8783	2.0841
007	Periph & cranial nerve & other nerv syst proc w CC[7]		1.7829	1.7829	1.5754
009	Spinal disorders & injuries		1.4118	1.4118	1.5025
012	Degenerative nervous system disorders		0.7773	0.7773	0.7485
013	Multiple sclerosis & cerebellar ataxia		0.7207	0.7207	0.7530
076	Other resp system OR procedures w CC		2.7674	2.7674	2.4382
087	Pulmonary edema & respiratory failure		1.6597	1.6597	1.6513
088	Chronic obstructive pulmonary disease		0.7532	0.7532	0.7653
148	Major small & large bowel procedures w CC[5]		2.8488	2.8488	2.0841
236	Fractures of hip & pelvis		0.7381	0.7381	0.7368

*Relative weights for these LTC-DRGs were determined by assigning these cases to the appropriate low-volume quintile because they had no LTCH cases in the FY 2001 MedPAR.

**Department of Health and Human Services. 2002 (August 30). *Federal Register.* Final rule. 67 (169): 56076–56084.

***Department of Health and Human Services. 2003 (June 6). *Federal Register.* Final rule. 68 (109): 34812–34190.

****Department of Health and Human Services. 2004 (May 7). *Federal Register.* Final rule. 69 (89): 25741–25749.

weight into a payment. In the LTCH PPS, the CF is known as the **standard federal rate.** The standard federal rate is based on the costs of a market basket of goods, such as operating costs and capital costs. The standard federal rate is updated annually. In 2003 and 2004, the standard federal rates were $34,956.15 and $35,726.18, respectively (DHHS 2003a, 34134; DHHS 2004b, 25682).

Generic payment formula:

LTC-DRG weight × Standard federal rate = Unadjusted LTCH PPS payment

For a patient discharged in 2006 with LTC-DRG 013 Multiple sclerosis & cerebellar ataxia (0.7820):

0.7820 × $37,975.53 [2006 standard federal rate] = $29,696.86 (DHHS 2005, 24180)

Implementation

The importance of accurate coding for the LTCH PPS cannot be overstated. Correct ICD-9-CM diagnosis and procedure coding play an important role, along with other factors, in the way Medicare pays the claim. The ICD-9-CM coding terminology and definitions of principal diagnosis, other diagnoses, and principal procedure follow the requirements of the Uniform Hospital Discharge Data Set (UHDDS). For example, coders must be careful to record the code that occasioned the admission to the LTCH and not the code that occasioned the admission to the acute care hospital. For the case depicted in figure 6.4, correct LTCH coding results in LTC-DRG 012. Incorrectly using the acute care codes would have resulted in LTC-DRG 015 (as LTC-DRGs match acute DRGs). Most important, the relative weights of the LTC-DRGs differ (DHHS 2005, 24248):

LTC-DRG 012 relative weight = 0.7416

LTC-DRG 015 relative weight = 0.7868

The difference is 0.0452; while seemingly insignificant, when multiplied by the standard federal rate, $37,957.53, the LTCH is overpaid $1,716.49 per incorrectly coded discharge.

Figure 6.4.   Case study to calculate long-term care prospective payment system reimbursement

Patient suffers a stroke (ICD-9-CM 436, Acute, but ill-defined cerebrovascular disease) and is admitted to an acute care hospital.

The inpatient DRG is 015, Nonspecific CVA & Precerebral occlusion w/o infarct.

Patient is discharged and then admitted to an LTC for further treatment of left-sided hemiparesis (ICD-9-CM 438.20, Late effects of cerebrovascular disease, hemiplegia affecting unspecified side) and dysphasia (ICD-9-CM 438.12, Late effects of cerebrovascular disease, dysphasia).

The LTC-DRG is 012, Degenerative nervous system disorders.

Source: Department of Health and Human Services. 2002 (August 30). Final Rule. *Federal Register.* 67 (169): 55981.

Summary

In summary, LTCHs are facilities certified under Medicare as acute-care hospitals that had been excluded from the federal inpatient prospective payment system. These facilities typically have an average inpatient length of stay of 25 days or more. The LTCH PPS, implemented October 1, 2002, replaced the previous reasonable cost-based payment system under which Medicare had previously reimbursed LTCHs.

Inpatient Rehabilitation Facility Prospective Payment System

Medicare has implemented a prospective payment system for Medicare beneficiaries residing in inpatient rehabilitation facilities: the inpatient rehabilitation facility (IRF) prospective payment system (PPS) or the IRF PPS.

According to CMS, the IRF PPS promotes:

- Quality of, access to, and continuity of care

- Efficient provision of rehabilitative services

- Fairness and equity to facilities, beneficiaries, and taxpayers. (DHHS 2001, 41320)

Background

In the past, Medicare paid rehabilitation services under a reasonable cost formula that factored in costs and demographic and geographic variations. Because inpatient rehabilitation services differ from acute care services, inpatient rehabilitation services had been excluded from the inpatient PPS that had been implemented in October 1983 and that used diagnosis related groups (DRGs). Both rehabilitation hospitals and rehabilitation units within acute care general hospitals were excluded from the DRG system.

Healthcare analysts recognized that to create a payment system for inpatient rehabilitation services, a special case mix classification was needed. This classification must account for the variation in resource use across patients in rehabilitation facilities. The Balanced Budget Act of 1997 (BBA) authorized the development of the IRF PPS and its concomitant classification. CMS phased in the IRF PPS as each inpatient rehabilitation facility began its new fiscal year on or after January 1, 2002. This implementation included the amendments to the IRF PPS from the Balanced Budget Refinement Act of 1999 (BBRA) and the Medicare, Medicaid, and SCHIP Benefits Improvement and Protection Act of 2000 (BIPA).

Today the IRF PPS applies to inpatient rehabilitation services that Medicare participating rehabilitation hospitals or distinct rehabilitation units in acute care hospitals provide to Medicare Part A fee-for-service patients. To meet CMS's definition of an IRF, facilities must have an inpatient population in which:

- At least a specified percentage of the patients require intensive rehabilitation services:

  —July 1, 2004 to June 30, 2005 = 50 percent

  —July 1, 2005 to June 30, 2006 = 60 percent

  —July 1, 2006 to June 30, 2007 = 65 percent

  —July 1, 2007 and thereafter = 75 percent
  (DHHS 2004a, 25762)

- For one of the following thirteen conditions:

  —Stroke

  —Spinal cord injury

  —Congenital deformity

  —Amputation

  —Major multiple trauma

  —Fracture of the femur (hip fracture)

  —Brain injury

  —Neurological disorders

  —Burns

  —Active, polyarticular rheumatoid arthritis, psoriatic arthritis, and seronegative arthropathies

  —Systematic vasculidities with joint inflammation (unresponsive to aggressive, sustained, and appropriate outpatient treatment)

  —Severe or advanced osteoarthritis involving two or more major weight-bearing joints

  —Knee or hip replacement with bilateral replacement, extreme obesity, or age eighty-five or older

Excluded from the IRF PPS are Department of Veterans Affairs (VA) hospitals, hospitals reimbursed under state cost-control systems or authorized demonstration projects, and nonparticipating hospitals furnishing emergency services to Medicare beneficiaries. There are approximately 1,200 facilities that meet the definition of a participating IRF.

Key components of the IRF PPS are data collection, grouping via case mix, single payment per discharge, and electronic data submission. The foundation of the IRF PPS is the case mix group (CMG). CMGs are classes of discharges in functional related groups.

Data Collection

The IRF PPS features an eighty-five-item, rehabilitation-specific tool. This tool is the inpatient rehabilitation facility patient assessment instrument (IRF PAI). The IRF PAI collects the information that drives payment.

Types of Patient Information

The IRF PAI consists of nine different types of patient information. These types are:

- Identification information
- Admission information
- Payer information
- Medical information
- Medical needs
- Function modifiers
- Functional independence assessment information
- Discharge information
- Quality measures (for example, pressure ulcers or patient falls)

Assignment of Codes

The IRF PAI must be completed for each Medicare patient twice, upon admission and again at discharge.

By the fourth day of the inpatient admission, the IRF PPS requires the assignment of codes. These codes reflect:

- The reason for admission to the rehabilitation facility (using impairment group codes)
- The etiology of the impairment (using ICD-9-CM codes)
- Comorbidities and complications (using ICD-9-CM codes)
- The reason for interruption, transfer, or death (using an ICD-9-CM code)

The functional abilities of the patient must be assigned using the functional independence assessment tool.

The codes on the IRF PAI are used for research, for grouping patients into CMGs, and for determining the payment tier. It must be emphasized that the codes on the IRF PAI do not follow the UHDDS and the UB-92 guidelines.

Impairment Group Code

The reason for admission is coded using an **impairment group code (IGC).** (See table 6.11). CMS provides these codes in the manual. There are eighty-five IGCs. The IGC structure consists of a two-digit ID number, a decimal point, and one to four digits representing the subgroups. The IGC describes the primary reason that the patient is being admitted to the rehabilitation program.

Etiologic Diagnosis

The IRF PAI also reports the code for the etiology of the problem that led to the condition requiring the inpatient rehabilitation admission. The **etiologic diagnosis** is an ICD-9-CM code. Therefore, a principal diagnosis, as defined by the Uniform Hospital Discharge Data Set (UHDDS), is not reported on the IRF PAI.

Complications and Comorbidities

A comorbidity is a specific condition that the patient had at admission to the IRF. Comorbidities affect patients in addition to their etiologic diagnoses and their impairments. Because of these comorbidities, the IRFs must use additional resources (costs) to treat these patients. Therefore, about 980 comorbid conditions affect the IRF PPS payment. ICD-9-CM coding of comorbid conditions is critical (Trela 2002, 48B). Up to ten ICD-9-CM codes for comorbid conditions may be reported on the PAI. Complications are comorbidities that occur after admission to the IRF (Trela 2002, 48B). Complications are reported both as comorbid conditions and as complications. Complications are also reported using ICD-9-CM codes.

These comorbid conditions are divided into three tiers by associated costs (table 6.12). CMS has linked the ICD-9-CM codes to their respective tiers. Tier 1 is high cost, tier 2 is medium cost, and tier 3 is low cost. On the table, a "1" is found in

Table 6.11.   Inpatient rehabilitation facility prospective payment system's impairment group code (IGC)

Example of Impairment Group Code (IGC)	
01.1	Stroke with left body involvement (right brain)
01.2	Stroke with right body involvement (left brain)
01.3	Stroke with bilateral involvement
01.4	Stroke with no paresis
01.9	Other stroke
02.21	Traumatic brain injury (TBI) with open injury
02.22	Traumatic brain injury (TBI) with closed injury
04.210	Traumatic spinal cord injury (TSCI) with paraplegia, unspecified
04.211	Traumatic spinal cord injury (TSCI) with paraplegia, incomplete
04.212	Traumatic spinal cord injury (TSCI) with paraplegia, complete
04.220	Traumatic spinal cord injury (TSCI) with quadriplegia, unspecified
04.2211	Traumatic spinal cord injury (TSCI) with quadriplegia, incomplete C1–4
04.2212	Traumatic spinal cord injury (TSCI) with quadriplegia, incomplete C5–8
04.2221	Traumatic spinal cord injury (TSCI) with quadriplegia, complete C1–4
04.2222	Traumatic spinal cord injury (TSCI) with quadriplegia, complete C5–8

Adapted Source: Department of Health and Human Services. 2001 (August 7). *Federal Register.* Final rule. 66 (152): 41342–41343.

Table 6.12.   Comorbidities in inpatient rehabilitation facility prospective payment system

Excerpt from List of Comorbidities and Tiers (2001)					
ICD-9-CM Code	Abbreviated Description	Tier 1	Tier 2	Tier 3	Excluded RIC
011.02	TB Lung Infiltr-Exm Unkn	0	1	0	15
093.20	Syphil Endocarditis NOS	0	0	1	14
112.4	Candidiasis of Lung	1	0	0	15
342.92	Unsp Hmiplga Nondominant Side	0	0	1	01
204.00	Acute Lym Leuk w/o Rmsion	0	0	1	—
787.2	Dysphagia	0	0	1	01
V49.75	Status Amput Below Knee	0	0	1	10

Source: Department of Health and Human Services. 2001 (August 7). *Federal Register.* Final rule. 66 (152): 41414–41427.

the respective tier. Conditions that are inherent to a specific **rehabilitation impairment category (RIC)** are excluded from the list of relevant comorbidities for that RIC. Excluded comorbidities do not affect the relative weight and, thus, do not increase the payment for that RIC.

Finally, the reason for transfer or death is reported by ICD-9-CM code on the IRF PAI.

Functional Independence Assessment

Another major element of the IRF PAI is the **functional independence assessment tool.** (See table 6.13). This is an eighteen-item, rehabilitation-specific instrument that reflects the characteristics of patients. It captures patients' functional status. **Functional status** is a patient's ability to perform activities of daily living. CMS has organized this assessment by motor and cognitive functioning.

The functional independence measure tool was developed in the 1980s. About 75 percent of U.S. IRFs use this standardized instrument to measure the severity of patients' impairments. The eighteen items are measured on a seven-level scale that classifies patients according to their ability to perform certain activities. A score of "7" indicates complete independence. Conversely, a score of "1" indicates complete dependence. The IRF PAI added an eighth level, "0," for not assessed. Therefore, a higher score means that the patient has more functional abilities; a lower score means that the patient has fewer functional abilities. Patients with fewer functional abilities (lower scores) need more assistance from facilities' personnel and, thus, require more resources.

All the patient's scores for the motor items are totaled and all the patient's scores for the cognitive items are totaled. With the patient's diagnosis, these two totals and the patient's age determine the exact case mix group. Completion of the indicators for medical needs and quality is voluntary.

IRF staff members must complete PAI within specific time frames. However, if entries are incorrect, facilities may update data at any time prior to transmission of the IRF PAI.

Grouping

Case mix groups (CMGs) are classes of patient discharges of rehabilitation facilities. These groups represent similar functional-related patient discharges based on impairment, functional capability of the patient, age, and comorbidities. The CMG is derived from:

- The rehabilitation impairment category (RIC)
- Motor and cognitive scores from the functional independence assessment tool
- Age
- Comorbid conditions

As previously noted, the IRF PAI is completed twice, one time with admission data and a second time with discharge data. The admission assessment assigns patients to a CMG. The discharge assessment determines the weighting factors associated with comorbidities (if they are present and applicable).

In the admission assessment, patients are assigned to a CMG based upon admission data and clinical characteristics. Patients are classified into CMGs based on the expected improvement of the patient's functional status as reflected by the functional independence assessment tool. IRFs must complete admission assessments that are the basis for CMG assignment according to a specific timetable (Trela 2002, 48C).

The CMS software that assigns patients to case mix groups is called the pricer. The pricer uses the impairment group codes (IGCs) on the PAI to classify patients into one of twenty-one RICs (table 6.14). RICs are clusters of similar impairments and diagnoses (table 6.15). It should be noted that staff members at IRFs enter the IGC on the PAI; they do not enter the RIC. The pricer calculates the RIC from the IGC. RICs, in turn, assign patients to CMGs (table 6.16). In RIC 1 Stroke (01), there are fourteen CMGs (0101, 0102 to 0114).

To summarize: IGC → RIC → CMG.

Table 6.13.   Functional independence measure (FIM™) and inpatient rehabilitation facility prospective payment system

Functional Independence Measure (FIM™) Instrument		
CMS Motor Items		**Min = 0, Max = 84**
No.	**Description**	**Score (0, 1 to 7)***
1.	Eating	
2.	Grooming	
3.	Bathing	
4.	Dressing-Upper	
5.	Dressing-Lower	
6.	Toileting	
7.	Bladder Control	
8.	Bowel Control	
9.	Bed, Chair, Wheelchair Transfer	
10.	Toilet Transfer	
11.	Tub, Shower Transfer (CMS Excludes)	▓▓▓▓▓▓▓▓▓
12.	Walk/Wheelchair Locomotion	
13.	Stairs Locomotion	
CMS Cognitive Items		**Min = 0, Max = 35**
14.	Comprehension	
15.	Expression	
16.	Social Interaction	
17.	Problem Solving	
18.	Memory	

*1 = complete dependence, 7 = complete independence, 0 = not assessed [0 score is unique to PAI].

Adapted Source: Department of Health and Human Services. 2001 (August 7). *Federal Register*. Final rule. 66 (152): 41333, 41349.

Within a RIC, the numbering of the CMGs is hierarchical. Therefore, a case mix group of 0101 is a less serious than a group 0102; 0102 is a less serious CMG than 0114. Moreover, lower CMGs tend to use fewer resources than higher CMGs.

There are one hundred CMGs. Ninety-five are clinical (typical) and five are administrative (special). CMGs are four-digit codes, such as 0101 and 5104. The CMGs are assigned relative weights to account for the comparative difference in resource use. Within a RIC (the two leading digits of the CMG number), higher CMG numbers are associated with higher weights.

Each of the ninety-five clinical CMGs has four payment weights. Comorbid conditions determine the payment weight. There is one rate for cases without a comorbid condition and three rates for cases with comorbid conditions (table 6.17). The three rates with comorbid conditions correspond to the three tiers. The pricer selects the condition that assigns the case to the tier with the highest payment.

The five administrative (special) CMGs are for case-level adjustments. There is one CMG for short-stay cases. Short stays comprise three days or less (including patient expirations) and do not meet the definition of a transfer. There are four CMGs for expired patients. These four CMGs are determined by the condition (orthopedic or nonorthopedic) and by the lengths of stay (≥ 4–13 or ≥ 14).

Reimbursement

CMS reimburses IRFs for each discharge, with all costs of covered inpatient services included (Trela

Table 6.14. Rehabilitation impairment categories (RICs) and associated impairment group codes (IGCs)

RIC	Description	IGC	Description
01	Stroke (Stroke)	01.1	Left body involvement (right brain)
		01.2	Right body involvement (left brain)
		01.3	Bilateral involvement
		01.4	No paresis
		01.9	Other stroke
02	Traumatic brain injury (TBI)	02.21	Open injury
		02.22	Closed injury
04	Traumatic spinal cord injury (TSCI)	04.210	Paraplegia, unspecified
		04.211	Paraplegia, incomplete
		04.212	Paraplegia, complete
		04.220	Quadriplegia, unspecified
		04.2211	Quadriplegia, incomplete C1–4
		04.2212	Quadriplegia, incomplete C5–8
		04.2221	Quadriplegia, complete C1–4
		04.2222	Quadriplegia, complete C5–8

Source: Department of Health and Human Services. 2001 (August 7). *Federal Register.* Final rule. 66 (152): 41342–41344.

Table 6.15.   Rehabilitation impairment categories (RICs)

RIC	Description
01	Stroke (Stroke)
02	Traumatic brain injury (TBI)
03	Nontraumatic brain injury (NTBI)
04	Traumatic spinal cord injury (TSCI)
05	Nontraumatic spinal cord injury (NTSCI)
06	Neurological (Neuro)
07	Fracture of lower extremity (FracLE)
08	Replacement of lower extremity joint (Rep1LE)
09	Other orthopedic (Ortho)
10	Amputation, lower extremity (AMPLE)
11	Amputation, other (AMP–NLE)
12	Osteoarthritis (OsteoA)
13	Rheumatoid, other arthritis (RheumA)
14	Cardiac (Cardiac)
15	Pulmonary (Pulmonary)
16	Pain syndrome (Pain)
17	Major multiple trauma, no brain injury or spinal cord injury (MMT–NBSCI)
18	Major multiple trauma, with brain injury or spinal cord injury (MMT–BSCI)
19	Guillain Barre (GB)
20	Miscellaneous (Misc)
21	Burns (Burns)

Information source: Department of Health and Human Services. 2001 (August 7). *Federal Register*. Final rule. 66 (152): 41342–41344.

Table 6.16.   Case mix groups (CMGs): numbers and descriptions

CMG	Description
0101	Stroke with motor score from 69–84 and cognitive score from 23–35.
0102	Stroke with motor score from 59–68 and cognitive score from 23–35.
0103	Stroke with motor score from 59–84 and cognitive score from 5–22.
0104	Stroke with motor score from 53–58.
0105	Stroke with motor score from 47–52.
0106	Stroke with motor score from 42–46.
0107	Stroke with motor score from 39–41.
0108	Stroke with motor score from 34–38 and patient is 83 years old or older.
0109	Stroke with motor score from 34–38 and patient is 82 years old or younger.
0110	Stroke with motor score from 12–33 and patient is 89 years old or older.
0111	Stroke with motor score from 27–33 and patient is between 82 and 88 years old.
0112	Stroke with motor score from 12–26 and patient is between 82 and 88 years old.
0113	Stroke with motor score from 27–33 and patient is 81 years old or younger.
0114	Stroke with motor score from 12–26 and patient is 81 years old or younger.

Source: Department of Health and Human Services. 2001 (August 7). *Federal Register*. Final rule. 66 (152): 41345–41347.

Table 6.17.   Comorbidity codes

A	Without comorbidities
B	Comorbidity in tier 1
C	Comorbidity in tier 2
D	Comorbidity in tier 3

2002, 48A). Thus, the unit of measure of the system is the discharge. There is a single payment for each discharge. CMS's pricer software also determines the payment.

Payments are based on the weight of the CMG. Higher CMGs are associated with higher relative weights. Therefore, the weight and associated payment for CMG 0114 is higher than the weight and associated payment for 0101. (See table 6.18.) Comorbid conditions increase the weight. The relative weights of the CMGs were calculated using cost report data from fiscal years 1996 through 1997. CMS may periodically adjust the case mix groups and weighting factors to reflect changes in:

- Treatment patterns
- Technology
- Number of discharges

- Other factors affecting the relative use of resources

IRFs report the health insurance prospective payment system (HIPPS) code on the claim. The HIPPS code collapses the information about the case mix group and comorbidity into one code. Only one HIPPS code is allowed per claim.

The HIPPS code is a five-character alphanumeric code. The first character is the letter designation of the comorbidity tier (A to D). The last four characters are the four-digit CMG. Therefore, the HIPPS code for a patient with a tier 1 comorbidity and a CMG of 0109 is B0109.

A **standardized payment** conversion factor (CF; formerly known as budget-neutral conversion factor) converts the CMG weight into a payment. In 2002 and 2003, the CF was $11,838.00 and $12,193.00,

Table 6.18. Excerpt from relative weights for case-mix groups and tiers

CMG	CMG Description (M = Motor, C = Cognitive, A = Age)	Tier 1	Tier 2	Tier 3	None
0101	Stroke; M = 69–84, C = 23–35	0.4778	0.4279	0.4078	0.3859
0102	Stroke; M = 59–68, C = 23–35	0.6506	0.5827	0.5553	0.5255
0103	Stroke; M = 59–84, C = 5–22	0.8296	0.7430	0.7080	0.6700
0104	Stroke; M = 53–58	0.9007	0.8067	0.7687	0.7275
0105	Stroke; M = 47–52	1.1339	1.0155	0.9677	0.9158
0106	Stroke; M = 42–46	1.3951	1.2494	1.1905	1.1267
0107	Stroke; M = 39–41	1.6159	1.4472	1.3790	1.3050
0108	Stroke; M = 34–38, A ≥ 83	1.7477	1.5653	1.4915	1.4115
0109	Stroke; M = 34–38, A ≤ 82	1.8901	1.6928	1.6130	1.5265
0110	Stroke; M = 12–33, A ≥ 89	2.0275	1.8159	1.7303	1.6375
0111	Stroke; M = 27–33, A = 82–88	2.0889	1.8709	1.7827	1.6871
0112	Stroke; M = 12–26, A = 82–88	2.4782	2.2195	2.1149	2.0015
0113	Stroke; M = 27–33, A ≤ 81	2.2375	2.0040	1.9095	1.8071
0114	Stroke; M = 12–26, A ≤ 81	2.7302	2.4452	2.3300	2.2050

Adapted source: Department of Health and Human Services. 2001 (August 7). *Federal Register.* Final rule. 66 (152): 41394–41396.

respectively. In 2005, the CF was $12,958 (DHHS 2004c, 45766).

Generic Payment Formula

The generic payment formula is as follows:

$$\text{CMG Weight} \times \text{CF} = \text{CMG Unadjusted Prospective Payment}$$

Calculating the payment for a patient with a HIPPS code of B0109 demonstrates the use of the formula (table 6.19):

$$\text{B0109} = \text{CMG 0109 and Tier 1 comorbidity}$$

$$\text{CMG 0109 and Tier 1 comorbidity} = \text{CMG relative weight of 1.8901}$$

$$\text{CF} = \$12,958.00$$
$$1.8901 \times \$12,958.00 = \$24,491.92$$

Therefore, in 2005, the unadjusted federal prospective payment was $24,491.92.

Wage-Related Adjustments

Wages vary among areas. This variation in wages is reflected in the wage index, specific to each area. The federal government adjusts the wage index each year. Another wage-related adjustment is the labor-related share (labor ratio). The labor-related share reflects facilities' costs related to wages and salaries, employee benefits, professional fees, and the labor-related share of capital costs. The labor-related share is standard across the United States and is also adjusted each year. For example, in 2002, the labor ratio was 0.72395 and in 2005, it was 0.72359; and the Greenville, North Carolina,

wage index was 0.9402 and 0.9098, respectively. These differences, although small, matter when multiplied across thousands of dollars and many discharges, as illustrated by the following calculations:

2005 Area wage adjustment: labor ratio, 0.72359; nonlabor ratio, 0.27641; Greenville, North Carolina wage index, 0.9098

Calculating the adjusted federal prospective payment for the local wage index in the urban area of Greenville, North Carolina results in (table 6.19):

$$\$24,491.92 \times 0.72359 \text{ (labor ratio)} = \$17,722.11 \text{ (labor portion)}$$

$$\$24,491.92 \times 0.27641 \text{ (nonlabor ratio)} = \$6,769.81 \text{ (nonlabor portion)}$$

$$\$17,722.11 \text{ (labor related portion)} \times 0.9098 \text{ (local wage index)} = \$16,123.57$$

Adding the portions back together to create a whole:

$$\$6,769.81 + \$16,123.57 = \$22,893.38.$$

It should be noted that the adjusted federal prospective payment of $22,893.39 is less than the unadjusted payment. This lowered payment occurs because the local wage index (0.9098) is less than 1.00. However, in some geographic areas of the country, the wage index is greater than 1.00. In those geographic areas, the adjustment increases the federal payment.

Payments are also adjusted to account for characteristics of the facility, such as cost outlier cases, rural areas, and percentage of low-income patients (LIP).

Table 6.19.   Calculation of payment under Inpatient Rehabilitation Facility Prospective Payment Systems (2005)

HIPPS Code	CMG and Tier	Weight	Std Pymt CF (FY 2005)	Unadjusted Rate ($)	Labor-Related Ratio	Local Wage Index	Adj Labor Portion (Unadj. Rate × Labor Ratio × Local Wage Index)	Nonlabor Related Ratio	Unadjusted Nonlabor Portion (Unadj. Rate × Nonlabor Ratio)	Wage Adj. Rate (Adj. Labor Portion + Unadj. Nonlabor Ratio) ($)
B0109	0109 Tier 1	1.8901	$12,958	$24,491.92	0.72359	0.9098	16123.57	0.27641	6769.81	$22,893.38

High-Cost Outliers

High-cost outliers are cases in which the costs exceed an adjusted threshold amount. The threshold amount is $11,211, adjusted for the IRF's wage adjustment, low-income patient adjustment, and rural adjustment, as applicable (DHHS 2004c, 45771). The outlier payment is 80 percent of the difference between the estimated cost of the case and the outlier threshold (Trela 2002, 48D).

Rural Adjustment

CMS defines *rural* as being located outside a core-based statistical area formerly known as a metropolitan statistical area (MSA). To increase payments to rural IRFs, their payments are multiplied by a rural adjustment. In 2002 through 2005, the rural adjustment was 1.1914.

Adjustment for Low-Income Patients

The adjustment for the percentage of low-income patients (LIP) is:

[1 + the disproportionate share percentage] raised to the power of .4838 (DHHS 2001, 41372).

Therefore, the calculation of the LIP for an IRF with a disproportionate share percentage of 5 percent is:

[1 + 5%] raised to .4838 power
[1 + .0500] raised to .4838 power
[1.0500] raised to .4838 power = 1.0239

Special Payments

Special payment arrangements are made for **interrupted stays** and transfer cases. In interrupted stays, the patient is discharged from the IRF and returns within three calendar days. Only one payment based on the CMG from the initial assessment is made. Transfer cases are paid on a per diem. This per diem is the facility-adjusted federal prospective payment (weight $\times$ CF) divided by the average length of stay for the tier (table 6.20).

Common Reimbursement Groups

Hospital leaders and financial analysts often use reimbursement reports to discern the financial viability of the organization. A typical report would provide aggregate data on the most common reimbursement groups (tables 6.21 and 6.22).

A representative IRF's overall reimbursement for 2002 was:

$3,773,487 (weight, 318.7605 $\times$ CF, $11,838)

and for 2005 was:

$4,130,499 (weight, 318.7605 $\times$ CF, $12,958).

The increase in the conversion factor between 2002 and 2005 accounts for $356.012 of the difference. However, increases in the level of dependence (higher relative weight) of the patients also affect overall reimbursement. In table 6.22, the effects of a hypothetical shift of ten patients are calculated. If ten more patients were discharged in the higher weight HIPPS A0404 (Traumatic spinal cord injury; 2.6212) rather than in the lower HIPPS of A0204 (Traumatic brain injury; 1.3269), the total HIPPS relative weight is increased to 331.7075 from 318.7605. This increase in total HIPSS relative weight results in an increase of $167,767, solely due to the increased case mix. Healthcare leaders carefully monitor the mix of patients to ensure the viability of their organizations.

Table 6.20.   Excerpt from average length of stay in days for case-mix groups and tiers

CMG	CMG Description (M = Motor, C = Cognitive, A = Age)	Tier 1	Tier 2	Tier 3	None
0101	Stroke; M = 69–84, C = 23–35	10	9	6	8
0102	Stroke; M = 59–68, C = 23–35	11	12	10	10
0114	Stroke; M = 12–26, A ≤ 81	37	34	32	33

Adapted source: Department of Health and Human Services. 2001 (August 7). *Federal Register.* Final rule. 66 (152): 41394–41396.

Table 6.21. Case study with change in conversion factor only: Our Town Inpatient Rehabilitation Facility top 10 HIPPS codes (2002 versus 2005)

HIPPS Code	Description (M = Motor, C = Cognitive, A = Age) and Tier	Relative Weight	2002			2005		
			No. of Pts	% of Tot	TOT HIPPS Relative Weight	No. of Pts	% of Tot	TOT HIPPS Relative Weight
A0103	Stroke; M = 59–84, C = 5–22; None	0.6700	15	5.0%	10.0500	15	5.0%	10.0500
D0103	Stroke; M = 59–84, C = 5–22; Tier 3	0.7080	16	5.3%	11.3280	16	5.3%	11.3280
A0108	Stroke; M = 34–38, A > 83, None	1.4115	30	10.0%	42.3450	30	10.0%	42.3450
D0108	Stroke; M = 34–38, A > 83; Tier 3	1.4915	23	7.7%	34.3045	23	7.7%	34.3045
A0204	Traumatic brain injury; M = 30–39; None	1.3269	59	19.7%	78.2871	59	19.7%	78.2871
A0404	Traumatic spinal cord injury; M = 12–18; None	2.6216	15	5.0%	39.3240	15	5.0%	39.3240
D0701	Fracture of lower extremity; M = 52–84; Tier 3	0.6710	65	21.7%	43.6150	65	21.7%	43.6150
A1701	Major multiple trauma without brain or spinal cord injury; M = 46–84; None	0.7205	45	15.0%	32.4225	45	15.0%	32.4225
D1701	Major multiple trauma without brain or spinal cord injury; M = 46–84; Tier 3	0.8138	20	6.7%	16.2760	20	6.7%	16.2760
A1802	Major multiple trauma with brain or spinal cord injury; M = 45–84, C = 5–32; None	0.9007	12	4.0%	10.8084	12	4.0%	10.8084
	TOTAL	11.3355	300	100%	318.7605	300	100%	318.7605
	2002 CF $11,838	$3,773,487						
	2005 CF $12,958	$4,130,499						
	Difference 2002 and 2005 due to change in CF	$357,012						

Table 6.22.   Case study with change in case mix: Our Town Inpatient Rehabilitation Facility top 10 HIPPS codes (2002 versus 2005)

HIPPS Code	Description (M = Motor, C = Cognitive, A = Age) and Tier	Relative Weight	2002			2005		
			No. of Pts	% of Tot	TOT HIPPS Relative Weight	No. of Pts	% of Tot	TOT HIPPS Relative Weight
A0103	Stroke; M = 59–84, C = 5–22; None	0.6700	15	5.0%	10.0500	15	5.0%	10.0500
D0103	Stroke; M = 59–84, C = 5–22; Tier 3	0.7080	16	5.3%	11.3280	16	5.3%	11.3280
A0108	Stroke; M = 34–38, A > 83, None	1.4115	30	10.0%	42.3450	30	10.0%	42.3450
D0108	Stroke; M = 34–38, A > 83; Tier 3	1.4915	23	7.7%	34.3045	23	7.7%	34.3045
A0204	Traumatic brain injury; M = 30–39; None	1.3269	59	19.7%	78.2871	49	16.3%	65.0181
A0404	Traumatic spinal cord injury; M = 12–18; None	2.6216	15	5.0%	39.3240	25	8.3%	65.5400
D0701	Fracture of lower extremity; M = 52–84; Tier 3	0.6710	65	21.7%	43.6150	65	21.7%	43.6150
A1701	Major multiple trauma without brain or spinal cord injury; M = 46–84; None	0.7205	45	15.0%	32.4225	45	15.0%	32.4225
D1701	Major multiple trauma without brain or spinal cord injury; M = 46–84; Tier 3	0.8138	20	6.7%	16.2760	20	6.7%	16.2760
A1802	Major multiple trauma with brain or spinal cord injury; M = 45–84, C = 5–32; None	0.9007	12	4.0%	10.8084	12	4.0%	10.8084
	TOTAL	11.3355	300	100%	318.7605	300	100%	331.7075
	2002 CF $11,838	$3,773,487	Portion of difference due to change in CF (see Table 6.21)		$357,012			
	2005 CF $12,958	$4,298,266	Portion of difference due to change in case mix		$167,767			
	Difference 2002 and 2005	$524,779						

Electronic Data Submission

Facilities must submit the IRF PAI to CMS electronically. The data must be encoded using CMS's free program, the **Inpatient Rehabilitation Validation and Entry (IRVEN)** software. There are strict time frames for submission (table 6.23). Failure to follow time frames results in a 25 percent reduction of the payment.

Implementation

Accuracy in coding and reporting the items of the IRF PAI is essential to generate correct Medicare payments. Documentation in the patient record should support the IGC and the ICD-9-CM codes. The guidelines for reporting codes on the IRF PAI need careful review.

The IRF and its agents must ensure the confidentiality of the information collected in accordance with the Conditions of Participation and HIPAA requirements. Patients must be informed of their rights regarding the collection of patient assessment data and the release of patient identifiable information.

An IRF must maintain all patient assessment data sets completed on Medicare Part A fee-for-service patients within the previous five years. The IRF may maintain these sets either in a paper format in the patient's clinical record or in an electronic computer file format that the IRF can easily obtain.

Summary

The key components of the prospective payment system for inpatient rehabilitation facilities are:

- Data collection through the inpatient rehabilitation facility patient assessment instrument
- Case mix grouping
- Per discharge unit of payment
- Electronic submission

Inpatient Psychiatric Facility Prospective Payment System

The Medicare Program provides benefits for inpatient psychiatric care provided to its beneficiaries. Psychiatric hospitals and psychiatric units in acute care hospitals referred to as **inpatient psychiatric facilities (IPFs)** for payment purposes were exempt from the inpatient prospective payment system from 1982 through 2004. Section 1886(ed)(1)(B) of the Social Security Act (the Act) created this exemption and established a reasonable cost payment scheme based on the Tax Equity and Fiscal Responsibility Act (TEFRA) payment methodology (DHHS 2004f, 66923).

The Balanced Budget Refinement Act of 1999 (BBRA) required the development of a per-diem prospective payment system (PPS) for inpatient psychiatric services provided in IPFs. Specifically, the BBRA charged CMS with developing a classification system that would reflect the resource consumption and, therefore, cost differences among various IPFs. The legislation gave CMS the

Table 6.23.   Inpatient rehabilitation facility prospective payment system time frames

Event	Admission	Discharge
Observation period	Days 1–3	Date of discharge or end of Medicare Part A fee-for-service coverage
Assessment reference date	Day 3	Date of discharge or discontinuation of covered services
Completion date	Day 4	Day 5 following discharge or discontinuation of covered services
Encoded date	Day 10	Day 7 following completion date (count completion date as day 1)
Transmission date	with discharge assessment	Day 7 following the encoded date

Source: Trela P. 2002. Inpatient rehabilitation PPS presents new challenges, opportunities. *Journal of the American Health Information Management Association.* 73 (1): 48A–48D.

authority to collect hospital data necessary for the development of the new PPS. The system was mandated to maintain budget neutrality and CMS instructed to submit a report of the proposed system to Congress. The initial implementation date was set to be October, 1, 2002. (DHHS 2004f, 66923).

Prior to the BBRA, CMS had researched several PPS options for IPFs. However, its research focus was a by-discharge payment methodology similar to other established PPSs, such as the IPPS and HOPPS. The research showed that a per-discharge system did not adequately explain the cost variations among psychiatric encounters (DHHS 2004f, 66923). Therefore a new approach was necessary. The BBRA gave CMS a three-year period to research and develop a per-diem system (DHHS 2004f, 66923).

More than a year after the initial implementation date of October 1, 2002, the proposed rule for the IPF PPS was released on November 28, 2003 (DHHS 2004f, 66920). The proposed rule outlined the new PPS based on a per-diem rate with several add-on payments to provide reimbursement for cost variations. The new PPS called for major changes in the way an IPF would be reimbursed for Medicare services and discussed complex cost issues. CMS received many comments on the proposed rule, and the public requested an extended period of time to review the proposed PPS. Therefore, the comment period was extended. On November 15, 2004, the final rule for the IPF PPS was released (DHHS 2004f, 66922).The final rule established a new implementation date of April 1, 2005.

The IPF PPS is based on a federal per-diem amount that represents the average daily operational, ancillary, and capital costs expended to care for Medicare beneficiaries. Adjustments to the payment are made at the facility and patient levels, as described in table 6.24. Although the large number of payment modifications creates a complex system, the payment methodology is designed to adequately reimburse facilities for the services provided to Medicare beneficiaries.

Table 6.24.   Facility and patient level adjustments

Facility-Level Adjustments	Patient-Level Adjustments
Wage index	Length of stay
Cost of living adjustment	DRG with principal diagnosis of mental disorder
Rural location	
Teaching status	Comorbidity
Full service emergency department	Age of patient
	Electroconvulsive therapy

CMS used a regression analysis model to determine the types and levels of adjustments that were necessary to create a payment system that would explain cost variation among IPFs. Regression analysis is a statistical methodology that uses an independent variable to predict the value of a dependent variable. In this case, patient demographics and length of stay (independent variables) were used to predict cost (dependent variable). The regression analysis performed for the IPF PPS proposed rule (2003) used data from the FY 1999 MedPAR file and the FY 1999 healthcare cost reporting information system (HCRIS). A revised regression analysis was performed for the Final Rule and used updated MedPAR data from 2002 and updated HCRIS data from 2001 and 2002.

Patient-Level Adjustments

Patient-level adjustments are made for length of stay, DRGs that contain a psychiatric ICD-9-CM code, comorbidity conditions, treatment of older patients, and encounters that include electroconvulsive therapy.

Length of Stay Adjustment

Cost regression, first based on 1999 claims data and then updated with 2002 data, showed that the per-diem cost for psychiatric cases decreased as the length of stay increased (DHHS 2004f, 66949). Therefore, the IPF PPS provides a length-of-stay adjustment factor for each day of the patient encounter. Table 6.25 shows the adjustment schedule by day.

Table 6.25.   Length-of-stay adjustment schedule

Day of Stay	Variable Per-Diem Payment Adjustment
Day 1	1.31/1.19*
Day 2	1.12
Day 3	1.08
Day 4	1.05
Day 5	1.04
Day 6	1.02
Day 7	1.01
Day 8	1.01
Day 9	1.00
Day 10	1.00
Day 11	0.99
Day 12	0.99
Day 13	0.99
Day 14	0.99
Day 15	0.98
Day 16	0.97
Day 17	0.97
Day 18	0.96
Day 19	0.95
Day 20	0.95
Day 21	0.95
Over 21	0.92

*The adjustment for day 1 would be 1.31 or 1.19, depending on whether the IPF has or is a psychiatric unit in an acute care hospital with a qualifying emergency department.

Source: Department of Health and Human Services. 2004 (November 15). *Federal Register.* 69 (216): 66949.

DRG Adjustment

The IPF PPS will provide reimbursement for DRGs that contain a psychiatric ICD-9-CM code as identified in chapter five of the code book as principal diagnosis. However, a payment adjustment will be made only for fifteen designated psychiatric DRGs. Table 6.26 provides a listing of the fifteen psychiatric DRGs.

Comorbidity Conditions

The regression analysis of 2002 cost data identified a need to provide a payment adjustment for some comorbidity conditions. Table 6.27 provides a listing of the comorbidity groupings that warrant

Table 6.26.   Psychiatric DRGs that qualify for payment adjustment

DRG Title	DRG Code	Adjustment Factor
Procedure with principal diagnosis of mental illness	DRG 424	1.22
Acute adjustment reaction	DRG 425	1.05
Depressive neurosis	DRG 426	0.99
Neurosis, except depressive	DRG 427	1.02
Disorders of personality	DRG 428	1.02
Organic disturbances	DRG 429	1.03
Psychosis	DRG 430	1.00
Childhood disorders	DRG 431	0.99
Other mental disorders	DRG 432	0.92
Alcohol/drug use, LAMA	DRG 433	0.97
Alcohol/drug, with CC	DRG 521	1.02
Alcohol/drug without CC	DRG 522	0.98
Alcohol/drug use, without rehab	DRG 523	0.88
Degenerative nervous system disorders	DRG 012	1.05
Nontraumatic stupor and coma	DRG 023	1.07

Source: Department of Health and Human Services. 2004 (November 15). *Federal Register.* 69 (216): 66938.

Table 6.27.   Comorbidity adjustment categories

Comorbidity Category	Applicable ICD-9-CM Codes	Adjustment Factor
Developmental disabilities	317, 318.0, 318.1, 318.2 and 319	1.04
Coagulation factor deficits	286.0 through 286.4	1.13
Tracheotomy	519.00 through 519.09 and V44.0	1.06
Renal failure, acute	584.5 through 584.9, 636.3, 637.3, 638.3, 639.3, 669.32, 669.34 and 958.5	1.11
Renal failure, chronic	403.01, 403.11, 403.91, 404.02, 404.03, 404.12, 404.13, 404.92, 404.93, 585, 586, V45.1, V56.0, V56.1 and V56.2	1.11
Oncology treatment	140.0 through 239.9 with either 92.21 through 92.29 or 99.25	1.07
Uncontrolled type I and type II diabetes mellitus with or without complications	250.02, 250.03, 250.12, 250.13, 250.22, 250.23, 250.32, 250.33, 250.42, 250.43, 250.52, 250.53, 250.62, 250.63, 250.72, 250.73, 250.82, 250.83, 250.92 and 250.93	1.05
Severe protein calorie malnutrition	260 through 262	1.13
Eating and conduct disorders	307.1, 307.50, 312.03, 312.33 and 312.34	1.12
Infectious disease	010.00 through 041.10, 042, 045.00 through 053.19, 054.40 through 054.49, 055.0 through 077.0, 078.2 through 078.89 and 079.50 through 079.59	1.07
Drug and/or alcohol induced mental disorders	291.0, 292.0, 292.2, 303.00 and 304.00	1.03
Cardiac conditions	391.0, 391.1, 391.2, 402.01, 404.03, 416.0, 421.0, 421.1 and 421.9	1.11
Gangrene	440.24 and 785.4	1.10
Chronic obstructive pulmonary disease	491.21, 494.1, 510.0, 518.83, 518.84, V46.11 and V46.12	1.12
Artificial openings—digestive and urinary	569.60 through 569.69, 997.5 and V44.1 through V44.6	1.08
Severe musculoskeletal and connective tissue diseases	696.0, 710.0, 730.00 through 730.09, 730.10 through 730.19 and 730.20 through 730.29	1.09
Poisoning	965.00 through 965.09, 965.4, 967.0 through 969.9, 977.0, 980.0 through 980.9, 983.0 through 983.9, 986 and 989.0 through 989.7	1.11

Source: Department of Health and Human Services. 2004 (November 15). *Federal Register.* 69 (216): 66944.

a payment adjustment in the IPF PPS system. This is not a complete list of comorbidities as used in the IPPS; rather, it is a listing of the conditions that were found to be more costly to treat for psychiatric patients in IPFs.

Older Patients

Reimbursement rates are altered to account for the additional costs incurred for treating older patients. Regression analysis showed that the cost per day increased with increasing patient age. Table 6.28 provides the age categories and the adjustment factors used for the IPF PPS.

Electroconvulsive Therapy

Providing electroconvulsive therapy (ECT) to Medicare beneficiaries is costly. Regression analysis showed that an encounter that included ECT was twice as expensive as an encounter that did not include ECT. The cost is mostly associated with the increased length of stay but is also a result of increased ancillary services (DHHS 2004f, 66951). The IPF PPS provides a patient-level adjustment for this service. Facilities will receive additional payment for each ECT session performed. For the implementation year (April 2005–June 2006)

Table 6.28.   Age adjustment categories

Age	Adjustment Factor
Under 45	1.00
45 and under 50	1.01
50 and under 55	1.02
55 and under 60	1.04
60 and under 65	1.07
65 and under 70	1.10
70 and under 75	1.13
75 and under 80	1.15
80 and over	1.17

Source: Department of Health and Human Services. 2004 (November 15). *Federal Register.* 69 (216): 66947.

the additional reimbursement equals \$247.96. The ECT amount is subject to cost of living (COLA) and wage index adjustments. ECT services should be reported with the CPT code 90870 and revenue code 901. The units of service must also be reported. ECT payments and charges are taken into account when fiscal intermediaries calculate the outlier threshold and outlier payment.

Facility-Level Adjustments

Payments are adjusted at the facility level to account for geographic variations such as wage differences, cost of living, and rural location. Adjustments are also made for teaching hospitals and facilities that provide emergency medical services. These adjustments are addressed in the following sections.

Wage Index Adjustment

A facility level adjustment is provided to account for wage differences among geographical areas. The labor portion of the federal per-diem base rate is 72.247 percent. The unadjusted, pre-reclassified IPPS hospital wage index based on 1993 metropolitan statistical area (MSA) definitions is used to make the adjustment. Figure 6.5 provides the IPF wage index adjustment formula. Please note that at implementation the IPFPPS wage index adjustment was not based on the newly reclassified CBSA values that are being used in the IPPS and HOPPS. CMS will review claims data in the future to determine if a conversion to the CBSA methodology is warranted under this system.

Cost-of-Living Adjustment

In addition to the wage index adjustment, a cost-of-living adjustment (COLA) will be made for IPFs in the states of Hawaii and Alaska. The nonlabor share portion (27.753 percent) of the federal per diem base rate will be adjusted by the adjustment factor provided for the county in which the facility

Figure 6.5.   Wage index adjustment formula

(Federal per diem base rate × Labor percent × Wage index) +
(Federal per diem base rate × Nonlabor percentage)

is located. Figure 6.6 provides the COLA formula. Table 6.29 provides a listing of the COLA adjustments.

Rural Location Adjustment

Regression analysis showed that IPFs incurred costs 17 percent greater when treating patients in rural locations than treating patients in urban locations. Many rural IPFs are small facilities that do not have the economy-of-scale advantages that larger facilities experience. Further, providing psychiatric services requires a set of minimum fixed costs that cannot be avoided or decreased. (DHHS 2004f, 66954). Therefore, the IPF PPS is providing a rural location adjustment of 1.17.

Teaching Hospital Adjustment

IPFs are granted a teaching hospital adjustment similar to the adjustment made for IPPS facilities. The adjustment is based on the number of full-time residents at the facility.

Emergency Facility Adjustment

Patients who receive emergency department (ED) care prior to admission are more costly to treat than

Figure 6.6.   COLA formula

(Federal per diem base rate × Labor percentage × Wage index)
+ (Federal per diem base rate × Nonlabor percentage × COLA)

Table 6.29.   COLA areas

State	Location	COLA
Alaska	All areas	1.25
Hawaii	Honolulu County	1.25
Hawaii	Hawaii County	1.165
Hawaii	Kauai County	1.2325
Hawaii	Maui County	1.2375
Hawaii	Kalawao County	1.2375

Source: Department of Health and Human Services. 2004 (November 15). *Federal Register.* 69 (216): 66958.

patients who do not receive such care. Therefore, CMS provides an adjustment to adequately reimburse facilities for this greater cost without creating an incentive to provide ED care when it is not medically necessary in order to receive additional payments. A facility-level adjustment is made for IPFs with full-service EDs. IPFs with qualifying EDs receive a greater per-diem adjustment for the first day of each stay for all patients. (See table 6.25, Day One.)

Provisions of the Inpatient Psychiatric Facility Prospective Payment System

The IPF PPS uses provisions to provide additional payments for unusual admissions that historically have added significant cost to patient care. Without the additional payments associated with these provisions, it may not be feasible for inpatient psychiatric facilities to provide all services to Medicare beneficiaries.

Outlier Payment Provision

The IPF PPS provides outlier payments for high cost encounters. Outlier payments are projected to account for 2 percent of the total payment for implementation year. In order to qualify for an outlier payment, the costs of an encounter must exceed the adjusted threshold amount. Cost is determined by converting charges to cost using cost-to-charge ratios (CCRs) from the facility's most recent settled or tentatively settled Medicare cost report. Facilities that have CCRs outside of the designated **trim points** will be required to use national rural/urban CCRs. The adjusted threshold amount is calculated by applying wage index, rural location, and teaching status adjustment to the national amount. The unadjusted threshold amount for implementation year is $5,700. In addition to reimbursement for the encounter, facilities will receive 80 percent of the difference between the IPF's estimated cost and the adjusted threshold amount for days one through nine, and 60 percent for days thereafter (DHHS 2004f, 66960).

Stop-Loss Provision

A stop-loss provision is a form of hold-harmless policy. A stop-loss schedule has been included in the implementation of the IPF PPS to assist facilities with changes in reimbursement levels that may occur. Multiple stop-loss levels were researched, but the 70 percent policy was adopted. IPF PPS payment can equal no less than 70 percent of the TEFRA payment had the IPF PPS not been implemented. In order to achieve the 70 percent policy, a four-year phase-in schedule was developed, as outlined in table 6.30.

Initial Stay and Readmission Provisions

The IPF PPS is designed to provide higher payment for initial days of a stay in order to adequately reimburse facilities for the higher costs associated with a new admission. CMS has expressed concern that this adjustment could provide an incentive for facilities to prematurely discharge patients and then subsequently readmit them in order to again receive the higher per-diem rates associated with the first days of a stay. Therefore, an interrupted stay provision was created. Patients discharged from an IPF who are then admitted to the same or another IPF within three consecutive days (before midnight on the third day) of the discharge from the original facility stay would be treated as continuous for purposes of the variable per-diem adjustment and outlier calculation (DHHS 2004f, 66963).

Table 6.30.   Stop-loss schedule

Year	TEFRA Payment	IPF PPS Payment
Year one (4/1/2005–6/30/2006)	75%	25%
Year two (7/1/2006–6/30/2007)	50%	50%
Year three (7/1/2007–6/30/2008)	25%	75%
Year four (7/1/2008–6/30/2009)	0%	100%

Example:

A patient is admitted to IPF A on March 1. The patient is discharged on March 5 (length of stay = four). The patient is then admitted to IPF B on March 7 and continues the hospital stay until March 10 (length of stay = three). The admission to IPF B is considered a continuation of the initial stay at IPF A. Therefore, day one of the readmission will be considered day five of the combined stay for the purposes of the length of stay adjustment and outlier calculation (see table 6.25).

Medical Necessity Provision

Medical necessity must be established for each patient upon admission to the IPF. Physician recertification to establish continued need for inpatient psychiatric care is required on the eighteenth day following admission. Inpatient care requires more intense service than outpatient. Inpatient admissions or continued stays are necessary when care requires intensive comprehensive multimodal treatments such as twenty-four hour supervision, safety concerns, diagnostic evaluations, monitoring for side effects of psychotropic medications, and evaluation of behaviors.

Payment Steps

Step One: Wage index adjust the labor portion of the per-diem rate.

Step Two: Apply COLA to the nonlabor portion of the per-diem rate if applicable.

Step Three: Add the results of step one and step two together to determine the wage adjusted per-diem rate.

Step Four: Apply the following patient-level and facility-level adjustments:
• Rural location
• Teaching
• Full-service ED
• DRG
• Comorbidity
• Age

Determine each level of adjustment for the case. Multiply the individual adjustments to determine the PPS adjustment factor.

Step Five: Multiply the PPS adjustment factor by the wage adjusted per-diem rate determined in step three to calculate the adjusted per diem.

Step Six: Identify whether the facility has a qualifying ED. If so, choose the appropriate (higher) adjustment factor for the first day of stay. Determine the patient's length of stay and LOS adjustment factor for each day.

Step Seven: Multiply the adjusted per-diem rate (step five) by the LOS adjustment factor for each day of the stay to calculate the per-diem payment amount.

Step Eight: Sum the per-diem payment amounts calculated for each day of the stay.

Step Nine: Calculate the adjusted ECT amount for the encounter if applicable. Multiply the national payment amount by the labor share and the area wage index. Then multiply the national payment amount by the nonlabor share and the applicable COLA. Sum these two products to calculate the adjusted ECT amount. Multiply the adjusted ECT amount by the units of service. Add the total ECT payment to the total per-diem payment amount (step eight).

Check Your Understanding 6.2

1. What cost-sharing applies to beneficiaries residing in a LTCH for ninety days?

2. Even though long-term care diagnosis related groups (LTC-DRGs) are based on the same six general factors as the acute care DRGs for the IPPS, LTC-DRGs differ from acute care DRGs because LTC-DRGs have higher weights, use quintiles for low volumes, and employ short-stay outliers. True or false?

3. The budget-neutral conversion factor (CF) that converts the LTC-DRG into a payment amount is the _____.

4. To collect information about Medicare patients that drives payment in the IRF PPS, the _____ is used.

5. IRF staff members record RICs on patients' PAIs to classify their impairment categories. True or false?

Summary

CMS has projected that Medicare will save at least $7.5 million during the next five years with implementation of the IPF PPS ((DHHS 2004f, 66974). Even though one of the primary objectives of implementing prospective payment systems is to control costs, CMS is dedicated to maintaining a PPS that not only focuses on cost and payment but also incorporates variables, such as quality and outcome measures, that influence cost and payment levels ((DHHS 2004f, 66968). CMS will continue to research various payment methods as it makes future refinements to the system.

Summary

The Medicare prospective payment system (PPS) was introduced by the federal government in October, 1983, as a way to change hospital behavior through financial incentives that encourage more cost-efficient management of medical care. Since that time, PPS has revolutionized healthcare reimbursement in settings across the continuum of care. Four more prospective payment systems for hospital settings in skilled nursing, long-term care, rehabilitation, and psychiatric facilities were designed and implemented between 1998 and 2005. As updates and revisions are required and/or warranted, CMS publishes proposed and final rules via the *Federal Register* to discuss and release updated information. Students and professionals should review final rules in order to obtain the most current payment values and provision specifications.

Chapter 6 Review Quiz

1. List at least two major reasons that Medicare administrators turned to the prospective payment concept for Medicare beneficiaries.

2. How do DRGs encourage inpatient facilities to practice cost management?

3. How are per-diem rates for SNF PPS patients determined for various cases?

4. When do temporary add-ons to RUGs terminate?

5. How are LTC-DRGs determined?

6. On the IRF PAI the patient's ability to perform activities of daily living, or _____ is recorded on the _____.

7. Why does the IPF PPS length-of-stay adjustment factor grow smaller during the patient encounter?

8. Describe at least two of the patient-level adjustments for IRF PPS claims and why they are used.

9. For inpatient rehabilitation facility patients, codes on the IRF PAI should follow the UHDDS and the UB-92 guidelines. True or false?

10. Facilities transmit IRF PAIs to the Centers for Medicare and Medicaid Services using CMS's free IRVEN software. True or false?

References and Bibliography

Averill, R. F., N. I. Goldfield, J. Eisenhandler, J. S. Hughes, and J. Muldoon. 2001. Clinical risk groups and the future of healthcare reimbursement. In *Reimbursement Methodologies for Healthcare Services* [CD-ROM], edited by L. M. Jones. Chicago: American Health Information Management Association.

Centers for Medicare and Medicaid Services. 2005. www.cms.hhs.gov.

Centers for Medicare and Medicaid Services. 2002a. Inpatient rehabilitation facility prospective payment system. Available online from www.cms.hhs.gov/medlearn/inpatref.asp.

Centers for Medicare and Medicaid Services. 2002b. LTCH PPS contractor training guide for providers. Available online from www.cms.hhs.gov/medlearn/trainguide.asp.

Centers for Medicare and Medicaid Services. 2003. Medicare Prescription Drug, Improvement, and Modernization Act of 2003. Section 626 (2)(B). Available online from www.cms.hhs.gov/medicarereform.

Centers for Medicare and Medicaid Services. 2004. *Expansion of Transfer Policy under Inpatient Prospective Payment System.* MedLearn Matters (MM2934), Medicare Learning Network. Available online from www.cms.hhs.gov/medlearn/matters/.

Department of Health and Human Services. 1999 (July 30). Medicare Program; Prospective Payment System and Consolidated Billing for Skilled Nursing Facilities—Update; Notices. *Federal Register* 64 (146). 41684–41701.

Department of Health and Human Services. 2001 (August 7). Medicare Program; Prospective Payment System for Inpatient Rehabilitation Facilities; Final Rule. *Federal Register* 66 (152): 41316–41347.

Department of Health and Human Services. 2002 (August 30). Medicare Program; Prospective Payment System for Long-Term Care Hospitals: Implementation and FY 2003 Rates; Final Rule. *Federal Register* 67 (169): 55953–56090.

Department of Health and Human Services. 2003a (June 6). Medicare Program; Prospective Payment System for Long-Term Care Hospitals: Annual Payment Rate Updates and Policy Changes; Final Rule. *Federal Register* 68 (109): 34122–34190.

Department of Health and Human Services. 2003b (November 28). Medicare Program; Prospective Payment System for Inpatient Psychiatric Facilities; Proposed Rule. *Federal Register* 68 (229): 66919–66978.

Department of Health and Human Services. 2004a (May 7). Medicare Program; Changes to the Criteria for Being Classified as an Inpatient Rehabilitation Facility; Final Rule. *Federal Register* 69 (89): 25751–25776.

Department of Health and Human Services. 2004b (May 7). Medicare Program; Prospective Payment System for Long-Term Care Hospitals: Annual Payment Rate Updates and Policy Changes; Final Rule. *Federal Register* 69 (89): 25674–25749.

Department of Health and Human Services 2004c (July 30). Medicare Program; Inpatient Rehabilitation Facility Prospective Payment System for Fiscal Year 2005; Notice. *Federal Register* 69 (146): 45721–45775.

Department of Health and Human Services 2004d (July 30). Medicare Program; Prospective Payment System and

Consolidated Billing for Skilled Nursing Facilities—Update; Notice. *Federal Register* 69 (146): 45775–45822.

Department of Health and Human Services. 2004e (August 11). Medicare Program; Changes to the Hospital Inpatient Prospective Payment Systems and Fiscal Year 2005 Rates; Final Rule. *Federal Register* 69 (154): 48915–48964.

Department of Health and Human Services. 2004f (November 15). Medicare Program; Prospective Payment System for Inpatient Psychiatric Facilities; Final Rule. *Federal Register* 69 (219): 66921–67015.

Department of Health and Human Services. 2004g (December 30). Medicare Program; Prospective Payment System and Consolidated Billing for Skilled Nursing Facilities; Corrections; Notices. *Federal Register* 69 (250): 78445–78464.

Department of Health and Human Services. 2005 (May 6). Medicare Program; Prospective Payment System for Long-Term Care Hospitals: Annual Payment Rate Updates, Policy Changes, and Clarification; Final Rule. *Federal Register* 70 (87): 24168–24261.

Dougherty, Michelle. 2002. New PPS proposed for LTC hospitals. *Journal of American Health Information Management Association* 73(7):72–73.

Gottlober, P., T. Brady, B. Robinson, T. Davis, S. Phillips, and A. Gruber. 2001 (August). *Medicare Hospital Prospective Payment System: How DRG Rates are Calculated and Updated.* Publication No. OEI-09-00-00200. Office of Inspector General, Office of Evaluation and Inspections, Region IX. Available online from www.oig.hhs.gov/oei/reports/oei-09-00-00200.pdf

Johns, Merida., ed. 2002. *Health Information Management Technology: An Applied Approach.* Chicago: American Health Information Management Association.

LaTour, K., and S. Eichenwald, eds. 2002. *Health Information Management: Concepts, Principles, and Practice.* Chicago: American Health Information Management Association.

Lave, J. R. 1989. The effect of the Medicare prospective payment system. *Annual Review of Public Health* 10:141–161.

Schraffenberger, L. 2005. *Basic ICD-9-CM Coding.* Chicago: American Health Information Management Association.

Trela, Patricia. 2002. Inpatient rehabilitation PPS presents new challenges, opportunities. *Journal of American Health Information Management Association.* 73 (January) (1): 48A–48D.

Chapter 7
Ambulatory and Other Medicare-Medicaid Reimbursement Systems

Objectives

- To differentiate major types of Medicare and Medicaid reimbursement systems for beneficiaries

- To define basic language associated with reimbursement under Medicare and Medicaid healthcare payment systems

- To explain common models and policies of payment for Medicare and Medicaid health-care payment systems for physicians and out-patient settings

Key Terms

Ambulatory payment classifications (APCs)
Ambulatory surgery center payment groups
Ambulatory surgical centers (ASCs)
Ancillary services
ASC list
Bundling
Calendar year (CY)
Carrier
Conversion factor (CF)
Core-based statistical area (CBSA)
Critical access hospitals (CAHs)
Critical care services
Discounted
Episode of care
Geographic practice cost index (GPCI)
Health insurance prospective payment system (HIPPS)
Hold-harmless status
Home assistance validation and entry (HAVEN)

Home health agencies (HHAs)
Home health resource group (HHRG)
Low-utilization payment adjustment (LUPA)
Metropolitan statistical area (MSA)
National standard episode amount
National unadjusted copayment amount
National unadjusted payment amount
Observation
Outcome Assessment Information Set (OASIS)
Outpatient Code Editor (OCE)
Packaging
Partial hospitalization
Pass-through
Payment status indicator
Relative value scale
Relative value units (RVUs)
Resource-based relative value scale (RBRVS)
Rural area

Introduction to Reimbursement Systems for Physicians and Ambulatory Settings

The first prospective payment system (PPS), the acute care PPS, was a successful initiative for Medicare reimbursement reform. However, as the rate of growth of Medicare inpatient payments was effectively curbed, the rate of growth of Medicare payments for ambulatory patients and to physicians escalated sharply. For example, in the 1980s, the average rate of growth for Medicare spending on physicians grew at an average rate of more than 12 percent (Scanlon 2002, 2). Therefore, Congress authorized the Department of Health and Human Services (DHHS) to develop and implement reformed fee systems and prospective payment systems across the continuum of care for Medicare beneficiaries. These payment systems include the resource-based relative value scale for physician services, the ambulance fee schedule, the ambulatory surgical center payment system, the hospital outpatient payment system, and the home health payment system.

Resource-Based Relative Value Scale for Physician Payments

A **resource-based relative value scale (RBRVS)** is a system of classifying health services based on the cost of furnishing physician services in different settings, the skill and training levels required to perform the services, and the time and risk involved. The RBRVS is the federal government's payment system for physicians.

Background

The concept of a **relative value scale** has existed since the mid-1940s. Such a system permits comparisons of the resources needed or appropriate prices for various units of service. It takes into account labor, skill, supplies, equipment, space, and other costs for each procedure or service.

In the 1940s, the Casualty Actuarial Society created a relative value scale for commercial insurance. In 1956, the California Medical Society devised one. Since 1956, medical societies of forty other states and six physician specialty groups have devised such scales. Antitrust actions in the 1970s slowed the adoption of relative value scales by professional groups. However, payers' interest in relative value scales continued.

Relative value scales attempt to represent the worth of healthcare services. Experts have used various ways to represent the worth of services. The different ways focus on the different qualities that people deem important. Some of the bases of these proposed ways have been:

- Historical charges for physician services (most popular and least difficult)

- Prices patients are willing to pay (consumerism)

- Physicians' assessments of the worth of different services and procedures

- Monetized benefits to society

- Consensus or negotiation process

- Estimates of the charges that would occur in a competitive market

- Micro-costing of physician services with time-and-motion studies or Delphi studies

The approach that eventually was adopted focused on the cost of furnishing physician services in different settings, the skill and training levels required to perform the services, and the time and risk involved.

History

In 1985, the Consolidated Omnibus Reconciliation Act (COBRA) directed the Department of Health and Human Services (DHHS) to develop a relative value scale for physician services. As a result of COBRA, in 1985, the Centers for Medicare and Medicaid Services (CMS; formerly the Health Care Financing Administration, [HCFA]) awarded a grant to Dr. William Hsaio of Harvard University to devise a system of classifying services using resource-based relative values. The purpose of this research was twofold. Primarily, the intent of the research was to address the issue of income disparity between physician specialists and general practitioners. Because specialists were higher paid than general practitioners, more medical students were entering specialty fields. The nation as a result had fewer family doctors; this shortage was especially severe in rural areas. To resolve this shortage, the federal government decided to increase the rate of reimbursement for services typical of general practitioners to rates comparable to those for services of specialists. Thus, services such as office visits and consultations were to be weighted more heavily than in the past. The additional purpose and side benefit of this new system of classification was to save the government Medicare funds.

In the 1989 Omnibus Budget Reconciliation Act, Congress required the government reform the physician payment system. Effective January 1, 1992, the federal government instituted RBRVS for reimbursement of physicians. RBRVS was phased in between 1992 and 1996. Although RBRVS is still a fee-for-service system of payment, the reimbursement is based on CMS's estimation of the value of a physician's service.

Structure of Relative Value Units

Relative value units (RVUs) exist for over four thousand types of health services, accounting for 85 percent of Medicare payments to physicians. The system assigns each service a value representing the true resources involved in producing it, including the time and intensity of work, the expenses of practice, and the risk of malpractice.

The RBRVS system applies to physician services, such as medical/surgical, diagnostic, and radiologic services. Physical and occupational therapy are also included. Laboratory tests are excluded. In addition, payments for the services of physician assistants, nurse practitioners, and nurse midwives are tied to the RBRVS payment amounts.

RBRVS is based on CPT coding. Each CPT code has been assigned a **relative value unit (RVU).** An RVU is a unit of measure designed to permit comparison of the amount of resources required to perform various provider services by assigning weights to such factors as personnel time, level of skill, and sophistication of equipment required to render service. In the RBRVS, the RVU reflects national averages and is the sum of the physician work, practice expenses, and malpractice costs. RVUs are adjusted to local costs through the geographic practice cost indexes (GPCIs).

Each RVU comprises three elements, each of which is a national average available in the *Federal Register:*

- Physician work (WORK)
- Physician practice expenses (PE)
- Malpractice (MP)

WORK is the element that covers the physician's salary. This work is the time the physician spends providing a service and the intensity with which that time is spent. The four aspects of intensity are:

- Mental effort and judgment
- Technical skill
- Physical effort
- Psychological stress

PE is the overhead costs of the practice, such as office rent, wages of nonphysician personnel, and supplies and equipment. PE is categorized as either facility or nonfacility. According to CMS experts, practice expenses differ for physicians when they perform services in facilities, such as hospitals, as opposed to nonfacilities, such as their own offices and clinics. In facilities, the organization incurs the overhead costs of personnel, supplies, equipment, and other costs, while in nonfacilities, the physician incurs the overhead expenses for such costs. Therefore, the PE is higher for nonfacilities. Some procedural codes do not have separate facility and nonfacility PEs. In these procedural codes, the description includes the setting (evaluation and management, initial hospital care) or the nature of the procedure restricts it to a particular site (major surgical procedures in hospitals).

Facilities include:

- Inpatient or outpatient hospital settings

- Emergency rooms

- Skilled nursing facilities

- Ambulatory surgical centers

- Inpatient psychiatric facilities

- Comprehensive inpatient rehabilitation facilities

- Community mental health centers

- Military treatment facilities

- Ambulance (land, air, or water)

- Psychiatric facility partial hospital

- Psychiatric resort treatment centers.

Nonfacilities include:

- Physicians' offices

- Clinics

- Dialysis centers

- Independent laboratories

- Nonskilled nursing facilities

- Patients' homes

- All other settings

Physicians can provide services in these multiple settings. Factors in choice of setting include:

- Patient's medical condition

- Type of procedure

- Patient's preference

- Geographic location

- Technology

- Regulation or healthcare insurance policies (Medicare Payment Advisory Commission 2004, 19)

The final decision of setting is a blend of the factors.

MP is the cost of the premiums for the professional liability insurance.

Payment Structure

Payments under the RBRVS system consist of three components. These three components are:

- The RVU

- A geographic adjustment

- A constant that converts a relative value into a payment

A payment amount results when the RVUs are adjusted for geographic variations, summed, and multiplied by the constant.

The elements of the RVU are national averages. A geographic adjustment is necessary because costs vary in different areas of the country. Therefore, each element of an RVU is adjusted for these differences. The adjustment component is called the **geographic practice cost index (GPCI).** This index is based on relative differences in the cost of a market basket of goods across geographic areas. GPCIs reflect local costs. Each element of the RVU—WORK, PE, and MP—has its own unique GPCI. The GPCIs can be found in the *Federal Register.*

The across-the-board multiplier is the **conversion factor (CF).** Unlike the GPCIs, the conversion factor is a constant that applies to the entire RVU. The conversion factor transforms the geographic-adjusted RVU into a national allowance for a Medicare payment. The conversion factor, as updated annually, can be found in the *Federal Register.*

The conversion factor is the government's most direct control on Medicare payments to physicians. CMS raises or lowers the conversion factor to raise or lower physician payments. For example, in 2001, CMS set the conversion factor at $38.2581 ($17.2600 for anesthesia). In 2002, in an effort to reduce costs, CMS set the conversion factor at $36.1992. In 2003 and 2005, Congress set the conversion factors at $36.7856 and $37.8975, respectively, to give physicians slight increases. Therefore, by adjusting one number, the CF, Congress can increase and decrease overall Medicare payments to physicians.

Payment Calculation

To calculate the national allowance for payments for various services, the following formula is used:

$$[(WORK\ RVU)\ (WORK\ GPCI) + \\ (PE\ RVU)\ (PE\ GPCI) + \\ (MP\ RVU)\ (MP\ GPCI)]\ = (SUM) \times CF = \\ National\ allowance$$

Table 7.1 dissects the general RBRVS formula, and table 7.2 shows the formula in action for a sample CPT code.

Finally, the actual Medicare payment is 80 percent of the national allowance. Medicare beneficiaries are responsible for 20 percent coinsurance and $100 Medicare Part B deductible.

Operational Issues

Poor coding and inadequate documentation negatively affect RBRVS reimbursement. For example, overlooking the removal of a polyp or lesion during an esophagoscopy can significantly reduce payment (table 7.3). Other examples illustrate the difference documentation and accurate coding make (tables 7.4 and 7.5).

Ambulance Fee Schedule

Section 1861(s)(7) of the Social Security Act (the Act) Medicare Part B provides beneficiary coverage for ambulance services. The benefit is intended to provide transportation services only if other means are inadvisable based on the beneficiary's medical condition. Transportation services are provided to the nearest facility that is able to provide services for the patient's condition. Beneficiaries may be transported from one hospital to another, to home, or to an extended care facility (DHHS 2002, 9100).

History

Prior to the prospective payment system implementation for ambulance services, providers and suppliers were reimbursed on a reasonable cost or charge methodology based on entity type. Providers were those ambulance service entities associated with a medical facility such as hospital, critical access hospital, skilled nursing facility, or home health agency, and were reimbursed based on retrospective reasonable cost payment. Providers used Health Care Common Procedure Coding System (HCPCS) Level II ambulance codes (A0030–A0999, excluding A0888) to report the type of service provided, and additional HCPCS Level II ambulance codes to report the type of mileage used. The charges associated with the HCPCS Level II codes selected for the case were converted to cost using the previous year's cost-to-charge ratio (CCR) for that entity.

Table 7.1.   Generic formula: Resource-based relative value scale

General RBRVS Formula		
Relative value (RVU) of service = sum of work value, practice expenses, malpractice, each adjusted for geographic practice cost index (GPCI)	× Conversion factor (Conv. Fact.)	= National allowance

Table 7.2.   Calculation of nonfacility payment under resource-based relative value scale

Specific Example of RBRVS Allowance Calculation in 2005*				
CPT code = 99202 (Office visit, new patient, expanded problem-focused)				
Element	RVU	GPCI	Geographic Adjustment (RVU × GPCI**)	Adjusted Payment [Adjusted RVU × Conv. Fact. ($37.8975)]
Work value (WORK)	.88	1.00	.88	
Practice expense (PE)	.79	0.925	.73075	
Malpractice (MP)	.05	0.64	.032	
Sum			1.64275	
Adjusted allowance				$62.26

*Data source: Centers for Medicare and Medicaid Services. 2004 (September 16). Medicare Physician Fee Schedule. Available online from www.cms.hhs.gov/physicians/mpfsapp/step0.asp).

**North Carolina payment locality (0553500).

Table 7.3.   Impact of coding on nonfacility reimbursement under resource-based relative value scale

Comparison of Nonfacility Payment Based on Coding (2005)*						
	CPT 43200, Esophagoscopy			CPT 43217, Esophagoscopy, with removal of tumor(s), polyp(s), or other lesion(s) by snare technique		
	RVU ×	GPCI**	=	RVU ×	GPCI**	=
Work value (WORK)	1.59	1.000	1.59	2.9	1.000	2.9
Practice expense (PE)	4.13	0.925	3.82025	6.95	0.925	6.42875
Malpractice (MP)	0.13	0.64	.0832	0.26	0.64	0.1664
Sum			5.49345			9.49515
× Conversion factor			$37.8975			$37.8975
Total			$208.19			$359.84
Loss due to incomplete coding			$121.65			

*Data source: CMS. 2004 (September 16). Medicare physician fee schedule. Available online from www.cms.hhs.gov/physicians/mpfsapp/step0.asp.

**North Carolina payment locality (0553500).

Table 7.4.   Effect of code selection on nonfacility revenue under resource-based relative value scale*

Examples of Lost Nonfacility Revenue** from Poor Coding or Inadequate Documentation						
Careless Coding or Incomplete Documentation			Accurate Coding with Complete Documentation			Lost Payment
Code	Description	$	Code	Description	$	
10060	Incision and drainage of abscess; simple or single	$89.67	10061	Incision and drainage of abscess; complicated or multiple	$161.06	$152.39
11400	Excision benign lesion; excised diameter 0.5 cm or less	$103.67	11406	Excision benign lesion; excised diameter over 4.0 cm	$219.63	$115.96
19100	Biopsy of breast; percutaneous, needle core, not using imaging guidance	$124.93	19101	Biopsy of breast; open, incisional	$287.48	$162.55
45378	Colonoscopy	$362.36	45382	Colonoscopy with control of bleeding	$574.14	$211.78

*Data source: CMS. 2004 (September 16). Medicare physician fee schedule. Available online from www.cms.hhs.gov/physicians/mpfsapp/step0.asp.
**North Carolina payment locality (0553500).

Table 7.5.   Comparison of sample Medicare fees by code: Nonfacility versus facility

2005 Medicare Allowables* for Selected Codes			
Code	Description	Nonfacility Fee**	Facility Fee**
99202	Office/outpatient visit, new patient	$62.26	$45.43
99211	Office/outpatient visit, established patient	20.36	8.79
99213	Office/outpatient visit, established patient	50.13	34.53
99243	Office consultation	117.06	90.42
33533	Coronary artery bypass, using arterial graft; single	NA	1817.44
43239	Upper gastrointestinal endoscopy, biopsy	314.27	155.28
66984	Extracapsular cataract removal with insertion of intraocular lens prosthesis (one stage procedure)	NA	657.23
71020	Chest x-ray	33.74	NA
93000	Electrocardiogram, routine ECG with at last 12 leads; with interpretation and report	25.05	NA

*Data source: CMS. 2004 (September 16). Medicare physician fee schedule. Available online from www.cms.hhs.gov/physicians/mpfsapp/step0.asp.
**North Carolina payment locality (0553500).

Suppliers were those ambulance service entities not associated with any medical facility. They were reimbursed on a reasonable charge payment mechanism. The supplier could choose to report ambulance services one of four ways, as described in table 7.6. Services, mileage, and supplies were reported with HCPCS Level II ambulance codes (A0030–A0999, excluding A0888), HCPCS Level I codes 93005 and 93041, and other applicable HCPCS Level II Codes (A0000–Z9999). Suppliers reported a charge with each service, mileage, or supply code selected for that case. Payment for services was based on the lowest of the customary, prevailing, actual, or inflation index charge.

Development of the Ambulance Fee Schedule

The Balanced Budget Act of 1997 (BBA) added a new section, 1834(l), to the Act. The section required the creation of a fee schedule to establish prospective payment rates for ambulance services. The fee schedule was to be devised through negotiated rulemaking, as delineated in the Negotiated Rulemaking Act of 1990. The Negotiated Rulemaking Committee on Medicare Ambulance Services Fee Schedule (the Committee) was instructed to:

- Control Medicare expenditures for ambulance services through a prospective payment system

- Establish service definitions to link payment to the type of service

- Consider regional and operational differences in setting payment rates

- Consider inflation in setting payment rates

- Construct a phase-in period for the implementation of the fee schedule

- Require ambulance providers and suppliers to accept Medicare assignment

- Reimburse providers and suppliers at the lower of the fee schedule amount or billed charges (DHHS 2002, 9103)

During the first year of the fee schedule, payment for services could be no more than payments under the current (reasonable cost/charge) system. Additionally, BBA established the paramedic intercept service type (discussed here under levels of service). The BBA set an implementation date of January 1, 2000, for the ambulance fee schedule and paramedic intercept services.

As with most Medicare payment systems, additional legislation influenced and modified the ambulance fee schedule. The Balanced Budget Refinement Act of 1999 (BBRA) and the Benefits Improvement and Protection Act of 2000 (BIPA) were enacted to provide protections in the Medicare and Medicaid programs and the State Child Health Insurance Program (SCHIP). The BBRA modified the definition of *rural* for the paramedic intercept service type. The BIPA excluded **critical access hospitals (CAHs)** from the fee schedule payment methodology when the CAH is the only supplier or provider of ambulance services within a 35-mile drive. This modification called for the creation of an application process for this exemption. A qualifying CAH would be reimbursed on a reasonable cost basis. BIPA added a provision to increase payment rates for rural ambulance mileage. The proviso called for at least one-half

Table 7.6.   Reporting methods for ambulance suppliers

Method	Reporting Requirements
1	A single, all-inclusive charge reflecting all services, supplies, and mileage
2	One charge reflecting all services and supplies (base rate) with a separate charge for mileage
3	One charge for all services and mileage, with a separate charge for supplies
4	Separate charges for services, mileage, and supplies

additional payment per mile for the first seventeen miles of a rural trip and specified that an add-on percent be considered for miles seventeen through fifty. Additionally, BIPA modified the inflation factor for services provided from July 1, 2001, through December 31, 2001. The inflation factor was increased by two percentage points and set at 4.7 percent. Lastly, BIPA eliminated the blended payment rate for mileage phase-in provision for suppliers. This elimination applied to any **carrier** in a state in which the carrier's payment to all suppliers did not include a separate payment for all in-county ambulance mileage prior to the fee schedule implementation (DHHS 2002, 9104).

Implementation of the Ambulance Fee Schedule

The effective date for the ambulance fee schedule was January 1, 2000. However, due to other CMS obligations, specifically the hospital outpatient prospective payment system, preparation for year 2000 (Y2K), and the large scope of this project, CMS delayed the implementation until April 1, 2002. Implementation methodology for the ambulance fee schedule includes a five-year phase-in plan for payment. Table 7.7 displays the implementation schedule.

Reimbursement for Ambulance Services

Reimbursement for ambulance services is based on the level of service provided to the beneficiary. The fee schedule consists of seven levels of service as defined in table 7.8. Each level specifies the EMT skill set necessary to provide services and care. The EMT skill sets are based on the National Emergency Medical Services Education and Practice Blueprint. (See table 7.9.)

Nonemergency Transport

Medical necessity must be established for nonemergency transport provided to Medicare beneficiaries. There are two categories of nonemergency

Table 7.7.   Ambulance fee schedule phase-in plan

Year	Former payment	Fee schedule
Year one (4/2002–12/2002)	80%	20%
Year two (CY 2003)	60%	40%
Year three (CY 2004)	40%	60%
Year four (CY 2005)	20%	80%
Year five (CY 2006)	0%	100%

Source: Department of Health and Human Services. 2004 (February 27). *Federal Register.* 67 (39): 9106.

transport: repetitive and nonrepetitive. For repetitive nonemergency transports, the ambulance provider or supplier may attain physician certification in advance for the transportation service. The certification should be obtained no earlier than sixty days prior to transport.

For reimbursement of nonrepetitive nonemergency transports, the ambulance provider or supplier must provide physician certification within 21 days after the service was provided. The physician certification is ideally collected from the attending physician. However, the certification may be provided by a physician assistant, nurse practitioner, clinical nurse specialist, registered nurse, or discharge planner who is employed by the facility, hospital, or physician. The service provider should have personal knowledge of the beneficiary's case. If the certification cannot be obtained from the physician or other service provider, the ambulance supplier or provider may submit a claim with documentation (that is, a signed return receipt from the U.S. Postal Service or similar delivery service) that shows all the attempts by the ambulance service to obtain certification (DHHS 2002, 9111).

Immediate Response Payment

Additional payment is made to ambulance providers and suppliers who furnish immediate response services in emergency situations. An *emergency*

Table 7.8.   Levels of ambulance services

Service	Acronym	Description
Basic Life Support	BLS	Service level of an Emergency Medical Technician (EMT)-Basic, including the establishment of a peripheral intravenous line.
Advanced Life Support, Level 1	ALS1	In emergency cases, an assessment provided by an EMT-Intermediate or Paramedic (ALS crew) to determine patient needs and the furnishing of one or more ALS interventions. An ALS intervention is a procedure beyond the scope of an EMT-Basic.
Advanced Life Support, Level 2	ALS2	The administration of at least three different medications or the provision of one or more ALS procedures.
Specialty Care Transport	SCT	For critically injured or ill patient, the level of interhospital service furnished is beyond the scope of a paramedic. Ongoing care must be furnished by one or more health professionals in an appropriate specialty area.
Paramedic ALS Intercept	PI	ALS services furnished by an entity that does not provide the ambulance transport.
Fixed Wing Air Ambulance	FW	Destination is inaccessible by land vehicle or great distances or other obstacles (heavy traffic) and the patient's condition is not appropriate for BLS or ALS ground transportation.
Rotary Wing Air Ambulance	RW	Helicopter transport. Destination is inaccessible by land vehicle or great distances or other obstacles (heavy traffic) and the patient's condition is not appropriate for BLS or ALS ground transportation.

Source: Department of Health and Human Services. 2004 (February 27). *Federal Register.* 67 (39): 9106.

response involves responding immediately at the basic life support (BLS) or advanced life support level 1 (ALS-1) level of service to a 911 or 911-type call. *Immediate response* is one in which the ambulance supplier/provider begins as quickly as possible to take the steps necessary to respond to a call (DHHS 2002, 9108). The additional payment is provided to compensate those providers/suppliers the extra overhead expenses that are incurred to stay prepared at all times for emergency services. Ambulance suppliers and providers indicate that an emergency response service was provided by selecting the appropriate HCPCS Level II ambulance code. (See table 7.10 for examples.)

Payment Adjustment for Regional Variations

The ambulance fee schedule provides a payment adjustment to account for regional variations. Based on the point of beneficiary pick-up (as indi-cated by zip code), a geographic adjustment factor is applied. The adjustment factor used for this payment system is equal to the practice expense portion of the geographic practice cost index (GPCI) established and maintained for the Medicare physician fee schedule. For ground transport services, 70 percent of the payment rate is adjusted by the GPCI. For air ambulance services, 50 percent of the payment rate is adjusted by the GPCI. Payments for mileage are not adjusted.

Rural Area Service Adjustment

A **rural area** service adjustment is made to the ambulance provider/supplier when the location at which the patient is picked up is a rural area. For purposes of this provision, a rural area is an area outside of a **core-based statistical area (CBSA)** (formerly known as a **metropolitan statistical area [MSA]**) or an area that is identified as rural

Table 7.9.   National Emergency Medical Services (EMS) education and practice blueprint

EMS Provider	Skill Set
First Responder Level	Personnel use a limited amount of equipment to perform initial assessments and interventions.
EMT-Basic	Has the knowledge and skill of the First Responder, but is also qualified to function as the minimum staff for an ambulance.
EMT-Intermediate	Knowledge and skills identified at the First Responder and EMT-Basic levels, but is also qualified to perform essential advanced techniques and to administer a limited number of medications.
EMT-Paramedic	In addition to having competencies of an EMT-Intermediate, has enhanced skills and can administer additional interventions and medications.

Source: Department of Health and Human Services. 2004 (February 27). *Federal Register.* 67 (39): 9106.

Table 7.10.   Sample of emergency response HCPCS Level II ambulance codes

HCPCS Code	Description
A0427	Ambulance service, ALS, emergency transport, specialized ALS services rendered, all inclusive (mileage and supplies)
A0429	Ambulance service, BLS, emergency transport, all inclusive (mileage and supplies)

(DHHS 2002, 9110). The patient pick-up location is established by reporting the zip code for that location. For ground transportation, a 50 percent add-on is applied to the mileage payment rate for the first seventeen loaded miles. A 25 percent add-on is applied to the mileage payment rate for miles eighteen through fifty. No adjustment is made to the base rate for the level of service provided. For air ambulance services, a 50 percent add-on is applied to the base rate and to all of the loaded mileage.

Multiple-Patient Transport

An ambulance supplier/provider may encounter a situation in which multiple patients must be transported (for example, in a traffic accident). In these situations, CMS prorates the payment rate for the ambulance service for each Medicare beneficiary. If two or more patients are transported, the payment rate for each Medicare beneficiary is 75 percent of the base rate for the level of service provided. If three or more patients are transported, the payment rate for each Medicare beneficiary equals 60 percent of the base rate for the level of service provided. A single payment is made for the mileage (DHHS 2002, 9113). HCPCS Level II modifier GM, multiple patients on one ambulance trip, must be reported with the ambulance level of service code.

Transport of Deceased Patients

There are specific rules for transport cases in which a Medicare beneficiary is pronounced dead. When a beneficiary is pronounced dead by an individual who is licensed to pronounce death in that state, the following rules apply:

- When a patient is pronounced dead prior to the ambulance being called, no payment is made to the ambulance supplier/provider.

- When a patient is pronounced dead after the ambulance has been called but prior to the ambulance arrival, a BLS base rate (for ground transport) or air ambulance base rate payment will be paid. Mileage will not be reimbursed.

- When a patient is pronounced dead during the ambulance transport, payment rules are followed as if the patient were alive (DHHS 2002, 9113).

HCPCS Level II modifier QL, Patient pronounced dead after ambulance called, should be reported with the ambulance level of service code.

Use of HCPCS Level II Modifiers

Providers must report HCPCS level II modifiers for services provided to Medicare beneficiaries. An origin and destination modifier must be reported for each ambulance trip. A two-character alpha code is designated for each line item on the claim. The first character of the modifier represents the origin of the trip. The second digit represents the destination of the trip. Table 7.11 provides a listing of the alpha characters. Additionally, a modifier must be reported to indicate whether the service was provided under arrangement by a provider of services (QM) or if the service was furnished directly by a provider of services (QN). Figure 7.1 displays example line items from an ambulance claim with correct use of origin/destination modifiers and service modifiers.

Payment Steps

A seven step process is used to determine payment for ambulance services. The process take into consideration patient service level, modifiers, zip codes, miles, and add-on payments.

Step One: Identify the level of service code for the transportation provided. Determine whether the case

Table 7.11. Ambulance-specific modifiers

Modifier	Definition
D	Diagnostic or therapeutic site other than "P" or "H" when these are used as origin codes
E	Residential, domiciliary, custodial facility (other than an 1819 facility, SNF)
H	Hospital
I	Site of transfer (e.g. airport or helicopter pad) between modes of ambulance transport
J	Nonhospital based dialysis facility
N	Skilled nursing facility (1819 facility)
P	Physician's office (includes HMO nonhospital facility, clinic, etc.)
R	Residence
S	Scene of accident or acute event
X	Intermediate stop at physician's office en route to the hospital (includes HMO nonhospital facility, clinic, etc.) Destination code only

Source: Centers for Medicare and Medicaid Services. 2005 (January 21). *Revisions and Corrections to the Medicare Claims Processing Manual*, Chapter 6, Section 30 and Various Sections in Chapter 15. Pub 100-04 Medicare Claims Processing. CMS Transmittal 437.

Figure 7.1. Ambulance origin and destination modifier example

Record Type	Revenue Code	HCPCS Code	Modifier #1	Modifier #2	Date of Service	Units	Total Charges
61	0540	A0428	RH	QN	082701	1 (trip)	100.00
61	0540	A0380	RH	QN	082701	4 (mileage)	8.00

meets the emergency response criteria before selecting the final code.

Step Two: Determine whether multiple patients were transported. If so, append modifier GM to the level of service code. Payment levels are adjusted to the prorated amounts: 75 percent per patient for two patients and 60 percent per patient for three or more patients.

Step Three: Determine whether the Medicare beneficiary was pronounced dead after the ambulance service was called. If so, append modifier QL to the level of service code. Payment levels are adjusted as outlined by this provision.

Step Four: Apply the regional variation adjustment. Identify the zip code for the location at which the patient was placed on the ambulance. Seventy percent of the service payment rate is adjusted for ground transportation and 50 percent of the service payment rate is adjusted for air ambulance.

Step Five: Identify the mileage code and number of miles for the transportation provided.

Step Six: Apply the rural area payment add-on. Determine whether the patient pick-up location is a rural area based on the CBSA methodology. If the area is rural, then add an additional 50 percent to miles one through seventeen and an additional 25 percent to miles eighteen through fifty for ground transportation. For air ambulance, add an additional 50 percent to the entire mileage for the trip.

Step Seven: Add together the level of service payment and the mileage payment to determine the total reimbursement for the ambulance service provided.

Expected Adjustments to the System

The move to prospective payment has been challenging for ambulance suppliers and providers. CMS states that it is dedicated to making necessary adjustments to the system as new claims data are analyzed. For example, many providers and suppliers have called for the use of medical condition lists to aid in determining the level of service required to transport patients. The proposed medical condition lists are broad in topic and do not use the mandated ICD-9-CM coding system as required by the Health Insurance Portability and Accountability Act of 1996 (HIPAA). Therefore, CMS, suppliers, and providers are researching alternatives to assist with the creation of these lists. Once fully implemented in 2006, Medicare expects the system to control ambulance costs while continuing to provide the ambulance benefit to its beneficiaries.

Ambulatory Surgical Center Prospective Payment System

Designated surgical services may be provided to Medicare beneficiaries in the outpatient setting at **ambulatory surgical centers (ASCs)** under the Medicare supplementary medical insurance program (Part B). In an effort to control healthcare costs, CMS introduced a prospective payment system for ambulatory surgery centers in 1982. Section 934 of the Omnibus Budget Reconciliation Act of 1980 amended sections 1832(a)(2) and 1833 of the Social Security Act (the Act) to specify procedures that would be covered under the prospective payment system, called the ASC List of Covered Procedures **(ASC list).**

Medicare Certification Standards

ASCs that choose to treat Medicare beneficiaries must be state-licensed and Medicare-certified and are considered a supplier of services rather than a provider. In order to qualify as a Medicare-certified ASC, several standards must be met. The surgical center must (Jones 2001, 13):

- Be a separate entity distinguishable from any other entity or type of facility

- Have its own national identifier or supplier number under Medicare

- Maintain its own licensure, accreditation, governance, professional supervision, administrative functions, clinical services, record keeping, and financial and accounting systems

- Have a sole purpose of delivering services in connection with surgical procedures that do not require inpatient hospitalization

- Meet all conditions and requirements set forth in Section 1832(a)(2)(F)(i) of the Act, in 42 CFR 416.25 and in 42 CFR 416, subpart C in the *Federal Register*

Payment for ASC Services

As a Medicare-certified ASC, the facility must accept Medicare reimbursement as payment in full for the services supplied to Medicare beneficiaries. Medicare payment equals 80 percent of the total reimbursement for services provided. Beneficiaries are responsible for the 20 percent copayment of the total payment and any deductible that is required.

Payment for the procedures included on the ASC list is intended to reimburse ASCs for the facility resources extended to provide surgical services in that locality. The costs of the physician's professional services are excluded from the ASC payment. Professional services must be separately reported and are reimbursed via the Medicare physician fee schedule. The ASC prospective payment is based on an overhead amount. CMS established the overhead amount by estimating a fair fee for the cost of providing specific services in the ASC setting. The overhead amount was calculated using sample survey data in combination with other, similar techniques that take into account volume of services (DHHS 2004c, 69178–69179). The payment rate is wage index-adjusted to account for regional differences among providers. The urban and rural wage index tables are used from the applicable year.

Criteria for ASC Procedures

By creating a list of applicable outpatient surgery procedures, CMS was able to influence the site of service for certain procedures. The ASC list created a motivation for surgical procedures to migrate from the more expensive inpatient setting to the less expensive outpatient surgery setting without creating a motivation to shift procedures from the less expensive physician office setting to the more expensive outpatient surgery setting (DHHS 2004c, 69179). The procedures and services included in the ASC list are reported using HCPCS codes. The ASC list criteria provided in 42 CFR 416.65(a) and (b) (DHHS 2004c, 69179) for procedures and services mandate that they:

- Be commonly performed in the inpatient setting but can be safely performed in an ASC

- Be limited to those requiring a dedicated OR or suite and generally requiring postoperative care

- Be limited to ones that have an OR time and local, regional, or general anesthesia with duration no greater than 90 minutes, and recovery room time no greater than four hours

- Include those not otherwise excluded from Medicare coverage

- Exclude ones that generally result in extensive blood loss, require major or prolonged invasion of body cavities, that directly involve major blood vessels, or that are generally emergency or life-threatening in nature

- Exclude those that are regularly and safely provided in the physician office setting

If an ASC performs a procedure not on the ASC list, it receives no reimbursement.

ASC List and Payment Rates

The ASC list is updated yearly to account for changes in the HCPCS coding system. Each year codes are added, deleted, and modified to account for changes in healthcare delivery practices. In addition to these changes, CMS implemented selection criteria in 1987 to assist with the ASC list maintenance. CMS used quantitative criteria to identify procedures to be added and deleted from the ASC list. If a procedure was performed on an inpatient basis 20 percent of the time or less, it would be excluded from the ASC list. Likewise, if a procedure was performed in a physician's office 50 percent of the time or more, it would be excluded from the ASC list. Applying these criteria resulted in the first major revision of the ASC list in 1987. (See table 7.12)

As the healthcare environment became ever more cost conscious, a growing number of procedure types were shifted from the inpatient setting to the outpatient setting. This trend created the need for a major revision to the ASC list. In 1995, CMS adopted a modified standard for ASC list maintenance that allowed for minor fluctuations in utilization across settings and account for site-

Table 7.12.   Release dates of the ASC List of Covered Procedures

Date	Reference	Action
August 5, 1982	47 FR 34082	Creation
April 21, 1987	52 FR 13176	Revision
June 1, 1989	54 FR 23540	Revision
December 31, 1991	56 FR 67666	Revision
January 26, 1995	60 FR 5185	Revision
March 28, 2003	68 FR 15268	Revision
November 26, 2004	69 FR 69178	Revision, proposed rule

Source: Department of Health and Human Services. 2004 (November 26). *Federal Register.* 69 (227): 69179.

of-service errors from the National Claims History File that was used to determine qualification for the list. Procedures that had a combined inpatient, outpatient, and ASC volume of less than 46 percent of the total procedure volume and were either performed 50 percent of the time or more in the physician office setting or 10 percent or less in the hospital inpatient setting would be deleted from the ASC list (DHHS 2004c, 69180). CMS retained the 20 percent inpatient/50 percent physician office criteria for additions to the ASC list.

Attempt to Implement Ambulatory Payment Classifications

In 1997, the Balanced Budget Act (BBA) proposed a new prospective payment system (PPS) for hospital outpatient services based on **ambulatory payment classifications (APCs).** Included in the BBA was the requirement that a new rate-setting methodology, APCs, be used for the ASC PPS. The new payment rates would be calculated using 1994 ASC survey data.

Several pieces of legislation modified the hospital outpatient prospective payment system (HOPPS) and the requirement for the transition to APCs for ASCs. The Balanced Budget Refinement Act of 1999 (BBRA) required that a three-year phase-in period be used for the implementation of the new APC system for ASCs. However, one year later, the Medicare, Medicaid and SCHIP Benefits Improvement and Protection Act of 2000 (BIPA) delayed the implementation of APCs for ASCs to January 1, 2002, or after and extended the phase-in period established by the BBRA to four years. Additionally, BIPA required that the payment rates for the ASC list be rebased with ASC survey data from 1999 or later by January 1, 2003. (DHHS 2003, 15270).

Implementation of the APC system for ASCs and the rebasing of payment rates for the ASC list did not occur. CMS was not able to focus on the ASC setting because the majority of the resources available were dedicated to the implementation of HOPPS. Further, preparation for Y2K changes tied up even more CMS resources.

Attempts to Resolve Rate-Setting Issues

In January of 2003, the Office of the Inspector General (OIG) issued results of the "Payments for Procedures in Outpatient Departments and Ambulatory Surgical Centers" study. The results showed that there was a need for greater similarity in payment rates between the hospital outpatient and ASC settings (DHHS 2004c, 69180). The study revealed that disparity in payments for the same services performed in the ASC setting versus the hospital outpatient setting resulted in additional costs of $1.1 billion to the Medicare system. The differences in reimbursement were not consistent. In 66 percent of the procedure codes examined, outpatient department rates were higher than ASC rates, with a median difference of $282.33. For the remaining 145 procedure codes, Medicare reimbursed ASCs more (DHHS 2003, 15270).

The OIG provided recommended that CMS should:

- Seek authority to set rates that are consistent across sites and reflect only the costs necessary for the efficient delivery of health services

- Conduct and use timely ASC survey data to reevaluate ASC payment rates

- Remove procedure codes that met deletion criteria (72 CPT codes were identified as meeting criteria for deletion)

CMS responded to the study in the March 28, 2003, ASC List of Covered Procedures Update Final Rule. CMS stated that it would consider assisting in the development of future legislation but expressed concerns with using survey data for rate setting. CMS administrators specifically responded that they wanted to be confident that the methodology

used to rebase the payment rates would not inadvertently result in disproportional reimbursement rates across the different ambulatory care sites of service (DHHS 2003, 15270). CMS administrators indicated that they would continue study alternatives for rate setting methodologies.

The Medicare Prescription Drug, Improvement and Modernization Act of 2003 (MMA) repealed the survey requirement or the need to collect updated ASC cost data to utilize for rebasing ASC payment rates set forth in BIPA. More importantly, MMA requires CMS to implement a revised prospective payment system for ASC services between January 1, 2006, and January 1, 2008. Therefore, updates to the current system that take place before the implementation of the new system will be based on the 1986 survey of ASC costs.

On November 26, 2004, CMS released a proposed rule for the Update of Ambulatory Surgical Center List of Covered Procedures. In the proposed rule, payment rates were updated for inflation. Several procedures were removed from the ASC list prompted by the 2003 OIG report and basic code updates were made based on the annual changes to the HCPCS Level I coding system. (DHHS 2004d, 69178).

Payment Groups

Reimbursement for the procedures included in the ASC list is distributed among nine **ambulatory surgery center payment groups.** The payment groups are not based on the patient severity of illness or medical condition; there is no clinical consistency within a group. A procedure is placed in a group based on the HCPCS code. Groups are formed for HCPCS codes that have similar average costs. The average costs for performing procedures were derived from the 1986 survey of ASC costs, updated for inflation. Originally in 1990, there were eight payment groups; however, in 1991 a ninth group was added to house extracorporeal shockwave lithotripsy (DHHS 2004c,

69180). Table 7.13 provides a listing of the groups and their proposed 2005 payment rates.

Multiple and Bilateral Procedures

When multiple procedures are performed during the same surgical session, a payment reduction is applied. The procedure in the highest level group is reimbursed at 100 percent and all remaining procedures are reimbursed at 50 percent. Bilateral procedures are reimbursed at 150 percent of the payment rate for their group.

Payment Steps

Coding and billing personnel follow five steps in obtaining payment for the ASC facility:

1. The procedure or service is coded using the HCPCS coding system.

2. The ASC Group (one through nine) is identified based on the HCPCS code reported.

Table 7.13.   ASC payment groups and proposed rates

Group	Payment Rate
Group 1	$333
Group 2	$446
Group 3	$510
Group 4	$630
Group 5	$717
Group 6	$826
Group 7	$995
Group 8	$973
Group 9	$1,339

Source: Department of Health and Human Services. 2004 (November 26). *Federal Register.* 69 (227): 69179.

3. Multiple procedure and bilateral procedure provisions are applied when applicable.

4. The payment for the established group is wage indexed.

5. Payment is made to the ASC facility.

New Payment System in 2006–2008

As mentioned earlier, even though the services provided in an ASC are currently reimbursed on a prospective basis, MMA has instructed CMS to implement a new payment system. CMS will be evaluating whether or not the current weighting and grouping system is adequate to reimburse facilities for specific types of procedures. Additionally CMS will determine whether there is a need to adjust payments for geographical differences, and if so, at what percentage the labor and nonlabor portions would be set (CMS 2005). Lastly, the new system will most likely strive to bring parity to outpatient payments across the varying service locations. The new system will be unveiled and implemented between 2006 and 2008.

Check Your Understanding 7.1

1. Claims for RBRVS physician payments are prepared by coding _____ that have associated RVUs.

2. What are the three elements of the RVU?

3. What are the bases for the seven levels of service used in the ambulance services fee schedule?

4. Medicare-certified ASCs may share record keeping and financial and accounting systems with hospitals in the same parent corporation. True or false?

5. CMS created a motivation for surgical procedures to migrate from the more expensive inpatient setting to the less expensive outpatient surgery setting without creating a motivation to shift procedures from the less expensive physician office setting to the more expensive outpatient surgery setting by creating _____.

Hospital Outpatient Prospective Payment System

In 1983, Medicare moved to a PPS for hospital inpatient services to help control increasing healthcare costs and Medicare expenditures. As CMS experienced savings by reducing Medicare expenditures for inpatient care by $17 billion per year from the payment system change, the program's administrators made efforts to incorporate prospective payment concepts into other healthcare settings (Averill 2001, 108). After more than thirteen years, CMS implemented a hospital outpatient prospective payment system (HOPPS) on August 1, 2000.

Legislative Influence and Background

The Omnibus Reconciliation Act (OBRA) of 1986 mandated that CMS move to a prospective payment system for hospital outpatient services. Congress instructed the Secretary of Health and Human Services (DHHS) to include facility costs for services provided in ambulatory surgery units, emergency departments, and hospital clinics in the system. Professional services, such as physician fees, were not intended to be included in the hospital outpatient PPS. The legislation prescribed that the system was to be based on the HCPCS levels I and II because that was the prevailing coding system in the outpatient setting. OBRA gave CMS five years to develop the system and projected implementation for 1991.

3M Information Systems

A grant was awarded to 3M Health Information Systems (3M HIS) in 1988 to develop a grouping system for the outpatient prospective payment system. In 1990, 3M HIS proposed version 1.0 ambulatory patient groups (APGs). The APG system is a visit-based classification that describes the amount and type of resources consumed during the visit. A *visit* is an encounter between a patient and any healthcare provider (Jones 2001, 64). In 1995, 3M HIS released an updated version of APG Version 2.0. Even though the 1991 deadline had come and gone, CMS had yet to implement APGs as the outpatient PPS for Medicare. However, many states were using APGs for Medicaid reimbursement.

1997 Balanced Budget Act

In 1997, the Balanced Budget Act (BBA) set new dates for Medicare to move to a prospective payment system. The implementation deadline for hospitals was January 1, 1999, and for IPPS exempt cancer centers was one year later. In September of 1998, CMS released the proposed rule for the outpatient prospective payment system. The grouping system introduced in the proposed rule was ambulatory payment classifications (APCs). APCs were developed by modifying the APG system (created by 3M HIS) using past claims data and clinical analysis.

1998 Balanced Budget Refinement Act

Prior to the implementation of the APC system proposed in 1998, the Balanced Budget Refinement Act (BBRA) of 1999 required several modifications to the system. The BBRA mandated that an annual review of groups, weights, and wage index adjustments should be made, similar to the review used in the inpatient prospective payment system (IPPS). CMS was instructed to develop a professional advisory panel to assist with maintenance of the system. The BBRA determined that the beneficiary coinsurance for any given procedure/service could not exceed the inpatient deductible for that year. Consequently, the **pass-through** APC category was developed for high-cost drugs, biologicals, and devices, and a high-cost outlier provision was added to the system. The BBRA also provided a phase-in financial assistance mechanism to facilitate hospitals' adjustment to the prospective payment system.

Implementation and Modification of the HOPPS

In April 2000, CMS released the final rule for APC implementation. The implementation date was set for August 1, 2000. Facilities worked feverishly to make system changes and provide education to prepare for APC changes. On August 1, 2000, CMS ended the cost-based reimbursement system and started HOPPS.

Shortly after the HOPPS system was implemented, the Medicare, Medicaid, and SCHIP Benefits Improvement Act (BIPA) of 2000 added supplementary modifications to the APC system. BIPA accelerated the reduction of beneficiary copayment amounts. The legislation granted children's hospitals **hold-harmless status,** and developed device categories for pass-through APCs.

The Medicare Prescription Drug, Improvement, and Modernization Act (MMA) of 2003 further modified the HOPPS system. MMA now allows payment for an initial preventive physical examination for beneficiaries whose coverage began after January 1, 2005. MMA changed the screening and diagnostic mammography payment from HOPPS to a fee schedule-based payment. MMA added radiopharmaceuticals to the drug and biological categories and reduced the threshold for establishment of separate APCs with respect to drugs and biologicals from $150 to $50 per administration. The high-cost outlier calculation was modified to exclude several separately payable drugs. Additionally, the legislation modified payment for brachytherapy devices (seeds) by instructing that these devices be paid on a reasonable cost basis from January 1, 2004, through January 1, 2007. Cost for brachytherapy seeds is calculated by adjusted hospital charges for each device to cost via ratio of cost to charge. Brachytherapy devices are also excluded from outlier calculations.

Hospital Outpatient Prospective Payment Methodology

Prior to HOPPS, Medicare payment for hospital outpatient services was cost-based. The cost of services was calculated by converting total charges for each encounter to cost by using department specific cost-to-charge ratios (CCRs) developed from cost report statistics. However, as healthcare costs continued to rise, CMS moved toward a prospective payment system to help encourage a more efficient delivery of care for outpatient beneficiaries (DHHS 2004a, 50450).

Reimbursement for Hospital Outpatient Services

CMS uses a variety of models to reimburse facilities for hospital outpatient services. The system uses two reimbursement methods: fee schedules and a prospective payment system. The primary standard that distinguishes a prospective payment system from a fee schedule system is that in the PPS the costs for certain items and secondary services associated with a primary procedure are packaged into the payment for that procedure. A fee schedule system establishes a separate payment amount for each item or service and no packaging occurs (DHHS 2004a, 50505). Certain items and services, such as acquisition of corneal tissue and influenza and pneumococcal pneumonia vaccines, continue to be paid on a reasonable cost basis.

Most procedures and services are reimbursed under APCs. Ambulance transportation, physical therapy, occupational therapy, and speech language pathology are reimbursed via various fee schedules. Physician and nonphysician practitioners are paid under the Medicare physician fee schedule. Laboratory services are paid via the clinical diagnostic laboratory fee schedule. End-stage renal disease services are reimbursed with a composite rate (DHHS 2004a, 50451).

Reporting of Services and Supplies under HOPPS

HOPPS uses Levels I and II HCPCS codes to report services/procedures performed and items/supplies provided for beneficiaries. Each code in HCPCS has been assigned a **payment status indicator.** The payment status indicator establishes how that service, procedure, or item is paid (that is, fee schedule, APC, reasonable cost, unpaid). Table 7.14 provides a listing of the payment status indicators and their definitions for **calendar year (CY)** 2005.

Table 7.14.   Payment status indicators for calendar year 2005

Payment Status Indicator	Reimbursement Method	Procedure or Service Example
A	Fee schedule payment	Durable medical equipment, prosthetics, orthotics, and supplies (DMEPOS)
B	Not reimbursed under HOPPS	Service not appropriate for Part B claim
C	Not reimbursed under HOPPS	Inpatient only services
D	Not reimbursed under HOPPS	Code is discontinued
E	Not reimbursed under HOPPS	Service not covered by Medicare
F	Reasonable cost payment	Acquisition of corneal tissue and certain CRNA services
G	Pass-through payment	Drugs, biologicals, and radiopharmaceutical agent
H	Pass-through payment	Devices and brachytherapy sources
K	APC payment	Drugs, biologicals (including blood and blood products), and radiopharmaceutical agents
L	Reasonable cost payment with no copayment amount	Flu and pneumococcal immunizations
M (via Medicare Program Transmittal R508CP, change request number 3756, dated March 18, 2005)	Services not billable to the fiscal intermediary and not payable under OPPS	Pharmacy dispensing fee, chemo assessment of nausea, pain, fatigue, etc.
N	Not reimbursed under HOPPS	Packaged into APC payment
P	Only reimbursed in partial hospitalization programs	Partial hospitalization
S	APC payment	Significant procedures, multiple procedure reduction does not apply
T	APC payment	Surgical procedures, multiple procedure reduction applies
V	APC payment	Medical visits
X	APC payment	Ancillary services
Y	Not reimbursed under HOPPS	Nonimplantable durable medical equipment that must be billed directly to the DME regional carrier

Source: Department of Health and Human Services. 2004 (August 16). *Federal Register.* 69 (157): 50531.

Because Level I HCPCS codes (CPT codes) were originally designed to report physician services, the system contains codes for inpatient and outpatient procedures. HOPPS only covers outpatient services. Each year the Secretary of Health and Human Services reviews claims data and determines which procedures are inpatient-only procedures and creates the "inpatient-only list" (payment status indicator C). In order to move off of the inpatient-only list, a procedure must be performed in noninpatient settings at least 60 percent of the time. Procedures indicated as inpatient-only must be provided to Medicare beneficiaries in an inpatient setting and are reimbursed under the IPPS.

Excluded Facilities

Excluded from HOPPS are Maryland hospital services that are part of a cost containment waiver, critical access hospitals (CAH), hospitals outside of the fifty states, District of Columbia, and Puerto Rico, and the Indian Health Service.

Maintenance of the HOPPS System

CMS maintains the HOPPS system. As mandated by the BBRA, CMS must perform an annual review of the APC groups and relative weights. The wage index amounts adjusted for the current IPPS system must also be incorporated into the HOPPS system each year.

BBRA also established the APC Advisory Panel to assist with the maintenance of HOPPS. The APC Advisory Panel is composed of fifteen experts from various healthcare settings. The panel is technical in nature and provides analysis and recommendations to CMS. CMS considers and addresses all panel recommendations, but does not have to accept them. CMS makes the final ruling for updates and changes to HOPPS. The panel has three subcommittees that focus on data issues, observation issues, and packaging issues.

Additionally, the Medicare Payment Advisory Commission (MedPAC) provides Congress and CMS with recommendations to improve HOPPS. Again, CMS considers and responds to all MedPAC recommendations, but does not have to accept or implement them. CMS has the final ruling for updates and changes to HOPPS. Revisions to HOPPS are released in the *Federal Register* within forty-five days of the start of the calendar year.

Ambulatory Payment Classification System

Each APC group comprises procedures or services that are clinically comparable with respect to resource use. All procedures and/or services assigned to an APC group must meet the "two-times rule," which establishes that the median cost of the most expensive item or service within a group cannot be more than two times greater than the median cost of the least expensive item or service within the same group (DHHS 2004a, 50454). CMS can propose exceptions to the two-times rule based on the following criteria (DHHS 2004a, 50463):

- Resource homogeneity
- Clinical homogeneity
- Hospital concentration
- Frequency of service (volume)
- Opportunity for upcoding and code fragments

Violations of the two-times rule are reviewed by the APC Advisory Panel. After analysis of each situation, the panel makes recommendations for each group that violated the rule. CMS uses the recommendations proposed by the panel and makes the final determination. For CY 2005, fifty-four APC groups violated the two-times rule.

Partially Packaged System Methodology

Packaging and **bundling** are a means to combine, into one lump sum payment, the costs of **ancillary services,** supplies, and pharmaceuticals with their associated major procedures or services (payment status indicator N). The logic of groupers in the ambulatory payment classification system includes ancillary packaging and bundling. Packaging and bundling give providers incentives to improve their efficiency by avoiding unnecessary ancillary services, supplies, and pharmaceuticals and by substituting less expensive, but equally effective, options.

In ancillary packaging, many ancillary service APC groups will automatically combine into a significant procedure APC group or a surgical service APC group, if one is present.

Example:

For a visit with an x-ray (APC group 0351) and fracture treatment (APC group 0059), payment is only made for APC group 0059.

Bundling combines supply and pharmaceutical costs or medical visits with associated procedures or services. APC systems have two methods of bundling:

- Supply and pharmaceutical cost bundling

- Medical visit bundling

Supply and pharmaceutical cost bundling involves supplies and drugs, except some expensive chemotherapy drugs. Medical visits may also be bundled in some situations. For example, if a simple laceration repair occurs during an encounter that also includes extensive medical and diagnostic services, the medical visit would be bundled into the laceration repair.

The APC system uses a partially packaged system methodology. Services or items, such as recovery room, anesthesia, and some pharmaceuticals, are packaged into the APC payment for the service or procedure with which they are associated. Bundled services that are reported with a HCPCS code have the payment status indicator N. Some services and items have not been assigned a HCPCS code and therefore are reported by revenue code. Table 7.15 provides a list of services that

are bundled into APC payment by revenue code. Although some services are packaged, many others are not. Ancillary services, such as x-rays, and MRI and minor procedures, such as injections, are not packaged, but rather paid separately via APC groups. For the inpatient setting, it is easier to predict which resources a patient will consume for a given clinical issue. However, in the outpatient setting treatment pathways greatly vary from patient to patient, making it much more difficult to determine the resources that will be consumed for a clinical issue. Consequently, average cost for a "typical" outpatient encounter cannot be accurately forecasted. Therefore, a partially packaged system provides adequate reimbursement and allows the treatment flexibility that is needed to appropriately care for patients in the outpatient setting.

Observation Services

Diagnosis coding plays a limited role in APC group determination. The exceptions are **partial hospitalization** and **observation** cases, for which qualification is restricted. Originally, the APC system bundled cost for observation services into the APC payment with which the procedure or visit the observation was associated. However, the CY 2002 revision added APC 0339 to pay separately for certain observation services associated with clinic visits, emergency department visits, or **critical care services.**

Three clinical conditions qualify an observation service for APC 0339: chest pain, congestive heart failure, and asthma. Several requirements must be met to bill appropriately for APC 0339 (DHHS 2004a, 50534):

- The correct ICD-9-CM diagnosis code for chest pain, congestive heart failure or asthma must be reported.

- An emergency department visit, clinic visit, or critical care service must be performed on the same day or day before the separately payable observation service.

Table 7.15.   Packaged services by revenue code

Revenue Code	Description	Revenue Code	Description
250	Pharmacy	390	Blood storage and processing
251	Generic pharmacy	399	Other blood storage and processing
252	Nongeneric pharmacy	560	Medical social services
254	Pharmacy incident to other diagnostic	569	Other medical social services
255	Pharmacy incident to radiology	621	Supplies incident to radiology
257	Nonprescription drugs	622	Supplies incident to other diagnostic
258	IV solutions	624	Investigational device (IDE)
259	Other pharmacy	630	Drugs requiring specific identification, general class
260	IV therapy, general class	631	Single source drugs
262	IV therapy/pharmacy services	632	Multiple source drugs
263	Supply/delivery	633	Restrictive prescription
264	IV therapy/supplies	637	Self-administered drug (insulin admin in emergency diabetic coma)
269	Other IV therapy	681	Trauma response, level I
270	M&S supplies	682	Trauma response, level II
271	Nonsterile supplies	683	Trauma response, level III
272	Sterile supplies	684	Trauma response, level IV
274	Prosthetic/orthotic devices	689	Trauma response, other
275	Pacemaker drug	700	Cast room
276	Intraocular lens source drug	709	Other cast room
278	Other implants	710	Recovery room
279	Other M&S supplies	719	Other recovery room
280	Oncology	720	Labor room
289	Other oncology	721	Labor
290	Durable medical equipment	762	Observation room
370	Anesthesia	810	Organ acquisition
371	Anesthesia incident to radiology	819	Other organ acquisition
372	Anesthesia incident to other diagnostic	942	Education/training

Source: Department of Health and Human Services. 2004a (August 16). *Federal Register.* 69 (157): 50488–50489.

- Direct admissions to observation must be reported with code G0263.

- HCPCS code G0244 (observation) must be billed for a minimum of eight hours.

- No procedures with a payment status indicator of T, except infusion therapy (other than chemotherapy drug), can be reported on the same day or day before the observation care is provided.

- Observation time must be recorded in the medical record. Observation time begins at admission and ends at discharge.

- The beneficiary must be under physician care during observation. Entries must be made and authenticated in the medical record by the managing physician(s).

- Medical record documentation must show that the physician assessed the patient risk and determined that the patient would benefit from observation care.

An observation associated with surgical procedures (payment status indicator T) is not separately reimbursed under APCs.

Partial Hospitalization

Partial hospitalization is an intensive outpatient program of psychiatric services provided to patients as an alternative to inpatient psychiatric care for patients who have an acute mental illness (DHHS 2004a, 50543). Partial hospitalization may be provided by hospital outpatient departments and Medicare-certified community mental health centers (CMHCs). Patients who receive psychiatric services and have a diagnosis of an acute mental health disorder are grouped to APC 0033, Partial hospitalization. The unit of service for partial hospitalization is one day. Therefore, the APC payment for APC 0033 is based on a per-diem amount. For CY 2005, the APC payment rate for APC 0033 is $281.33, of which $56.27 is the beneficiary copayment amount.

Structure of the APC System

In the APC system there are six classification types that represent the various services procedures and supplies used in the hospital outpatient setting. The classification type for any APC can be identified by the payment status indicator assigned to the procedures and/or services in the group. All procedures or services in an APC have the same payment status indicator. The six classification types are:

- Medical (payment status indicator V)

- Surgical procedure (payment status indicator T)

- Significant procedure (payment status indicator S)

- Ancillary service (payment status indicator X)

- Drugs and biological (payment status indicator K)

- Pass-through drug, biological, and device (payment status indicators G and H)

Each HCPCS code is assigned to one and only one APC. The APC assignment for a procedure or service does not change based on the patient's medical condition or the severity of illness. There may be an unlimited number of APCs per encounter for a single patient. The number of APC assignments is based on the number of reimbursable procedures or services provided for that patient.

Each APC contains the same components that drive the APC assignment (see figure 7.2):

- Title

- Payment status indicator

- Relative weight

- **National unadjusted payment amount**

- **National unadjusted copayment amount**

- **Code range**

Figure 7.2.   APC components

APC 0610 Title: Low Level Emergency Visits	
Payment Status Indicator	V
Relative Weight	1.3544
National Unadjusted Payment Amount	$77.18
National Unadjusted Co-payment Amount	$19.57
Minimum Co-payment Amount	$15.44
HCPCS Procedure Code(s) 99281 Emergency Department Visit 99282 Emergency Department Visit	

The relative weight is a measure of the resource intensity of a particular procedure or service. The national unadjusted payment amount is the total amount a hospital will receive for a procedure or service in that APC. Hospital outpatient claims data from 1996 were used to determine the APC payment rates for implementation in 2000. The national unadjusted payment amount is divided into two components: Medicare facility amount and beneficiary copayment amount.

Copayment

CMS wanted to move to a prospective payment system to ensure that the beneficiary copayment amount from hospital to hospital is consistent. Prior to PPS, beneficiaries were responsible for 20 percent of total charges and charges for procedures varied from hospital to hospital. Therefore, if hospital A charged $3,000 for a colonoscopy, the beneficiary amount would be $600, but if hospital B charged $3500 for the same colonoscopy, the beneficiary would be responsible for $700.

Again using 1996 data, CMS established the historical average copayment amount as the starting copayment amount in the APC system. However, the intent of the HOPPS for all copayment amounts to be only 20 percent of the total APC payment amount. Section 1833(t)(8)(C)(ii) of the Social Security Act requires CMS to reduce the national unadjusted copayment amount to meet reduction requirements mandated in BIPA (DHHS 2004a, 50544). For CY 2005, the national unadjusted copayment amount cannot exceed 45 percent of the total APC payment. Any newly created APC (those added to the system after August 1, 2000) must be added with a copayment amount equal to 20 percent of the total APC payment. The copayment amount may be collected from the beneficiary at the time of service or on a retrospective basis.

Both the Medicare facility component and the beneficiary copayment components are adjusted for differences in wage indexes. This is the only adjustment made to APC payment rates to account for differences among hospitals. Sixty percent of the facility amount is wage index adjusted. The wage index amount for the facility location based on CBSA is determined in the IPPS update for the corresponding federal fiscal year.

New Technology APCs

New technology APCs were created to allow new procedures and services to enter HOPPS quickly, even though their complete cost and payment information is not known. New technology APCs house modern procedures and services until enough data is collected to properly place the new procedure in an existing APC or to create a new APC for the service/procedure. A procedure/ service can remain in a new technology APC for an indefinite amount of time.

The APC system contains seventy-four new technology APCs. Thirty-seven groups have payment status indicator S and are not subject to multiple procedure discounting. The remaining thirty-seven groups have payment status indicator T and are subject to the multiple-procedure discount provision. Placement into new technology APCs is based on cost bands. For example, APC 1501, New Technology–Level I, contains procedures whose average cost is $0–$50. The payment for the group is $25.

Provisions of the APC System

The APC system uses provisions to provide additional payments for high-cost items and unusual admissions that historically have added significant cost to patient care. Without the additional payments associated with these provisions, it may not be feasible for hospital outpatient facilities to provide all services to Medicare beneficiaries.

Discounting

Multiple surgical procedures with payment status indicator T performed during the same operative session are **discounted.** The highest weighted procedure is fully reimbursed. All other procedures with payment status indicator T are reimbursed at 50 percent. (See figure 7.3.) This reduction is made to account for resource saving that hospitals experience by performing multiple procedures together. For example, OR surgical instruments are only prepped once, anesthesia is administered once, and recovery room is used once for all of the procedures performed.

High-Cost Outlier

Established by the BBRA, this provision is intended to provide financial assistance for unusually high cost services. The equations for case qualification and additional payment levels are adjusted each year. Medicare limits the percentage of total payments that can be attributed to outlier payments to 2 percent. For CY 2005, two requirements must be met to be eligible for outlier payment. The cost for a service must exceed 1.75 times the APC payment. The cost must also exceed the APC payment plus a fixed dollar threshold of $1,175. If these two conditions are met, the outlier payment is 50 percent of the cost that exceeds 1.75 the APC payment. Most separately paid drugs, biologicals, radiopharmaceuticals, and brachytherapy sources (payment status indicator G) are excluded from the outlier calculation.

Pass-Through Payments

Pass-throughs are exceptions to the Medicare prospective payment systems. These exceptions exist for high-cost services. Pass-throughs are not included in the prospective payment systems and are "passed-through" to other payment mechanisms that attempt to adjust for the high cost of pass-throughs. Therefore, pass-throughs minimize the negative financial impact of combining all services into one lump-sum payment. Pass-throughs occur in both the inpatient prospective payment system and the HOPPS.

Pass-through payments were established by the BBRA to provide hospitals with additional payment for high-cost drugs, biologicals, and devices. This specification was added to ensure the use of new and innovative drugs and supplies for Medicare beneficiaries when medically appropriate. Such drugs and supplies are often costly. If cost exceeds the payment for a new and innovative drug, a hospital might be motivated through cost containment practices to use a less expensive and potentially less effective drug for Medicare beneficiaries.

Pass-through payments cannot exceed 2 percent of the total payments for the year. CMS uses historical claims data to project whether pass-through payments will exceed this limit. If so, CMS can put a pro rata reduction in place for that calendar year. The pro rata reduction decreases all pass-through payments by a selected percentage so that the total pass-through payments will not exceed 2 percent for the year.

Drugs, biologicals, radiopharmaceuticals, and devices qualify for pass-through status if they were not being paid for as a hospital outpatient drug as of

Figure 7.3.   Discounting provision illustration for HOPPS

APC	Payment Status Indicator	Payment Rate
1	T	100%
2	T	50%
3	T	50%
4	S	100%
5	S	100%

December 31, 1996, and their cost is "not insignificant" in relation to the HOPPS payment for the procedures or services associated with their use (DHHS 2004a, 50502). An item can have pass-through status for at least two years, but not more than three years. After three years, the cost of the item will be bundled into the APC payment for the procedure in which the item is used or be transitioned into an individual APC group. The pass-through status application process is described on the CMS Web site (CMS 2005).

Pass-through device APCs (payment status indicator H) are paid on a reasonable cost basis less the device offset amount. The device offset amount is the portion of the APC payment amount that CMS has determined is associated with the cost of the device (DHHS 2004a, 50501). This amount is deducted from the pass-through payment because it is already reimbursed as part of the surgical APC payment. Drug, biological, and radiopharmaceutical pass-through APCs (payment status indicator G) are reimbursed by using an average sales price (ASP) methodology. The average sales price is equivalent to the dollar amount at which these drugs and biologicals would be reimbursed in the physician office setting (DHHS 2004a, 50503). From this amount the portion of the applicable fee schedule amount (APC payment rate) is subtracted. The result is the pass-through payment.

Transitional Corridor and Hold-Harmless Payments
The BBRA provided a mechanism for hospitals to decrease the financial burden of the implementation of HOPPS. This phase-in period provided the transitional corridor payments. Transitional corridor payments were provided beginning in 2000 and were discontinued December 31, 2003. However, hold-harmless payments are permanent for IPPS-exempt cancer centers and children's hospitals. Small rural hospitals (having less than one hundred beds) and sole community hospitals located in rural areas will receive hold-harmless payments through the end of CY 2005 (DHHS 2004a, 50530).

Eligible facilities receive a quarterly interim hold-harmless payment that provides additional reimbursement when the payment received under HOPPS is less than the payment the facility would have received for the same services under the prior reasonable cost-based system in 1996 (DHHS 2004a, 50530). The interim payment is based on ratios of cost to charge from their most recently closed Medicare cost report and their assigned pre-BBRA payment-to-cost ratio determined from their 1996 cost report. Payment-to-cost ratios average around 80 percent. Figure 7.4 displays the formula for hold-harmless payment calculation. The final hold-harmless amount is determined at the settlement of the cost report for that facility's fiscal year.

APC Assignment

The APC system is primarily based on the HCPCS code(s) assigned for each service or procedure performed and for devices, drugs, and reimbursable items provided to the patient. The first step in APC assignment is to code the encounter accurately and completely. The APC system is a partially packaged system and several items/services are separately reimbursed; therefore, failure to capture all reimbursable charges with HCPCS codes will result in lost revenue for the facility. Once all HCPCS codes have been assigned, the payment status indicator is identified for each code. Payment status indicators

Figure 7.4.   Hold harmless formula for HOPPS

For specified quarter:

Department charges × Department-specific ratios of cost-to-charge = Department cost

Sum department cost for all departments = Total cost

Total cost × Payment to cost ratio from 1996 = Pre-HOPPS reimbursement

HOPPS reimbursement from current quarter − Pre-HOPPS reimbursement = Hold-harmless payment

When current HOPPS exceeds Pre-HOPPS reimbursement, no hold harmless payment is made.

that are assigned to an APC and indicate APC payment are F, G, H, K, S, T, X, V, and P. There may be multiple APCs with the same or different payment status indicator per claim.

For two exceptions to this process the ICD-9-CM diagnosis code assignment is crucial. In partial hospitalizations (APC 0033), an acute mental health disorder diagnosis must be assigned with an ICD-9-CM code. For observation services (APC 0339), a diagnosis of chest pain, congestive heart failure, or asthma must be assigned with an ICD-9-CM code. This code must be reported as either the first reported diagnosis or the reason for admission. If the appropriate ICD-9-CM diagnosis code is not assigned, the procedure/service will not group to the correct APC and may result in incorrect reimbursement.

Payment Determination

HOPPS payment for outpatient services is determined by using a seven-step methodology:

1. *APC assigned.* Hospitals submit a claim to Medicare for payment. Claims are sent electronically to the designated fiscal intermediary. Each claim contains visit information, patient information, facility information, detailed charges by procedure code, and diagnosis codes. The fiscal intermediary performs an audit of the claim to ensure that the claim contains complete and accurate information based on the edits found in the **Outpatient Code Editor (OCE).** During the editing process, APC(s) are assigned using grouper software as appropriate based on the HCPCS codes submitted.

2. *APC Payment rate established.* The payment rate is calculated by multiplying the relative weight for the assigned APC by the conversion factor for the current calendar year (CY). The conversion factor is the dollar amount that is equal to the relative weight of 1.000 and is updated each CY. For CY 2005, the conversion factor is $56.983.

3. *Wage index adjusted to national unadjusted facility component.* The facility component of the APC payment rate is wage-index adjusted. The formula for this adjustment is displayed in figure 7.5.

4. *Fee schedule amounts applied.* HCPCS codes with payment status indicator A are paid under a designated fee schedule. The fee schedule amounts for these procedures, services, and items are applied by the pricer software.

5. *Reasonable cost amounts applied.* HCPCS codes with payment status indicators F or L are reimbursed at a reasonable cost level. To calculate reasonable cost, the charge for the item or services is converted to cost by applying a department-specific ratio of cost to charge determined by historical cost report data for that hospital. These amounts are calculated and applied by the pricer software.

6. *Medicare payments summed.* All Medicare payments (APC, fee schedule, and reasonable cost) are summed for the claim.

7. *Outlier add-on applied.* The outlier calculation is completed in the pricer software for all eligible procedures and services. The amount is added to the total Medicare payments.

Figure 7.5.   Wage Index Adjustment Formula for HOPPS

[(National Unadjusted Payment Amount × 60%) × Wage index] + (National Unadjusted Payment Amount × 40%) = Locality payment

The pricer software completes steps two through seven. When the seven steps are completed, payment is made to the facility and the data from the encounter is included in the national claims history file. The outpatient standard analytical file and the hospital outpatient prospective payment system file, extracts from the national claims history file, are used for statistical analysis and research.

Summary

The hospital outpatient prospective payment system for hospital outpatient services provided to Medicare beneficiaries was successfully implemented in 2000. HOPPS has influenced hospitals to practice cost analysis and containment practices for their outpatient service areas. Additionally it has successfully lowered Medicare expenditures to hospitals for outpatient services. Hospitals continue to struggle with the intricacies of this complex reimbursement system and the numerous pieces of legislation that continue to modify the system.

Home Health Prospective Payment System

Since October 1, 2000, Medicare has reimbursed **home health agencies (HHAs)** under a PPS based on the **home health resource group (HHRG)** classification. The system is known as the home health prospective payment system (HHPPS). The legal authorization for the HHPPS comes from the Balanced Budget Act (BBA) of 1997 and the Omnibus Consolidated and Emergency Supplemental Appropriations Act (OCESAA) of 1999. Section 4603(a) of the BBA of 1997 amended the Social Security Act by adding Section 1895, entitled "Prospective Payment for Homes Health Services." The OCESAA amended Section 1895 by making the effective date October 1, 2000, and by stating that all Medicare services under the Medicare home health benefit that previously had been covered and paid on the basis of reasonable cost

would now be paid on the basis of a prospective payment amount. The final rule implementing the HHPPS was published in the *Federal Register* of July 3, 2000 (DHHS 2000).

Data Collection

The payment is based on data elements in the **Outcome Assessment Information Set (OASIS).** OASIS uses ICD-9-CM codes to represent the health status of patients. In addition, for tracking purposes, HCPCS codes may be used to report non-routine supplies. Medicare Program Memorandum, Transmittal A-00-71 (October 2, 2000; Change Request 1356) describes in detail the required data elements on CMS Form 485 (Youmans, Scichilone, and Dougherty 2001, 76).

One data element in addition to the OASIS is also collected: the number of therapy hours that the patient has received in the sixty-day episode that forms the basic unit of service under HHPPS.

CMS defines the principal diagnosis for the HHPPS as the diagnosis most related to the current plan of care. The diagnosis may or may not be related to the patient's most recent hospital stay, but must relate to the services rendered by the HHA. If more than one diagnosis is treated concurrently, the diagnosis that represents the most acute condition and requires the most intensive services should be entered (Youmans, Scichilone, and Dougherty 2001, 77). The ICD-9-CM guidelines dictate that a certain specific diagnosis is only to be used when a specific secondary diagnosis is present.

> The principal diagnosis must match the diagnosis reported on the physician certified plan of care, the OASIS, and the UB-92 (CMS 1450) form. In addition, V codes are not acceptable as either principal or additional diagnoses, but could be reported in item 21, Orders for Discipline and Treatments."

Examples:

A Medicare beneficiary was surgically treated for a subtrochanteric fracture (code 820.22) with an admission to a home care agency for rehabilitation services

(V57.1). The HHA must use 820.22 as the principal diagnosis and may enter V57.1 in field 21.

A patient is immediate post bowel resection for adenocarcinoma of the descending colon (code 153.2) with exteriorization of the colon. Admission to home care is ordered for surgical follow-up and instruction in care of the colostomy (V55.3). Even though code V55.3 is more specific to the nature of the proposed service, the HHA must assign code 153.2 as the principal diagnosis, but may assign code V55.3 in field 21. (Youmans, Scichilone, and Dougherty 2001, 77).

The OASIS data set is completed and submitted electronically. Special software called the **home assistance validation and entry (HAVEN)** system is used for the collection and submission of the OASIS data, with a new OASIS data set completed whenever an unexpected decline or improvement in the patient's situation occurs.

Episode-Based Payment

The unit of payment is the **episode of care.** The per-episode home health payment covers all home care services and nonroutine medical supplies delivered to the patient during a sixty-day period. Claims for episodes of care usually include more than one date of service.

A special adjustment accounts for the circumstance in which an agency provides minimal care. The special adjustment is termed a **low-utilization payment adjustment (LUPA).** The LUPA is applied when an agency provides four or fewer visits in an episode. Under LUPA, the agency is reimbursed for each visit rather than for the sixty-day episode (Dougherty 2000, 84). The episode-based payment system consolidates payments. Types of services consolidated into the single payment include all therapy (speech, physical and occupational), skilled nursing visits, home health aide visits, medical social services, and nonroutine medical supplies. Durable medical equipment (DME) is excluded from the per-episode payment and is reimbursed under another payment method (DME fee schedule).

Grouping and Payment

The case-mix system for the HHPPS combines twenty data elements from the OASIS to measure the three domains of the case mix. These three domains are:

- Clinical severity (C)

- Functional status (F)

- Service utilization (S)

The HHPPS defines eighty HHRGs based on these three domains, which are derived from all possible combinations of the severity levels across the three domains. The grouper program reviews selected data to assign the HHRG. This grouper program is embedded in the HAVEN software. This embedded grouper program is sometimes called the Pricer.

The HHRG is a six-character alphanumeric code that represents a severity level in the three domains: C, F, and S (Dougherty 2000, 86). These domains form the core of the **health insurance prospective payment system (HIPPS)** codes (table 7.16). A patient with the lowest severity in all three domains would be C0F0S0. This score is the minimum score.

From the HHRG the health insurance prospective payment system (HIPPS) code is derived (table 7.16). There are eight HIPPS codes for each HHRG. HIPPS codes are five-character alphanumeric codes:

- The first character is an H.

- The second, third, and fourth characters represent the HHRG.

- The fifth character indicates what elements were computed or derived. Computed elements are output from the grouper based on complete OASIS data. Derived elements are output from the grouper based on a system of defaults where OASIS data are incomplete.

Table 7.16.   Basics of health insurance prospective payment system code and home health resource group classification

Coding Scheme for Home Health Resource Group (HHRG) Classification				
(Clinical) Position #2	**(Functional) Position #3**	**(Service) Position #4**	**Position #5**	**Domain Level**
A (C0)	E (F0)	J (S0)	1 = all positions computed	= min
B(C1)	F (F1)	K (S1)	2 = 2nd position derived	= low
C (C2)	G (F2)	L (S2)	3 = 3rd position derived	= mod
D (C3)	H (F3)	M (S3)	4 = 4th position derived	= high
	I (F4)		5 = 2nd & 3rd positions derived	= max
			6 = 3rd & 4th positions derived	
			7 = 2nd and 4th positions derived	
			8 = 2nd, 3rd & 4th positions derived	
	N through Z	9, 0		expansion values

Health Care Financing Administration (HCFA; now known as Centers for Medicare and Medicaid Services, CMS). 2000 (July 27). Program Memorandum Intermediaries Transmittal A-00-41, Change Request 1264. p. 4. Available online from www.cms.hhs.gov/manuals/pm_trans/A0041.pdf.

Therefore, the HIPPS code for the HHRG, C0F0S0, would be HAEJ1.

- First character = H

- Second, third, and fourth characters are: C0 = A, F0 = E, S0 = J

- 1 = all positions are computed

The HIPPS code is submitted on the claim to the regional home health intermediary (RHHI). The weight of the applicable HIPPS code is multiplied by the **national standard episode amount,** or conversion factor (table 7.17). The national standard episode amount is an across-the-board multiplier or a constant. The national standard episode amount is changed from year to year. In 2000, the national standard episode rate was $2,115.30; in 2005, the national rate was $2,264.28 (DHHS 2000, 41190–41191; DHHS 2004b, 62133).

The product resulting from the multiplication of the weight by the national standard episode amount is also adjusted for geographic wage differences. Adjusting for geographic wage differences is a two-step process:

1. In order to calculate this adjustment, the labor and nonlabor portions must be computed. The labor and nonlabor portions are computed from ratios. These ratios also vary from year to year. For example, in 2000 the ratio for the labor portion was 0.77668 and the ratio for the nonlabor portion was 0.22332 (DHHS 2000, 41191). In 2005, though, the ratio for the labor portion was 0.76775 and the ratio for the nonlabor portion was 0.23225 (DHHS 2004b, 62133).

Table 7.17.   Sample listing of home health resource groups (HHRGs), health insurance prospective payment system (HIPPS) codes, and weights

Excerpt from Listing of HHRGs, HIPPS Codes, and Weights			
HHRG Description	**Case Mix Description of Domains**	**HIPPS Code**	**Weight**
C0F0S0—all computed	Clinical = Min, Functional = Min, Services = Min	HAEJ1	0.5265
2nd position derived		HAEJ2	0.5265
3rd position derived		HAEJ3	0.5265
4th position derived		HAEJ4	0.5265
2nd & 3rd position derived		HAEJ5	0.5265
3rd & 4th position derived		HAEJ6	0.5265
2nd & 4th position derived		HAEJ7	0.5265
All derived		HAEJ8	0.5265
C0F0S1—all computed	Clinical = Min, Functional = Min, Services = Low	HAEK1	0.6074
2nd position derived		HAEK2	0.6074
3rd position derived		HAEK3	0.6074
4th position derived		HAEK4	0.6074
2nd & 3rd position derived		HAEK5	0.6074
3rd & 4th position derived		HAEK6	0.6074
2nd & 4th position derived		HAEK7	0.6074
All derived		HAEK8	0.6074
C3F4S3—all computed	Clinical = High, Functional = Max, Services = High	HDIM1	2.8113
2nd position derived		HDIM2	2.8113
3rd position derived		HDIM3	2.8113
4th position derived		HDIM4	2.8113
2nd & 3rd position derived		HDIM5	2.8113
3rd & 4th position derived		HDIM6	2.8113
2nd & 4th position derived		HDIM7	2.8113
All derived		HDIM8	2.8113

Source: CMS. Available online from www.cms.hhs.gov/medlearn/hhppsa1.pdf or www.cms.hhs.gov/medlearn/addendc.pdf.

2. The labor portion is then adjusted for the wage index of the geographic area. Urban geographic areas use the wage index of the corresponding **core-based statistical area (CBSA)** (similar to the former metropolitan statistical area [MSA]). Rural areas use the nonurban area wage index of the respective state (sometimes called non-MSA). Again, the wage indexes vary from year to year. For example, in 2000 the wage index for Greenville, North Carolina (MSA 3150) was 0.9501 (DHHS 2000, 41176). In 2005, the wage index for Greenville, North Carolina was 0.9183 (DHHS 2004d, 69699). To calculate this adjustment, the labor portion of the product is multiplied by the wage index of the CBSA. The product of the labor portion multiplied by the MSA wage index is then added back to the nonlabor portion to produce the total possible episode payment (table 7.18).

Case Study of HHPPS Calculations

With key data and the formulae, readers can calculate the wage-adjusted episode payment for an HHA patient in Greenville, North Carolina. The patient is receiving home health services following discharge from an acute care hospital. The patient's HIPPS code (HDIM1) reflects the highest severity in all three domains.

Key Data

HHRG = C3F4S3 and the OASIS is complete (all computed)

HIPPS = HDIM1

Weight = 2.8113

National standard episode amount = $2,264.28

Labor ratio = 0.76775

Nonlabor ratio = 0.23225

CBSA wage index = 0.9183

Generic Formula

Weight × constant = Unadjusted payment

2.8113 × $2,264.28 = $6,365.57

Geographic Wage Adjustment

Unadjusted payment × 0.76775 (labor ratio) = Labor portion

$6,365.57 × 0.76775 (labor ratio) = $4,887.17

Labor portion × 0.9183 (CBSA wage index)

$4,887.17 × 0.9183 (CBSA wage index)

$4,887.17 × 0.9183 = $4,487.89

Unadjusted payment × 0.23225 (nonlabor ratio) = Nonlabor portion

$6,365.57 × 0.23225 (nonlabor ration) = $1,478.40

Wage-index adjusted labor portion + Nonlabor portion = Total possible episode payment

$4,487.89 + $1,478.40 = $5,966.29

Table 7.18 illustrates this process.

To allow for patients who have a significant change in condition, the HHA may resubmit an updated OASIS data set for a revised HHRG to appropriately adjust reimbursement.

Implementation

Abraham (2001) provides the major steps of the payment process:

1. Complete OASIS within seven days of start of care (SOC), resumption of care (ROC), significant change in condition (SCIC), or end of care (EOC). A regulatory interpretation changed this reporting requirement to within forty-eight hours for discharges, transfers, or deaths.

2. Calculate the HHRG with grouper software.

3. Convert the HHRG into health insurance prospective payment system (HIPPS) code for payment.

Table 7.18.   Calculation of home health payments

Sample Calculation of Wage-Adjusted Federal Payment (2005)							
A	B	C	D	E	F	G	H
HIPPS Code	Weight	Nat'l. Stnd. Epi. Amt. (NSAE) ($)*	Unadj. Rate [Weight × NSEA] ($)	Local Wage Index**	Adjusted Labor Portion [Unadj. Rate × Labor Ratio (.76775) × Local Wage Index] ($)	Nonlabor Portion [Unadj. Rate × Nonlabor Ratio (.23225)] ($)	Wage-Adjusted Rate [Adj. Labor Portion + Nonlabor Portion]($)
HAEJ1	0.5265	2264.28	1192.14	0.9183	840.49	276.88	1117.37
HDIM1	2.8113	2264.28	6365.57	0.9183	4487.89	1478.40	5966.29

*National 60-day episode rate. Department of Health and Human Services. 2004 (October 22). *Federal Register.* 69 (204): 62133.

**Greenville, NC, is in the Metropolitan Statistical Area [MSA] 3150. Department of Health and Human Services. 2004 (November 30). *Federal Register.* 69 (229): 69699.

4. Send request for anticipated payment (RAP), low-utilization payment adjustment (LUPA), or final claims to regional home health intermediary (RHHI).

5. Extract and transmit OASIS data to state survey agency once monthly.

6. Retrieve and analyze outcome-based quality improvement management (OBQM) reports to identify quality improvement opportunities.

Coding accuracy and completeness are critical. Some ICD-9-CM diagnosis codes affect payment (DHHS 2000). CMS is tracking the HCPCS codes used for the nonroutine supplies (Youmans, Scichilone, and Dougherty 2001, 76).

Check Your Understanding 7.2

1. Ambulatory payment classifications (APCs) were developed by modifying _____.

2. Name the two reimbursement methods used by HOPPS.

3. Procedures in HOPPS with a status indicator of C are indicated as inpatient-only; they must be provided to Medicare beneficiaries in an inpatient setting and are reimbursed under the IPPS. True or false?

4. When is LUPA used and how does it affect reimbursement?

5. Name the three domains of case mix measured using data elements from OASIS for the home health prospective payment system.

Summary

Reform of reimbursement systems for healthcare services provided to ambulatory patients began in 1992. Spurred by effective curbs in the acute care setting, Congress authorized the Department of Health and Human Services to design and implement reformed payment systems in many settings for ambulatory patients. These settings include physician offices, ambulance services, ambulatory surgery centers, hospital outpatient services, and home health agencies. To the credit of lawmakers and CMS analysts, these systems combine a focus on cost savings and an attention to quality outcomes. Updates and revisions for these payment systems are released each year in the *Federal Register* via proposed and final rules. Students and professionals should reference these documents to obtain yearly payment rates and to examine revised or new payment provisions and policies.

Review Quiz

1. How can physician payments be adjusted for the price differences among various parts of the country?

2. What is the control mechanism the government uses on Medicare payments to physicians, and how is it applied?

3. Describe at least two issues that delayed implementation of the APC system for ambulatory surgical centers.

4. What is the current status of the ASC PPS?

5. How is the "two-times rule" applied to APC groups?

6. In the HHPPS, the _____ software is used to collect and submit OASIS data.

7. How is durable medical equipment (DME) reimbursed in the HHPPS?

8. When a patient is pronounced dead during ambulance transport, Medicare payment rules are followed as if the patient were alive. True or false?

9. CMS, not the APC Advisory Panel or MedPAC, makes the final ruling for updates and changes to HOPPS. True or false?

10. The number of APCs per encounter for a single patient is limited to ten. True or false?

References and Bibliography

Abraham, P. 2001 (October). HIPPS table for pricer. Home health prospective payment systems (HHPPSs). AHIMA Convention Proceedings. Centers for Medicare and Medicaid Services. Available online from www.cms.hhs.gov/medlearn/addendc.pdf.

Averill, R. F., N. I. Goldfield, J. Eisenhandler, J. S. Hughes, and J. Muldoon. 2001. Clinical risk groups and the future of healthcare reimbursement. In *Reimbursement Methodologies for Healthcare Services* [CD-ROM], edited by L. M. Jones. Chicago: American Health Information Management Association.

Centers for Medicare and Medicaid Services. 2005. Listing of HHRGs, HIPPS codes and weights. Available online from www.cms.hhs.gov/medlearn/hhppsa1.pdf.

Department of Health and Human Services. 2000 (July 3). Medicare Program; Prospective Payment System for Home Health Agencies; Final Rule. *Federal Register* 65 (128): 41127–41214.

Department of Health and Human Services. 2002 (February 27). Medicare Program; Fee Schedule for Payment of Ambulance Services and Revisions to the Physician Certification Requirements for Coverage of Nonemergency Ambulance Services; Final Rule. *Federal Register* 67 (39): 9099–9135.

Department of Health and Human Services. 2003a (March 28). Medicare Program; Update of Ambulatory Surgical Center List of Covered Procedures Effective July 1, 2003; Final Rule. *Federal Register* 68 (60): 15267–15312.

Department of Health and Human Services. 2003b. Payments for procedures in outpatient departments and ambulatory surgical centers. Report of a study from the Office of the Inspector General. Available online from oig.hhs.gov/oei/reports/oei-05-00-00340.pdf.

Department of Health and Human Services. 2004a (August 16). Medicare Program; Proposed Changes to the Hospital Outpatient Prospective Payment System and Calendar Year 2005 Payment Rates; Proposed Rule. *Federal Register* 69 (157): 50447–50546.

Department of Health and Human Services. 2004b (October 22). Medicare Program; Home Health Prospective Payment System Rate Update for Calendar Year 2005; Final Rule. *Federal Register* 69 (204): 62123–62162.

Department of Health and Human Services. 2004c (November 26). Medicare Program; Update of Ambulatory Surgical Center List of Covered Procedures; Proposed Rule. *Federal Register* 69 (227): 69178–69180.

Department of Health and Human Services. 2004d (November 30). Medicare Program; Home Health Prospective

Payment System Rate Update for Calendar Year 2005; Correction; Final Rule. *Federal Register* 69 (229) 69685–69727.

Dougherty, Michelle. 2000. New home care PPS brings major changes. *Journal of the American Health Information Management Association* 71(9):84–86.

Health Care Financing Administration (HCFA; now the Centers for Medicare and Medicaid Services, CMS). 2000 (July 27). Program Memorandum Intermediaries Transmittal A-00-41. Change Request 1264, 4. Available online from www.cms.hhs.gov/manuals/pm_trans/A0041.pdf.

Jones, L. M. ed. 2001. Ambulatory payment classifications for freestanding ambulatory surgery centers. In *Reimbursement Methodologies for Healthcare Services*

[CD-ROM]. Chicago: American Health Information Management Association.

Medicare Payment Advisory Commission. 2004 (December). *Report to the Congress: Growth in the Volume of Physician Services.* Available online from www.medpac.gov/publications/congressional_reports/Dec04_PhysVolume.pdf.

Scanlon, W. J. 2002 (February). *Medicare Physician Payments: Spending Targets Encourage Fiscal Discipline, Modifications Could Stabilize Fees.* Publication No. GAO-02-441T. Government Accounting Office. Available online from www.gao.gov/cgi-bin/getrpt?GAO-02-441T.pdf.

Youmans, Karen, Rita Scichilone, and Michelle Dougherty. 2001. Another look at home care PPS. *Journal of American Health Information Management Association* 72(2):78–78.

Chapter 8
Revenue Cycle Management

Objectives

- To understand the components of the revenue cycle

- To define revenue cycle management

- To describe the importance of effective revenue cycle management in a provider's fiscal stability

Key Terms

Accounts receivable
Charge capture
Charge description master
Copayment
Deductible
Explanation of benefits
Fiscal Intermediary
Hard coding
Key performance indicator
Medicare carrier
Medicare Summary Notice
Remittance advice
Revenue cycle
Revenue cycle management

Introduction to Revenue Cycle Management

Prospective payment systems have been implemented in virtually every service area in the healthcare arena. In order to maintain profitability under the prospective payment systems, healthcare facilities must constantly examine and implement methods to either increase reimbursement or decrease costs. Managers of many facilities understand the importance of decreasing payment delays and lost revenue through **revenue cycle management (RCM).** RCM is the supervision of all administrative and clinical functions that contribute to the capture, management, and collection of patient service revenue.

Multidisciplinary Approach

Traditionally, RCM used a silo approach where each clinical department was responsible for its own functions and contributions to the **revenue cycle.** However, this linear approach was often reactive in nature, and rather than promoting communication between departments, it tended to foster hostility and division. The twenty-first century approach is for healthcare facilities to take a new multidisciplinary approach to RCM. This recent, dynamic approach promotes teamwork among various clinical departments by creating an RCM team composed of representatives from all revenue cycle areas. An emphasis on education encourages all team members to be updated on changing market forces such as payer trends, government and regulatory modifications, and organization strategy. As result of higher understanding of all members' contributions and importance to the revenue cycle, this modern management style has influenced the team to take a proactive approach to reimbursement issues.

Components of the Revenue Cycle

Each section of the revenue cycle is vital to creating efficient and compliant reimbursement processes. Although each area is responsible for its own functions and tasks, cooperation from outside departments and clinical areas is often critical for timely and accurate completion and submission of healthcare claims. The major components of the revenue cycle are:

- Preclaims submission activities
- Claim processing activities
- **Accounts receivable**
- Claims reconciliation and collections

Preclaims Submission Activities

Preclaims submission activities comprise tasks and functions from the admitting and case management areas. Specifically, this portion of the revenue cycle is responsible for collecting the patient's and responsible parties' information completely and accurately for determining the appropriate financial class, educating the patient as to his or her ultimate financial responsibility for services rendered, collecting waivers when appropriate, and verifying data prior to procedures/services being performed and submitted for payment. For example, when a Medicare patient arrives for admission into the cardiology unit for a coronary artery stent placement, the admitting representative is responsible for collecting the patient demographic data including the individual's Medicare healthcare identification claim number (HICN). Additionally, the Medicare patient may need to be educated about any annual **deductible** amount or **copayment** responsibilities if the inpatient stay were to last longer than 60 days.

Claims Processing Activities

Claims processing activities include the capture of all billable services, claim generation, and claim corrections. **Charge capture** is a vital component of the revenue cycle. All clinical areas that provide services to a patient must report charges for the services that they have performed. Failure to report charges for these services will result in lost reimbursement for the healthcare facility. Charge capture can be accomplished in a variety of ways depending on the technological capabilities of the healthcare facility.

Order Entry

Electronic order entry systems have been implemented at hospitals to help capture the charge at the point of service delivery. With an electronic order entry system, the charge for the service or supply is automatically transferred to the patient accounting system and posted to the patient's claim. Facilities without electronic systems use paper-based processes such as charge tickets, superbills, or encounter forms to assist in charge collection. With a paper-based process, the paper forms are collected and then entered into the patient accounting system, where the charge is then transferred to the claim. The paper system leaves more room for error as charges can be posted to the wrong patient's account, digits can be transposed during data entry, and backlogs can occur when data entry clerks are absent or pulled off task.

Charge Description Master

Coding is a major portion of charge capture. Claims submission regulations require ICD-9-CM and/or HCPCS codes to be reported on a patient's claim. Several types of visits, such as clinic visits, or services, such as laboratory or radiology, are designed to have procedure codes posted to the claim via the **charge description master (CDM).** During order entry, electronic or paper-based, a unique identifier for each service is entered. This unique identifier triggers a charge from the CDM to be posted to the patient's account. This process is known as **hard coding.**

Different facilities use different terminology for the CDM. Some more common synonyms include: chargemaster, charge compendium, service master, price list, service item master, and charge list

(Schraffenberger 2005, 117). The CDM is a large database maintained by the facility, which houses the price list for all services provided to patients. The basic CDM model contains the revenue code, HCPCS code, service description, and price/charge for services and procedures. However, facilities do house other pieces of charge information in the CDM based on their individual needs, such as general ledger key, activity status, and department number. Table 8.1 provides a sample CDM. The CDM is typically under the responsibility of the finance department.

With the growing complexity of coding and billing regulations, many facilities have created a CDM coordinator position. A CDM coordinator should have coding and claims processing knowledge. Many HIM professionals that are interested in revenue cycle management are entering this arena via the CDM coordinator position.

CDM Maintenance

Although the CDM is managed by one individual at most facilities, CDM maintenance is a joint effort. Influenced by the multidisciplinary approach taken by many RCM teams, each ancillary area and revenue cycle area participates in the maintenance process. Because code sets are modified each year, basic yearly maintenance of the CDM is critical. All code changes must be incorporated into the CDM to ensure proper reimbursement will be obtained. Inclusion of new codes must be coordinated with the ancillary department to ensure that services are properly reported. Further, code changes should be communicated to the ancillary areas so that proper education can be provided to order/charge entry staff.

In addition to yearly maintenance, several other updates may be necessary throughout the year. The Centers for Medicare and Medicaid Services (CMS) releases coding and billing guidance at various times during the fiscal year that may include information that warrants CDM updates. As new services are introduced at a facility, line

Table 8.1.   Sample charge description master

Department Number	Item Number*	Item Description	Revenue Code	HCPCS Code**	Price***	Active/Inactive Status
700	7008989	Dermagraft (Synth skin graft)	252	C9201	$1,525.00	Active
700	7005202	Minor surgery – $1/2$ hour	360		$1,203.00	Active
700	7005203	Regular OR – 1st hour	360		$4,687.00	Active
700	7005205	Regular OR – $1/2$ hour	360		$1,682.00	Active
715	7157059	Open heart – 1st hour	360		$5,589.00	Active
715	7157060	Open heart – $1/2$ hour	360		$2,782.00	Active
760	7605161	OB/GYN surgery	360		$1,975.00	Active
800	8004557	Rabies Vaccine-IM use	450	90675	$632.00	Active
822	8224210	Albumin 5% saline	250	P9045	$265.00	Active
367	3675839	Speech screening	440	V5362	$298.00	Active
367	3675840	Language screening	440	V5363	$298.00	Active
367	3675841	Dysphagia screening	440	V5364	$298.00	Active
200	2578961	Venipuncture	300	G0001	$18.00	Inactive
200	2578989	Venipuncture	300	36415	$18.00	Active
110	1478951	MRI upper extremity w/o dye	610	73218	$817.00	Active
110	1478952	MRI upper extremity with dye	610	73219	$857.00	Active
110	1478953	MRI upper extremity w/o & with dye	610	73220	$897.00	Active

*Also called charge code, charge number, item code, service code and service number.

**When blank, HCPCS code is determined via coding in HIM department.

***Price is fictitious and should not be used for rate setting.

items will need to be added to the CDM so that services and procedures may be billed for payment. And when claims processing improvements are made, the CDM should always be reviewed and modified to ensure that the components are up-to-date and will efficiently facilitate the claims processing changes.

Many healthcare facilities have contracted with maintenance companies to help keep the CDM up-to-date. Many consulting companies provide Web-based or software-based updating systems that allow the facility to easily make changes to the CDM. In addition to providing up-to-date codes sets and regulations, many of these companies provide consultation services that assist facilities in the charge capture process.

Failure to effectively maintain the CDM puts a facility at risk for compliance violations and lost reimbursement as outlined in table 8.2. With the implementation of PPS in various healthcare settings, it is vital that the correct information be reported to third party payers. Because key information used to determine payment is transmitted to the claim via the CDM, it is critical that the CDM always be precise. Whereas the focus of the CDM may have been simply the charge value in the past, it is clearly now the accuracy of the entire line item.

Table 8.2.   Charge description master maintenance issues

Issue	Possible Result	Risk Area
Undercharging for services	Under payment	Lost revenue
Overcharging for services	Over payment	Compliance
Incorrect HCPCS or diagnosis code	Claims rejection/denial	Lost revenue
Incorrect revenue code	Claims rejection/denial	Lost revenue

Coding by HIM

Other types of visits, such as inpatient or complex ambulatory surgery, require the diagnoses and operating room procedures to be coded by health information management (HIM) professionals. During the coding process, medical records are viewed and read by the coding staff. All diagnoses and procedures are identified, coded, and then abstracted into the HIM coding system. This system then transfers the diagnoses and procedure codes to the patient accounting system where they are posted to the patient's claim prior to submission for payment.

Auditing and Review

Once all data have been posted to a patient's account, the claim can be reviewed for accuracy and completeness. Many facilities have internal auditing systems known as *scrubbers*. The auditing system runs each claim through a set of edits specifically designed for that third party payer. The auditing system identifies data that has failed edits and flags the claim for correction. Examples of errors that cause claim rejections or denials if not caught by the scrubber are:

- Incompatible dates of service

- Nonspecific or inaccurate diagnosis and procedure codes

- Lack of medical necessity

- Inaccurate revenue code assignment

The auditing process prevents facilities from sending incomplete or inaccurate claims to the payer. Facilities that do not have an editing system may perform a hand audit of a sample of claims. HIM and reimbursement specialists review claims with the medical record to determine if all services, diagnoses, and procedures were accurately reported. If errors are found, they can be corrected before claim submission.

Submission of Claims

Once reviewed and corrected, the claim can be submitted to the third party payer for payment. The Health Insurance Portability and Accountability Act of 1996 (HIPAA) added a new part to the Social Security Act titled Administrative Simplification. The purpose of this section is to improve the efficiency and effectiveness of the healthcare delivery system. Through this section, Medicare has established standards and requirements for the electronic exchange of certain health information (DHHS 2003a, 8381). The Final Rule on Standards for Electronic Transactions and Code Sets, also known as the Transactions Rule, identified eight electronic transactions and six code sets (see tables 8.3 and 8.4). This Rule ensures that all providers, third party payers, claims clearinghouses, and so forth, use the same sets of codes to communicate coded health information, therefore ensuring standardization for systems and applications across the healthcare continuum. Not only does this support standardization, but it also supports administrative simplification. Providers can now maintain a select number of code sets at their current version, rather than maintaining different versions (current and old) of many code sets based on payer specification as required in the past.

Healthcare claims, healthcare payment and **remittance advice,** and coordination of benefits are included in the electronic transactions. As of October 16, 2003, all healthcare facilities were required to electronically submit and receive healthcare claims, remittance advices, and coordination of benefits. Thus, today facilities submit claims via the 837I electronic format, which replaces the UB-04 or CMS-1450 billing form. Physicians submit claims via the 837P electronic format, which takes the place of the CMS-1500 billing form.

Accounts Receivable

The accounts receivable department manages the amounts owed to a facility by customers who

Table 8.3. HIPAA electronic transactions

Healthcare claims or equivalent encounter information
Eligibility for a health plan
Referral certification and authorization
Healthcare claim status
Enrollment and disenrollment in a health plan
Healthcare payment and remittance advice
Health plan premium payments
Coordination of benefits

Source: Department of Health and Human Services. 2003 (February 20). *Federal Register.* 68 (34): 8382.

Table 8.4. HIPAA code sets

International Classification of Diseases, 9th Edition, Clinical Modification, Volumes 1 and 2
International Classification of Diseases, 9th Edition, Clinical Modification, Volume 3
National Drug Codes
Code on Dental Procedures and Nomenclature
Health Care Financing Administration Common Procedure Coding System
Current Procedural Terminology, 4th Edition

Source: Department of Health and Human Services. 2003 (February 20). *Federal Register.* 68 (34): 8382.

received services but whose payment will be made at a later date by the patient or his or her third party payer. Once the claim is submitted to the third party payer for reimbursement, the accounts receivable clock begins to tick. Typical performance statistics maintained by the accounts receivable department include days in accounts receivable and aging of accounts. Days in accounts receivable is calculated by dividing the ending accounts receivable balance for a given period by the average revenue per day. Facilities typically set performance goals for this standard. Aging of accounts is maintained in 30-day increments (0–30 days, 31–60 days, and so forth). Facilities monitor the number of accounts and the total dollar value in each increment. The older the account or the longer the account remains unpaid, the less of a chance that the facility will receive reimbursement for the encounter.

Insurance Processing

Once a claim is received by the third party payer (TPP), the insurance processing of the claim begins. Medicare claims for Part A services and hospital-based Medicare Part B services are submitted to a designated **fiscal intermediary.** Fiscal intermediaries (FIs) contract with Medicare to process claims for a specific area or region. The FI determines costs and reimbursement amounts, conducts reviews and audits, and makes payments to providers for covered services on behalf of Medicare. Part B claims for services rendered by physicians and for medical supplies are submitted to a designated **Medicare carrier.** Like the FI, the carrier determines charges allowed by Medicare and makes payment to physicians and suppliers on behalf of Medicare.

Benefits Statements

In addition to processing the claim for payment, TPPs prepare an **explanation of benefits (EOB)** that is delivered to the patient. The EOB is a statement that describes services rendered, payment covered, and benefits limits and denials. Specifically for Medicare patients, FIs and carriers prepare **Medicare Summary Notices (MSNs).** The MSN details amounts billed by the provider, amounts approved by Medicare, how much Medicare reimbursed the provider, and what the patient must pay the provider by way of deductible and copayments. EOBs and MSNs are part of the Transactions Rule and are provided to the facility via electronic data interchange (EDI) and are sent to the patient via postal mail.

Remittance Advice

Once the claim is processed by the TPP, a remittance advice (RA) is electronically returned to the provider via the 835A or 835B electronic format. Payments are typically made in batches with the RA sent to the facility and payments electronically transferred to the provider's bank. The RA reports claim rejections, denials, and payments to the facility via EDI.

Claims Reconciliation and Collection

The last component of the revenue cycle is reconciliation and collections. The healthcare facility uses the EOB, MSN, and RA to reconcile accounts. EOBs and MSNs identify the amount owed by the patient to the facility. Collections can contact the patient to collect outstanding deductibles and copayments. RAs indicate rejected or denied line items or claims. Facilities can review the RAs and determine whether the claim error can be corrected and resubmitted for additional payment. If a correction is not warranted, reconciliation can be made via a write-off or adjustment to the patient's account. Once the account has been settled, the revenue cycle is completed. Figure 8.1 provides a flow chart of the revenue cycle.

Check Your Understanding 8.1

1. The first step in the revenue cycle is _____.

2. How are charges for healthcare at all of the points of services collected and reported to the appropriate patient account for entry onto the provider's claim?

3. What do scrubbers do?

Revenue Cycle Management Team

The purpose of a revenue cycle management (RCM) team is to improve the efficiency and effectiveness of the revenue cycle process. Each team will develop different goals and objectives to guide their focus and discussions. Some sample objectives are:

- To identify issues to improve accounts receivable

Figure 8.1.   Flow chart of the revenue cycle

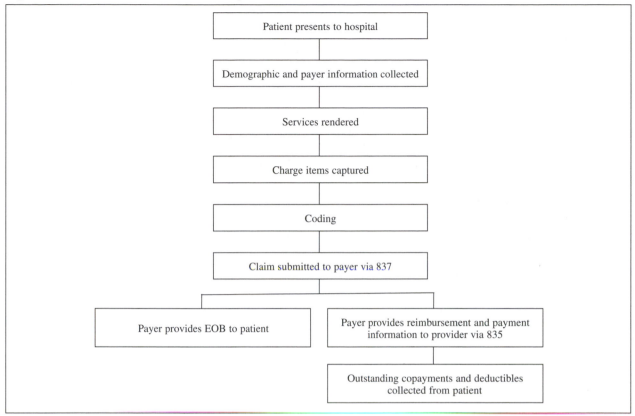

- To communicate issues with appropriate areas

- To develop educational materials such as a revenue cycle manual

- To create a map or blueprint on how to bring up new services

- To review denials and actively discuss the appeal process and successes

- To discuss **key performance indicators** and measures

Once an RCM team establishes goals and objectives, team members must define optimal performance for their facility. Many teams define opti-

mal performance by establishing key performance indicators and by setting a standard for each indicator. Key performance indicators should represent areas that need improvement. The facility should design indicators so that they can be measured to gauge performance improvement. Some sample key performance indicators are:

- Dollar value of discharged not final billed encounters

- Days from discharge to coded

- Number of accounts receivable days

- Percentage and amount of write-offs

- Percentage of nonerror claims (clean claims)

- Percentage of claims returned to provider for correction by third party payers

- Percentage of denials by third party payers

- Percentage of late charges

- Percentage of accurate registrations

Current levels for each key indicator should be determined and compared to the standard. For example, if the standard for key performance indicator "Dollar value of discharged not final billed encounters" is $2 million and the current value is $10 million, the facility is exceeding the standard by $8 million. Therefore, significant focus should be placed on reducing that total. Perhaps the facility is experiencing a coder shortage or there is a backlog in the prepping and scanning area so the coders are unable to review the records online. The HIM management team must investigate the issues and practice performance improvement techniques to improve the coding and/or record processing procedures so that the standard can be met. Key indicators should be continuously monitored until their related standard is consistently met. Once met, facilities typically review the indicator quarterly or semiannually to ensure continued optimal performance.

RCM Case Study

Facility A submitted one month of Medicare outpatient claims for auditing by the Medicare Outpatient Code Editor (OCE). The data set contained 2,530 claims, 17,710 line items, and $5,457,513 in charges. The results of an OCE audit are displayed in table 8.5.

Table 8.5.   Hospital A OCE Audit Results

OCE Edit	Edit Description	Violations	Claims Processing Area
01	Invalid diagnosis code	23	Coding
06	Invalid procedure code	21	Coding/CDM
15	Service unit out of range for procedure	46	Order entry
27	Only incidental services reported	16	Order entry/coding/CDM
28	Code not recognized by Medicare; alternate code for same service may be available	54	Coding/CDM
38	Inconsistency between implanted device and implantation procedure	47	Order entry/CDM
41	Invalid revenue code	65	CDM
43	Transfusion or blood product exchange without specification of blood product	15	Order entry/CDM
44	Invalid use of observation revenue code	49	Order entry/CDM
48	Revenue center requires HCPCS code	29	CDM
61	Service can only be billed to the DMERC	14	Order entry/CDM
68	Service provided prior to date of National Coverage Determination (NCD) approval	32	Coding/CDM
71	Claim lacks required device code	28	Order entry/CDM

Several edits were evoked during the audit. In order to improve the revenue cycle process, the RCM team investigates each edit to uncover its root problems.

OCE Edit 41

OCE edit 41 (Invalid revenue code) has been evoked, which usually arises when the revenue code reported on the claim is not in the list of valid revenue codes for HOPPS. When this edit is activated, the claim is returned to the provider for correction. Therefore, this error is delaying payment of several claims and is also costing the facility staff time in rework. Each claim must be corrected and resubmitted to the fiscal intermediary for payment.

Clearly, this situation raises revenue code issues. Revenue codes are stored in the charge description master (CDM) and are placed on the claim via charge/order entry. Therefore, a CDM review is warranted because several line items obviously are stored with incorrect revenue codes. Perhaps a program transmittal was incorrectly interpreted or a typing mistake was made during data entry in the CDM.

A review of the sixty-five error claims shows that two line items in the ancillary section of physical therapy have incorrect information. The two line items represent physical therapy evaluation services, which should be reported with revenue code 0424. However, these line items had been assigned revenue code 0425—not a valid revenue code. This was a simple data entry mistake, but it resulted in delayed payment for several claims. This error is easy to correct, but it reveals the need for the CDM update process to be reviewed to identify risk areas for typing errors. Facility A subsequently implements a review component as part of its CDM update process.

OCE Edit 48

OCE edit 48 (Revenue center requires HCPCS code) is triggered when an HCPCS code is not reported with a revenue code on the claim and the revenue center status indicator is not bundled. This edit is not applicable for revenue codes 100x, 210x, 310x, or 905–907. Because this edit is activated, claims are being returned to the facility for correction. Like OCE edit 41, this error is also delaying the payment of several claims and is costing facility A staff time for rework.

Review of these twenty-nine claims reveals they all included the line item number 3268916, which is used to report lithotripsy. Facility A had recently hard coded the lithotripsy services in the CDM, so the RCM team could not understand why the HCPCS code was not appearing on the claim. Further, the lithotripsy unit was contacted and its staff confirmed that they performed thirty-five procedures last month, so why did only twenty-nine claims evoke this edit? What happened to the other six claims? The RCM team asked the CDM coordinator to review all line items for lithotripsy services.

The CDM review revealed that there were duplicate line items for this service. Apparently the old line item for this service was not marked as inactive when the hard-coding update occurred. Therefore, the CDM contained two active line items for the same service. However, the RCM team was still puzzled because they thought that they had thoroughly educated the charge entry staff about the line item changes. After further investigation the RCM team discovered that one charge entry staff member was on vacation during the training, and upon return to work she was not informed about the line item changes. She had continued to use the old line item number.

Two fixes were implemented. First, line item number 3268916 was marked inactive. Second, the charge entry staff member was scheduled for training immediately. Additionally, the RCM team and coding manager learned two lessons. An additional component was needed to the hard-coding conversion plan to review all old line items for inactive status, and a sign-in sheet was needed to be used for training sessions and followed up for missing attendees to ensure that all staff members would be educated in the future.

OCE Edit 38

OCE edit 38 (Inconsistency between implanted device and implantation procedure) is triggered when an HCPCS code with APC payment status indicator H (pass-through device) is present on the claim, but no APC with a payment status indicator of S (significant), T (surgical), X (ancillary—non-implant) is reported. This edit causes the claim to be returned to the provider for correction.

To determine whether this situation resulted from a CDM error or a flaw in the order entry process, facility A required a claim analysis. Claim review showed that the forty-seven cases evoking OCE edit 38 were all cardiac pacemaker claims. Further investigation of the cardiac encounters revealed that the order entry process included reporting the device code via the CDM, but the facility's chart flow process was bypassing the HIM department. Therefore, the code for the pacemaker insertion procedure was not being coded or reported on the claim.

Not only did facility A require rework and resubmission for these forty-seven claims, but the HIM and cardiac departments had to learn through the RCM team to work together to change claims processing flow.

This case study shows that each claim that evokes an edit from an internal or external auditing system or process should be investigated and corrected if warranted. Facilities should resubmit all possible claims in order to achieve optimal reimbursement. Failure to review and rework error claims will result in significant lost payment. A facility's RCM team should facilitate this process so that efforts can be coordinated and streamlined.

Check Your Understanding 8.2

1. Healthcare facilities should design key performance indicators so they _____.

2. What system is typically used to audit Medicare claims?

3. Describe at least two problems uncovered during the claims audit at facility A.

Summary

The revenue cycle and the management of the processes contained within are vital to obtaining accurate reimbursement. Every piece of healthcare information collected during the cycle contributes to the production of an error-free claim. Effective management of the revenue cycle results in efficient processes that meet key performance indicator standards defining optimal performance. Achieving and maintaining optimal performance levels not only improves revenue but allows the healthcare facility to focus on other areas for improved profitability.

Review Quiz

1. Which provider order entry system is usually more reliable, paper-based or electronic? Why?

2. What are two sources of new charge description master codes?

3. What risk areas are concerns when the charge description master is not properly maintained and revised?

4. How has HIPAA changed claims processing?

5. What are two roles of EDI in claims processing?

6. List the ways discrepancies between submitted charges and paid charges are reconciled by the provider.

7. How do providers decide what optimal performance is for units of their facility?

8. Facility B just completed an analysis of its alarmingly high balance of unpaid claim amounts. What are some key performance indicators a provider's RCM team could use to learn the reason(s) for the surge in unpaid balances?

9. Describe at least three sources of errors that cause claim denials.

10. Use of the charge description master has made manual coding by HIM coders obsolete. True or false?

References and Bibliography

3M Health Information Systems. 2005. *Outpatient Code Editor with Ambulatory Payment Classification Software: Installation and User's Manual.* Software version 6.2.

AHIMA. 1999. Practice Brief: The Care and Maintenance of Charge Masters. *Journal of American Health Information Management Association* 70 (7) 80A–B.

Berkey, Tim. 1998. Reducing accounts receivable through benchmarking and best practices identification. *Journal of American Health Information Management Association* 69:10, 30–34.

Department of Health and Human Services. 2003a (February 20). Health Insurance Reform: Security Standards; Final Rule. *Federal Register* 68 (34): 8333–8381.

Department of Health and Human Services. 2003b (February 20). Health Insurance Reform: Modifications to Electronic Data Transaction Standards and Code Sets. *Federal Register* 68 (34): 8381–8399.

Schraffenberger, Lou Ann. 2005. *Effective Management of Coding Services.* Chicago: American Health Information Management Association.

VHA: 2002. Revenue Cycle Management: The Paradigm Shift to Success. VHA, Inc. Available online from www.vha.com.

Work, M. 2005. Best practices in revenue cycle management. *Journal of American Health Information Management Association* 76:7, 31.

Youmans, Karen. 2004. An HIM spin on the revenue cycle. *Journal of American Health Information Management Association* 75:3, 32–36.

Appendix A
Glossary

Abuse: Unknowing or unintentional submission of an inaccurate claim for payment.

Accounts receivable: Department in a healthcare facility that manages the amounts owed to the facility by customers who have received services but whose payment is made at a later date.

Actual charge: Amount provider actually bills a patient, which may differ from the allowable charge.

AHA *Coding Clinic for HCPCS:* Official coding guidance for HCPCS Level II procedure, service, and supply codes.

AHIMA Standards of Ethical Coding: Standards developed by the Council on Coding and Classification of the American Health Information Management Association to give health information coding professionals ethical guidelines for performing their coding and grouping tasks.

Allowable charge: Average or maximum amount the third party payer will reimburse providers for the service.

Allowable fee: *See* Allowable charge.

Ambulatory payment classification (APC): Hospital outpatient prospective payment system (HOPPS). The classification is a resource-based reimbursement system. The payment unit is the ambulatory payment classification group (APC group).

Ambulatory payment classification group (APC group): Basic unit of the ambulatory payment classification (APC) system. Within a group, the diagnoses and procedures are similar in terms of resources used, complexity of illness, and conditions represented. A single payment is made for the outpatient services provided. APC groups are based on HCPCS/CPT codes. A single visit can result in multiple APC groups. APC groups consist of five types of service: significant procedures, surgical services, medical visits, ancillary services, and partial hospitalization. The APC group was formerly known as ambulatory visit group (AVG) and ambulatory patient group (APG).

Ambulatory surgery center (ASC): Free-standing, outpatient facility in which outpatient surgeries are performed.

Ambulatory surgery center (ASC) payment group: Payment made to an ambulatory surgery center (ASC) for facility-related costs. A fixed payment rate for procedures designated to be ASC procedures. ASC procedures are classified into nine payment groups. A fixed payment rate is designated for each group. The ASC facility payment in each group is a single rate adjusted for geographic variation. This prospectively determined rate covers the cost of standard overhead items (nursing care, supplies, equipment, and use of facility). It does not include physicians' fees and some other medical items and services (such as prostheses).

Ambulatory surgery center list (ASC list): Procedures that Medicare will cover when they are performed in the ambulatory setting.

Ancillary services: Professional healthcare services such as radiology, laboratory, or physical therapy.

Appeal: Request for reconsideration of denial of coverage or rejection of claim.

Arithmetic mean length of stay (AMLOS): Sum of all lengths of stay in a set of cases divided by the number of cases. The national average number of days patients within a given diagnosis related group (DRG) are hospitalized.

Average length of stay (ALOS): Average number of days patients are hospitalized. Statistic is calculated by dividing the total number of hospital bed days in a certain period by the admissions or discharges during the same period.

Balanced Budget Act of 1997 (BBA): Legislation that effected several aspects of the healthcare industry including the hospital outpatient prospective payment system (HOPPS), fraud and abuse, and programs of all-inclusive care for elderly (PACE).

Base (payment) rate: Rate per discharge for operating and capital-related components for an acute care hospital.

Base year: Cost reporting period upon which a rate is based.

Benchmarking: The process of comparing performance to a preestablished standard or performance of another facility or group.

Beneficiary: An individual who is eligible for benefits from a health plan.

Benefit: Healthcare service for which the healthcare insurance company will pay. *See also* Covered service.

Benefit cap: Total dollar amount that a healthcare insurance company will pay for covered healthcare services during a specified period, such as a year or lifetime.

Block grant: Fixed amount of money given or allocated for a specific purpose, such as a transfer of governmental funds to cover health services.

Budget neutrality: Adjustment of payment rates when policies change so that total spending under the new rules is the same as it would have been under the previous payment rules.

Bundling: Combination of supply and pharmaceutical costs or medical visits with associated procedures or services for one lump sum payment.

Calendar year (CY): Twelve-month period (year) that begins January 1 and ends December 31.

Capitation: Method of payment for health services in which an individual or institutional provider is paid a fixed, per capita amount for each person enrolled without regard to the actual number or nature of services provided or number of persons served.

Carrier: Entity that has a contract with the Centers for Medicare and Medicaid Services (CMS) to determine and make Medicare payments for Part B benefits.

Case: Patient, resident, or client with a given condition or disease.

Case management: Coordination of individuals' care over time and across multiple sites and providers, especially in complex and high-cost cases. Goals include continuity of care, cost-effectiveness, quality, and appropriate utilization.

Case mix: Set of categories of patients (type and volume) treated by a healthcare organization and representing the complexity of the organization's case load.

Case mix group (CMG): Class of functionally similar discharges in the inpatient rehabilitation facility prospective payment system (IRF PPS). Basis of similarity is impairment, functional capability, age, and comorbidities.

Case mix index (CMI): Single number that compares the overall complexity of the healthcare organization's patients to the complexity of the average of all hospitals. Typically, the CMI is for a specific period and is derived from the sum of all diagnosis related group (DRG) weights, divided by the number of Medicare cases.

Case-based payment: Type of prospective payment method in which the third party payer reimburses the provider a fixed, preestablished payment for each case.

Catastrophic expense limit: Specific amount, in a certain time frame such as one year, beyond which all covered healthcare services for that policyholder or dependent are paid at 100 percent by the healthcare insurance plan. (*See also* Maximum out-of-pocket cost *and* Stop-loss benefit.)

Centers for Medicare and Medicaid Services (CMS): A division of the Department of Health and Human Services (DHHS) that is responsible for administering the Medicare program and the federal portion of the Medicaid program; responsible for maintaining the procedure portion of the International Classification of Diseases, 9th revision, Clinical Modification (ICD-9-CM). Prior to 2001 was named the Health Care Financing Administration (HCFA).

Certificate holder: Member of a group for which the employer or association has purchased group healthcare insurance. *See also* Insured, Member, Policyholder, *and* Subscriber.

Charge: Price assigned to a unit of medical or health service, such as a visit to a physician or a day in a hospital. The charge for a service may be unrelated to the actual cost of providing the service. *See also* Fee.

Charge capture: The process of collecting all services, procedures, and supplies provided during patient care.

Charge description master: Database used by healthcare facilities to house the price list for all services provided to patients.

Civilian Health and Medical Program: Veterans Administration (CHAMPVA): A benefits program administered by the Department of Veterans Affairs for the spouse or widow(er) and for the children of a veteran who meets specified criteria.

Claim: Request for payment, or itemized statement of healthcare services and their costs provided by a hospital, physician's office, or other healthcare provider. Claims are submitted for reimbursement to the healthcare insurance plan by either the policy or certificate holder or the provider. Also called bills for Medicare Part A and Part B services billed through fiscal intermediaries and for Part B physician or supplier services billed through carriers.

Clean claim: Request for payment that contains only accurate information (no errors in data).

Clinical risk group (CRG): Capitated, prospective payment system that predicts future healthcare expenditures for populations.

Closed panel: Type of health maintenance organization that provides hospitalization and physicians' services through its own staff and facilities (also known as staff model or group model).

Code range: Applicable set of diagnosis or procedure codes.

Coding Clinic for ICD-9-CM: Official coding guidance for the International Classification of Diseases, 9th revision, Clinical Modification (ICD-9-CM) diagnosis and procedure codes.

Coding compliance plan: A component of an HIM compliance plan or a corporate compliance plan that focuses on the unique regulations and guidelines with which coding professionals must comply.

Cognitive: Related to mental abilities, such as talking, memory, and problem solving.

Coinsurance: Cost-sharing in which the policy or certificate holder pays a preestablished percentage of eligible expenses after the deductible has been met. The percentage may vary by type or site of service.

Community (-based premium) rating: Method of determining healthcare premium rates by geographic area (community) rather than by age, health status, or company size. This method increases the size of the risk pool. Costs are increased to younger, healthier individuals who are, in effect, subsidizing older or less healthy individuals.

Comorbidity: Preexisting condition that, because of its presence with a specific diagnosis, causes an increase in length of stay by at least one day in approximately 75 percent of the cases (as in complication and comorbidity [CC]).

Compliance: Managing a coding or billing department according to the laws, regulations, and guidelines that govern it.

Compliance officer: Designated individual who monitors the compliance process at a healthcare facility.

Compliance program guidance: Information provided by the Office of Inspector General (OIG) of the Department of Health and Human Services (DHHS) to assist healthcare organizations with the development of compliance plans and programs.

Complication: Condition that arises during the hospital stay that prolongs the length of stay at least one day in approximately 75 percent of the cases (as in complication and comorbidity [CC]).

Consumer-directed (driven) healthcare plan (CDHP): Managed care organization characterized by influencing patients and clients to select cost-efficient healthcare through the provision of information about health benefit packages and through financial incentives.

Contracted discount rate: Type of fee-for-service reimbursement in which the third party payer has negotiated a reduced (discounted) fee for its covered insureds. *See also* Discounted fee-for-service.

Conversion factor (CF): National dollar multiplier which sets the allowance for the relative values; a constant.

Coordination of benefits (COB): Method of integrating benefits payments from all health insurance sources to ensure that payments do not exceed 100 percent of the covered healthcare expenses.

Copayment: Cost-sharing measure in which the policy or certificate holder pays a fixed dollar amount (flat fee) per service, supply, or procedure that is owed to the healthcare facility by the patient. The fixed amount that the policyholder pays may vary by type of service, such as $20.00 per prescription or $15.00 per physician office visit.

Core-based statistical area (CSBA): Statistical geographic entity consisting of the county or counties associated with at least one core (urbanized area or urban cluster) of at least 10,000 population, plus adjacent counties having a high degree of social and economic integration with the core as measured through commuting ties with the counties containing the core. Metropolitan and micropolitan statistical areas are two components of CBSAs.

Cost-of-living adjustment (COLA): Alteration that reflects a change in the consumer price index (CPI), which measures purchasing power between time periods. The CPI is based on a market basket of goods and services that a typical consumer buys.

Cost report: Report required from providers on an annual basis in order for the Medicare program to make a proper determination of amounts payable to providers under its provisions.

Cost-sharing: Provision of a healthcare insurance policy that requires policyholders to pay for a portion of their healthcare services; a cost-control mechanism.

Covered condition: Health condition, illness, injury, disease, or symptom for which the healthcare insurance company will pay.

Covered service (expense): Specific service for which a healthcare insurance company will pay. *See also* Benefit.

Customary, prevailing, and reasonable (CPR): Type of retrospective fee-for-service payment method in which the third party payer pays for fees that are customary, prevailing, and reasonable.

CPT Assistant: Official coding guidance for CPT codes.

Creditable coverage: Prior health care coverage that is taken into account to determine the allowable length of preexisting condition exclusion periods (for individuals entering group health plan coverage).

Includes healthcare insurance through a group health plan or health maintenance organization (HMO), federal employees health benefits program, military healthcare plan (TRICARE), Indian Health Service (IHS), state high risk pools, Medicare, Medicaid, coverage under the Consolidated Omnibus Budget Reconciliation Act (COBRA), or other public health plan. Excluded from creditable coverage are accidental death and dismemberment plan, automobile medical payment insurance, disability insurance, and workers' compensation.

Credited coverage: Reduction of waiting period for preexisting condition based on previous creditable coverage. Credited coverage may be calculated on a day-by-day basis or other method that is at least as favorable to the individual. To receive credit for previous creditable coverage, the lapse (break) in coverage cannot exceed 63 days.

Critical access hospital (CAH): Small facility that gives limited outpatient and inpatient hospital services to people in rural areas.

Critical care services: Evaluation and management of critically ill or critically injured patients.

Current Procedural Terminology (CPT): Coding system created and maintained by the American Medical Association that is used to report diagnostic and surgical services and procedures.

Current Procedural Terminology (CPT) Category I Code: A CPT code that represents a procedure or service that is consistent with contemporary medical practice and is performed by many physicians in clinical practice in multiple locations.

Current Procedural Terminology (CPT) Category II Code: A CPT code that represents services and/or test results that contribute to positive health outcomes and quality patient care.

Current Procedural Terminology (CPT) Category III Code: A CPT code that represents emerging technologies for which a Category I Code has yet to be established.

Deductible: Annual amount of money that the policyholder must incur (and pay) before the health insurance will assume liability for the remaining charges or covered expenses.

Dependent: An insured's spouse and unmarried children, claimed on income tax. The maximum age of dependent children varies by policy. A common ceiling is 19 years of age, with continuation to age 23 provided the child is a full-time student at an accredited school, primarily dependent upon the covered employee for support and maintenance, and is unmarried. Some healthcare insurance polices also allow same sex domestic partners to be listed as dependents.

Diagnosis related group (DRG): Inpatient classification that categorizes patients who are similar in terms of diagnoses and treatments, age, resources used, and lengths of stay. Under the prospective payment system (PPS), hospitals are paid a set fee for treating patients in a single DRG category, regardless of the actual cost of care for the individual.

Discounted fee-for-service: Type of fee-for-service reimbursement in which the third party payer has negotiated a reduced ("discounted") fee for its covered insureds. *See also* Contracted discount rate.

Discounting: Reducing the payment in the hospital outpatient prospective payment system (HOPPS) (payment status indicator = T). In the CMS's discounting schedule, Medicare will pay 100 percent of the Medicare allowance for the principle procedure (exclusive of deductible and copayment) and 50 percent (50 percent discount) of the Medicare allowance for each additional procedure. For example, if two CT scans (APC group 0349) are performed in the same visit, the first is reimbursed at the full APC group rate, the second at 50 percent of the APC group rate.

Disease management: Program focused on preventing exacerbations of chronic diseases and on promoting healthier life styles for patients and clients with chronic diseases.

Disproportionate share hospital (DSH): Healthcare organizations that meet governmental criteria for percentages of indigent patients.

Editor: Logic (algorithms) within computer software that evaluates data. Medicare's Standard Claims Processing System (or PSC Supplemental Edit Software) and its Outpatient Code Editor (OCE) contain editors that select certain claims, evaluate, or compare information on the selected claims or other accessible source, and depending on the evaluation, take action on the claims, such as pay in full, pay in part, or suspend for manual review. Also known as a code editor.

Encounter: Professional, direct personal contact between a patient and a provider who delivers services or is professionally responsible for services delivered to a patient. Face-to-face contact between a patient and a provider who has primary responsibility for assessing and treating the condition of the patient at a given contact and exercises independent judgment in the care of the patient.

Endorsement: Language or statements within a healthcare insurance policy providing additional details about coverage or lack of coverage for special situations that are not usually included in standard policies. May function as a limitation or exclusion.

Episode of care: One or more healthcare services given by a provider during a specific period of relatively continuous care in relation to a particular health or medical problem or situation. In home health, the episode of care is all home care services and nonroutine medical supplies delivered to a patient during a 60-day period. In the home health prospective payment system (HHPPS), the episode of care is the unit of payment.

Episode-of-care reimbursement: Healthcare payment method in which providers receive one lump sum for all the care they provide related to a condition or disease. *See also* Episode of care.

Etiologic diagnosis: Underlying cause of the problem that led to the condition requiring admission to an inpatient rehabilitation facility.

Evidence of insurability: Statement or proof of a health status necessary to obtain healthcare insurance, especially private healthcare insurance.

Evidence-based clinical practice guideline: Explicit statement that guides clinical decision making and has been systematically developed from scientific evidence and clinical expertise to answer clinical questions. Systematic use of guidelines is termed evidence-based medicine.

Exclusion: Situation, instance, condition, injury, or treatment that the healthcare plan states will not be covered and for which the healthcare plan will pay no benefits (synonym is impairment rider).

Exclusive provider organization (EPO): Hybrid managed care organization that is sponsored by self-insured (self-funded) employers or associations and exhibits characteristics of both health maintenance organizations and preferred provider organizations.

Explanation of benefits (EOB): Report sent from a healthcare insurer to the policyholder and to the provider that describes the healthcare service, its cost, applicable cost-sharing, and the amount the healthcare insurer will cover. The remainder is the policyholder's responsibility.

False Claims Act: Legislation passed during the Civil War that prohibits contractors from making a false claim to a governmental program; used to reinforce healthcare fraud and abuse.

Federal Employees' Compensation Act of 1916 (FECA): A benefit program that ensures that civilian employees of the federal government are provided medical, death, and income benefits for work-related injuries and illnesses.

Fee: Price assigned to a unit of medical or health service, such as a visit to a physician or a day in a hospital. A fee for a service may be unrelated to the actual cost of providing the service. *See also* Charge.

Fee schedule: Third party payer's predetermined list of maximum allowable fees for each healthcare service.

Fee-for-service (FFS) reimbursement: Healthcare payment method in which providers retrospectively receive payment for each service rendered.

Fiscal intermediary (FI): Local payment branch of the Medicare program. Intermediaries are public or private insurance companies that contract with the Centers for Medicare and Medicaid Services (CMS) to act as agents of the federal government in dealing directly with participating providers of Medicare services. An intermediary is usually, but not necessarily, an insurance company, such as Blue Cross. FIs reimburse for inpatient or hospital services (Part A Medicare) and some Part B services.

Fiscal year: Yearly accounting period; the twelve month period on which a budget is planned. The federal fiscal year is October 1st through September 30th of the next year. Some state fiscal years are July 1st through June 30th of the next year. Often, agencies and companies match their fiscal years to the state and federal governments with which they contract.

Formulary: List of preferred drugs including brand-name and generic.

Fraud: Intentionally making a claim for payment that one knows to be false.

Functional independent assessment tool: Standardized tool to measure the severity of patients' impairments in rehabilitation settings. The tool captures characteristics that reflect the functional status of patients. Patients with lower scores on the tool have less independence and need more assistance than patients with higher scores.

Functional status: Patient's ability to perform the activities of daily living.

Gatekeeper: Health care provider or entity responsible for determining the healthcare services a patient or client may access. May be a primary care provider, a utilization review or case management agency, or a managed care organization.

Geographic practice cost index (GPCI): Index based on relative difference in the cost of a market basket of goods across geographical areas. A separate GPCI exists for each element of the relative value unit (RVU), which includes physician work, practice expenses, and malpractice. GPCIs are a means to adjust the RVUs, which are national averages, to reflect local costs of service.

Geometric mean length of stay (GMLOS): Statistically adjusted value of all cases of a given diagnosis related group (DRG), allowing for the outliers, transfer cases, and negative outlier cases that would normally skew the data. The GMLOS is used to compute hospital reimbursement for transfer cases.

Global payment method: Method of payment in which the third party payer makes one consolidated payment to cover the services of multiple providers who are treating a single episode of care.

Group practice model: Type of health maintenance organization (HMO) in which the HMO contracts with a medical group and reimburses the group on a fee-for-service or capitation basis. *See also* Closed panel.

Group practice without walls (PWW): Type of integrated delivery system in which the individual physicians share administrative systems but maintain their separate practices and offices distributed over a geographic area. (Also known as clinic without walls [CWW]).

Grouper: Computer program that uses specific data elements to assign patients, clients, or residents to groups, categories, or classes.

Guarantor: Person who is responsible for paying the bill or guarantees payment for healthcare services. Patients who are adults are often their own guarantor. Parents guarantee payments for the healthcare costs of their children.

Hard coding: Use of the charge description master to code repetitive services.

Health Care Procedure Coding System (HCPCS): Coding system created and maintained by the Centers for Medicare and Medicaid Services (CMS) that provides codes for procedures, services, and supplies not represented by a Current Procedural Terminology (CPT) code.

Health Information Technology (HIT): The use of electronic devices and media to collect, store, and retrieve healthcare information.

Health Insurance Portability and Accountability Act of 1996 (HIPAA): Significant piece of legislation aimed at improving healthcare data transmission among providers and insurers; designated code sets to be used for electronic transmission of claims.

Health insurance prospective payment system (HIPPS) code: Five-character alphanumeric code used in the home health prospective payment system (HHPPS) and in the inpatient rehabilitation facility prospective payment system (IRF PPS). In the HHPPS, the HIPPS code is derived or computed from the home health resource group (HHRG). In the IRF PPS, the HIPPS code is derived from the case mix group and comorbidity. Reimbursement weights for each HIPSS code correspond to the levels of care provided.

Health maintenance organization (HMO): Entity that combines the provision of healthcare insurance and the delivery of healthcare services. Characterized by: (1) organized healthcare delivery system to a geographic area, (2) set of basic and supplemental health maintenance and treatment services, (3) voluntarily enrolled members, and (4) predetermined fixed, periodic prepayments for members' coverage. Prepayments are fixed without regard to actual costs of healthcare services provided to members.

High-cost outlier. *See* Outlier.

High-cost threshold: Criterion to assess whether technologies would be inadequately paid under the inpatient prospective payment system (IPPS). The sum of the geometric mean and the lesser of .75 of the national adjusted operating standardized payment amount (increased to reflect the difference between costs and charges) or .75 of one standard deviation of mean charges by diagnosis related group (DRG).

Hold harmless: Status in which one party does not hold the other party responsible.

Home Assistance Validation and Entry (HAVEN) System: Computer software for the collection and submission of the data elements in the Outcome Assessment Information Set (OASIS). HAVEN is used in the home health prospective payment system (HHPPS).

Home health agency (HHA): Organization that provides services in the home. These services include skilled nursing care, physical therapy, occupational therapy, speech therapy, and personal care by home health aides.

Home health resource group (HHRG): Classifications (groups) for the home health prospective payment system (HHPPS) derived from the data elements in the Outcome Assessment Information Set (OASIS). The HHRG is a six-character alphanumeric code that represents a severity level in three domains.

Hospital Outpatient Prospective Payment System (HOPPS): The reimbursement system created by the Balanced Budget Act of 1997 for hospital outpatient services rendered to Medicare beneficiaries; maintained by the Centers for Medicare and Medicaid Services (CMS).

Hospital Payment Monitoring Program (HPMP): Coding compliance monitoring program created by the 7th Scope of Work which ensures that proper payment is made for Medicare beneficiary admissions; administered by regional Quality Improvement Organizations (QIOs).

ICD-9-CM Coordination and Maintenance Committee: Committee composed of representatives from the National Center for Health Statistics (NCHS) and the Centers for Medicare and Medicaid Services (CMS) that is responsible for maintaining the United States' clinical modification version of the International Classification of Diseases, 9th revision (ICD-9-CM) code sets.

Impairment group code (IGC): Multidigit code that represents the primary reason for a patient's admission to an inpatient rehabilitation facility.

Indemnity health insurance: Traditional, fee-for-service healthcare plan in which the policyholder pays a monthly premium and a percentage of the usual, customary, and reasonable healthcare costs, and the patient can select the provider.

Independent practice association (IPA) or organization (IPO): Type of health maintenance organization (HMO) in which participating physicians maintain their private practices, and the HMO contracts with the independent practice association. The HMO reimburses the IPA on a capitated basis; the IPA may reimburse the physicians on a fee-for-service or a capitated basis.

Indian Health Service (IHS): An agency within the Department of Health and Human Services (DHHS) responsible for upholding the federal government's obligation to promote healthy American Indian and Alaskan native people, communities, and cultures.

Indirect medical education (IME) adjustment: Percentage increase in Medicare reimbursement to offset the costs of medical education that a teaching hospital incurs.

Inpatient rehabilitation facility patient assessment instrument (IRF PAI): Data collection tool specific to rehabilitation facilities.

Inpatient Rehabilitation Validation and Entry (IRVEN): Computer software for data entry in inpatient rehabilitation facilities (IRFs). Captures data for the IRF Patient Assessment Instrument (IRF PAI) and supports electronic submission of the IRF PAI. Also allows data import and export in the standard record format of the Centers for Medicare and Medicaid Services (CMS).

Insurance: Reduction of a person's (insured's) exposure to risk of loss by having another party (insurer) assume the risk.

Insured: Individual or entity that purchases healthcare insurance coverage. *See also* Certificate holder, Member, Policyholder, *and* Subscriber.

Integrated delivery system (IDS): Generic term for the separate legal entity that healthcare providers form to offer a comprehensive set of healthcare services to a population. Other terms are health delivery network, horizontally integrated system, integrated services network (ISN), and vertically integrated system.

Integrated provider organization (IPO): Corporate, managerial entity that includes one or more hospitals, a large physician group practice, other healthcare organizations, or various configurations of these businesses.

International Classification of Diseases, 9th Revision, Clinical Modification (ICD-9-CM): Coding and classification system used to report diagnoses in all healthcare settings and inpatient procedures and services.

Interrupted stay: Discharge in which the patient was discharged from the inpatient rehabilitation facility and returned within three calendar days.

Key performance indicator: Area identified for needed improvement through benchmarking and continuous quality improvement.

Labor-related share (portion, ratio): Sum of facilities' relative proportion of wages and salaries, employee benefits, professional fees, postal services, other labor-intensive services, and the labor-related share of capital costs from the appropriate market basket. Labor-related share is typically 70 to 75 percent of healthcare facilities' costs. Adjusted annually and published in the *Federal Register.*

Late enrollee: Individual who does not enroll in a group healthcare plan at the first opportunity, but enrolls later if the plan has a general open enrollment period.

Length of stay (LOS): Number of days a patient remains in a healthcare organization. The statistic is the number of calendar days from admission to discharge including the day of admission, but not the day of discharge. This statistic may have an impact on prospective reimbursement.

Limitation: Qualification or other specification that reduces or restricts the extent of the health-care benefit.

Local Coverage Determination (LCD): Reimbursement and medical necessity policies established by regional fiscal intermediaries. New format for Local Medical Review Policies (LMRPs). LCDs and LMRPs vary from state to state.

Local Medical Review Policy (LMRP): *See* Local Coverage Determination (LCD).

Long-term care diagnosis related group (LTC-DRG): Inpatient classification that categorizes patients who are similar in terms of diagnoses and treatments, age, resources used, and lengths of stay. Under the prospective payment system (PPS), hospitals are paid a set fee for treating patients in a single DRG category, regardless of the actual cost of care for the individual. LTC-DRGs are exactly the same as the DRGs for the inpatient prospective payment system (IPPS). *See also* Diagnosis related group (DRG).

Long-term care hospital (LTCH): Hospitals that provide general acute care and specialized services to patients who have longer than average lengths of stay. These patients may have chronic diseases or acute diseases that require long-term therapies. The Centers for Medicare and Medicaid Services (CMS) has two ways to categorize hospitals as LTCHs. First, an LTCH has an average length of stay for Medicare patients that is twenty-five days or longer. Second, an LTCH can be a hospital excluded from the inpatient prospective payment system and that has an average length of stay for all patients that is twenty days or longer.

Low-utilization payment adjustment (LUPA): Payment adjustment applied when a home health agency provides four or fewer visits in an episode of care.

Major diagnostic category (MDC): Highest level in hierarchical structure of the federal inpatient prospective payment system (IPPS). The twenty-five MDCs are primarily based on body system involvement, such as MDC No. 06, Diseases and Disorders of the Digestive System. However, a few categories are based on disease etiology, for example, Human Immunodeficiency Virus Infections.

Malpractice (MP): Element of the relative value unit (RVU); costs of the premiums for professional liability insurance.

Managed care: Payment method in which the third party payer has implemented some provisions to control the costs of healthcare while maintaining quality care. Systematic merger of clinical, financial, and administrative processes to manage access, cost, and quality of healthcare.

Managed care organization (MCO): Entity that integrates the financing and delivery of specified healthcare services. Characterized by (1) arrangements with specific providers to deliver a comprehensive set of healthcare services, (2) criteria for selecting providers, (3) quality assessment and utilization review, and (4) incentives for members to use plan providers. Also known as coordinated care organization.

Management (medical) service organization (MSO): Specialized entity that provides management services and administrative and information systems to one or more physician group practices or small hospitals. An MSO may be owned by a hospital, physician group, physician-hospital organization, integrated delivery system, or investors.

Market basket: Mix of goods and services.

Market basket index: Relative measure that averages the costs of a mix of goods and services.

Maximum out-of-pocket cost: Specific amount, in a certain time frame such as one year, beyond which all covered healthcare services for that policyholder or dependent are paid at 100 percent by the healthcare insurance plan. *See also* Catastrophic expense limit *and* Stop-loss benefit.

Medicaid: Part of the Social Security Act, a joint program between state and federal governments to provide healthcare benefits to low-income persons and families.

Medical emergency: Severe injury or illness (including pain); definition depends upon the healthcare insurer.

Medical foundation: Multipurpose, nonprofit service organization for physicians and other healthcare providers at the local and county levels. As managed care organizations, medical foundations have established preferred provider organizations, exclusive provider organizations, and management service organizations. Emphases are freedom of choice and preservation of the physician–patient relationship.

Medical necessity: Healthcare services and supplies that are proven or acknowledged to be effective in the diagnosis, treatment, cure, or relief of a health condition, illness, injury, disease, or its symptoms and to be consistent with the community's accepted standard of care. Under medical necessity, only those services, procedures, and patient care are provided that are warranted by the patient's condition.

Medicare: Federally funded healthcare benefits program for those persons sixty-five years of age and older, as well as for those entitled to Social Security benefits.

Medicare Advantage (Part C): Optional managed care plan for Medicare beneficiaries who are entitled to Part A, are enrolled in Part B, and live in an area with a plan. Types of plans available include health maintenance organization, point-of-service plan, preferred provider organization, and provider-sponsored organization (formerly Medicare+Choice).

Medicare carrier: Contractor with Medicare to process Medicare Part B claims; determines charges allowed by Medicare and makes payment to physicians and suppliers on behalf of Medicare.

Medicare Modernization Act of 2003 (MMA): Most significant legislative change to the Medicare Program since its creation; the law created the outpatient prescription drug benefit and provided expanded coverage choices and improved benefits.

Medicare Part A: The portion of Medicare that provides benefits for inpatient hospital services.

Medicare Part B: An optional and supplemental portion of Medicare that provides benefits for physician services, medical services, and medical supplies not covered by Medicare Part A.

Medicare Part C: Also known as Medicare Advantage, this is a managed care option that includes services under Parts A, B and D and additional services that are not typically covered by Medicare; Medicare Part C requires an additional premium; plan known formerly as Medicare+Choice.

Medicare Part D: Medicare drug benefit created by the Medicare Modernization Act of 2003 (MMA) that offers outpatient drug coverage to beneficiaries for an additional premium.

Medicare Summary Notice: Statement that describes services rendered, payment covered, and benefits limits and denials for Medicare beneficiaries.

Medigap: Type of private insurance policy available for Medicare beneficiaries to supplement Medicare Part A and or Part B coverage.

Member: Individual or entity that purchases healthcare insurance coverage. *See also* Certificate holder, Insured, Policyholder, *and* Subscriber.

Metropolitan division: County or group of counties within a core-based statistical area (CBSA) that contains a core with a population of at least 2.5 million. A metropolitan division consists of one or more main/secondary counties that represent an employment center or centers, plus adjacent counties associated with the main county or counties through commuting ties. *See also* Core-based statistical area.

Metropolitan statistical area (MSA): Core-based statistical area associated with at least one urbanized area that has a population of at least 50,000. The MSA comprises the central county or counties containing the core, plus adjacent outlying counties. *See also* Core-based statistical area (CBSA).

Minimum data set (MDS): Standardized, comprehensive assessment instrument that the Centers for Medicare and Medicaid Services (CMS) requires be completed for residents of skilled nursing facilities. The MDS collects administrative and clinical information. States have the option of having supplemental data collected with the approval of CMS.

Modifier: Two-digit alpha/alphanumeric/numeric code that provides the means by which a physician or facility can indicate that a service provided to the patient has been altered by some special circumstance(s), but for which the basic code description itself has not changed.

Mortality: The incidence of death.

Motor: Related to movement of muscles and coordination and includes both large motor skills, such as walking, and fine motor skills, such as buttoning and zipping clothing.

National Center for Health Statistics (NCHS): Organization that developed the clinical modification to the International Classification of Diseases, Ninth Revision (ICD-9); responsible for maintaining and updating the diagnosis portion of the International Classification of Diseases, 9th revision, Clinical Modification (ICD-9-CM).

National Correct Coding Initiative (NCCI): A set of coding regulations to prevent fraud and abuse in physician and hospital outpatient coding; specifically addresses unbundling and mutually exclusive procedures.

National Coverage Determination (NCD): National medical necessity and reimbursement regulations.

National standard episode amount: Set dollar amount (conversion factor, constant, across-the-board multiplier), unadjusted for geographic differences, that is multiplied with the weights of the health insurance prospective payment system (HIPPS) codes in the home health prospective payment system (HHPPS). The amount for each year is published in the *Federal Register.*

National unadjusted copayment: Set dollar amount, unadjusted for geographic differences, that beneficiaries pay under the hospital outpatient prospective payment system (HOPPS).

National unadjusted payment: Product of the conversion factor multiplied by the relative weight, unadjusted for geographic differences.

Network: Physicians, hospitals, and other providers who provide healthcare services to members of a managed care organization. Providers may be associated through formal or informal contracts and agreements.

Network model: Type of health maintenance organization (HMO) in which the HMO contracts with two or more medical groups and reimburses the groups on a fee-for-service or capitation basis. (*See also* Group practice model.)

New technology: Advance in medical technology that substantially improves, relative to technologies previously available, the diagnosis or treatment of Medicare beneficiaries. Applicants for the status in new technology must submit a formal request, including a full description of the clinical applications of the technology and the results of any clinical evaluations demonstrating that the new technology represents a substantial clinical improvement, along with data to demonstrate the technology meets the high cost threshold.

Nonlabor share (portion, ratio): Facilities' operating costs not related to labor (typically 25 to 30 percent). *See also* Labor-related share.

Observation: Service in which providers observe and monitor a patient to decide whether the patient needs to be admitted to inpatient care or can be discharged to home or an outpatient area, usually charged by the hour.

Office of Inspector General (OIG): A division of the Department of Health and Human Services (DHHS) that investigates issues of noncompliance in the Medicare and Medicaid programs such as fraud and abuse.

Office of Inspector General (OIG) Workplan: Yearly plan released by the OIG that outlines the focus for reviews and investigates in various healthcare settings.

Operating room (OR) procedure: Procedure that physician panel classified as occurring in the operating room in most hospitals. Presence of an OR procedure groups a case to a surgical diagnosis related group (DRG).

Operation Restore Trust: A 1995 joint effort of the Department of Health and Human Services (DHHS), Office of Inspector General (OIG), the Centers for Medicare and Medicaid Services (CMS), and the Administration of Aging (AOA) to target fraud and abuse among healthcare providers.

Out-of-pocket: Payment made by the policyholder or member.

Outcome Assessment Information Set (OASIS): Set of data elements that represent core items of a comprehensive assessment for an adult home care patient. OASIS is used to measure patient outcomes in outcome-based quality improvement (OBQI). This assessment is performed on every patient who receives services from home health agencies that participate in the Medicare or Medicaid programs. The OASIS is the basis of the home health prospective payment system (HHPPS).

Outlier: Cases in prospective payment systems with unusually long lengths of stay or exceptionally high costs; day outlier or cost outlier, respectively.

Outpatient code editor (OCE): *See* Editor.

Outpatient Service Mix Index (SMI): The sum of the weights of ambulatory payment classification groups for patients treated during a given period divided by the total volume of patients treated.

Packaging: Combination of an ancillary service with its related procedure or service for one lump-sum payment in the hospital outpatient prospective payment system.

Partial hospitalization: Program of intensive psychotherapy that is provided in a day outpatient setting and is designed to keep patients with severe mental conditions from being hospitalized in an inpatient unit.

Pass-through: Exception to the Medicare prospective payment systems (PPSs) for a high-cost service. The exception minimizes the negative financial impact of the lump-sum payments of the PPSs. Pass-throughs are not included in the PPSs and are passed through to cost-based (retrospective) payment mechanisms. In the hospital outpatient prospective payment system (HOPPS), the Centers for Medicare and Medicaid Services (CMS) created exceptions for some expensive drugs, pharmaceuticals, biologicals, and devices. Rather than being bundled or packaged, these exceptions to the CMS's HOPPS are "passed-through" the HOPPS to other payment mechanisms (payment status indicators F, G, H, and J). The inpatient prospective payment system (IPPS) passes through the costs of medical education and organ acquisition and some capital costs.

Payment Error Prevention Program (PEPP): Payment compliance program established under the 6th Scope of Work to help healthcare facilities identify simple mistakes that are causing payment errors; monitored by Quality Improvement Organizations (QIOs).

Payment status indictor (PSI). Alphabetic code that provides payment information in the hospital outpatient prospective payment system (HOPPS).

There are two types of indicators. The first type designates one of three major categories of reimbursement *outside* the ambulatory patient classification (APC) system (A, C, and E). The second type gives directions related to payment rules for APC payments (D, F, G, H, K, L, N, P, S, T, V, and X).

Per diem (per day): Type of prospective payment method in which the third party payer reimburses the provider a fixed rate for each day a covered member is hospitalized.

Per member per month (PMPM): Amount of money paid monthly for each individual enrolled in a capitation-based health insurance plan.

Physician care group (PCG): Type of outpatient prospective payment method for physician services in which patients are classified into similar, homogenous categories.

Physician work (WORK): Component or element of the relative value unit (RVU) that should cover the physician's salary. This work is the time the physician spends providing a service and the intensity with which that time is spent. The four elements of intensity are: (a) mental effort and judgment, (b) technical skill, (c) physical effort, and (d) psychological stress.

Physician-hospital organization (PHO): Hybrid type of integrated delivery system that is a legal entity formed by a hospital and a group of physicians.

Point-of-service (POS) healthcare insurance plan: Plan in which members choose how to receive services at the time they need the services, also known as open-ended HMOs.

Policy: Binding contract issued by a healthcare insurance company to an individual or group in which the company promises to pay for healthcare to treat illness or injury (also known as health plan agreement and evidence of coverage).

Policyholder: Individual or entity that purchases healthcare insurance coverage. *See also* Insured, Certificate holder, Member, *and* Subscriber.

Practice expenses (PE): Element of the relative value unit (RVU) that covers the physician's overhead costs, such as employee wages, office rent, supplies, and equipment. There are two types, facility and nonfacility.

Practice without walls (PWW): *See* Group practice without walls (PWW).

Preadmission certification: *See* Prior approval (authorization).

Preadmission review: *See* Prior approval (authorization).

Preauthorization: *See* Prior approval (authorization).

Preauthorization (precertification) number: Control number issued when a healthcare service is approved.

Precertification: *See* Prior approval (authorization).

Preexisting condition: Disease, illness, ailment, or other condition (whether physical or mental) for which, within six months before the insured's enrollment date of coverage, medical advice, diagnosis, care, or treatment was recommended or received. Healthcare coverage may be denied for a period of time for a preexisting condition. The Health Insurance Portability and Accountability Act (HIPAA) constrains the use of exclusions for preexisting conditions and establishes requirements exclusions for preexisting conditions must satisfy.

Preferred provider organization (PPO): Entity that contracts with employers and insurers to render, through a network of providers, healthcare services to a group of members. Members can choose to use the healthcare services of any physician, hospital, or other healthcare provider. Members who choose to use the services of in-network (in-plan) providers have lower out-of-pocket expenses than members who choose to use the services of out-of-network (out-of-plan) providers.

Premium: Amount of money that policyholder or certificate holder must periodically pay a healthcare insurance plan in return for healthcare coverage.

Prescription management: Cost control measure that expands the use of a formulary to include patient education; electronic screening, alert, and decision-support tools; expert and referent systems; criteria for drug utilization; point-of-service order entry; electronic prescription transmission; and patient-specific medication profiles.

Pricer: Software module in Medicare claims processing systems, specific to certain benefits, used in pricing claims and calculating payment rates and payments, most often under prospective payment systems.

Primary care physician (PCP): Physician who provides, supervises, and coordinates the healthcare of a member. Family and general practitioners, internists, pediatricians, and obstetricians/gynecologists are primary care physicians. *See also* Primary care provider.

Primary care provider (PCP): Healthcare provider who provides, supervises, and coordinates the healthcare of a member. The PCP makes referrals to specialists and for advanced diagnostic testing. Family and general practitioners, internists, pediatricians, and obstetricians/gynecologists are primary care physicians. Other PCPs include nurse practitioners and physician assistants. *See also* Primary care physician.

Primary insurer (payer): Entity responsible for the greatest proportion or majority of the healthcare expenses. *See* Secondary insurer.

Principal diagnosis: Reason established after study to be chiefly responsible for occasioning the admission of the patient to the hospital for care.

Prior approval (authorization): Process of obtaining approval from a healthcare insurance company before receiving healthcare services (also known as precertification).

Program for Evaluation Payment Patterns Electronic Report (PEPPER): A benchmarking database maintained by the Texas Medical Foundation that supplies individual QIOs with hospital data to determine state benchmarks and monitor hospital compliance.

Programs of All-Inclusive Care for Elderly (PACE): A joint Medicare–Medicaid venture that allows states to choose a managed care option for providing benefits to the frail elderly population.

Prospective payment method: Type of episode-of-care reimbursement in which the third party payer establishes the payment rates for healthcare services in advance for a specific time period.

Prospective payment system (PPS): Method of reimbursement in which payment rates for healthcare services are established in advance for a specific time period. The predetermined rates are based on average levels of resource use for certain types of healthcare.

Provider: Physician, clinic, hospital, nursing home, or other healthcare entity (second party) rendering the care.

Provider-sponsored organization (PSO): Type of point-of-service plan in which the physicians that practice in a regional or community hospital organize the plan.

Quality Improvement Organization (QIO): Medicare contractor that is responsible for carrying a specified scope of work during a three-year period; monitors and assists healthcare facilities with quality, payment, treatment denial, and health information technology issues.

Quintile: Portion of a frequency distribution containing one-fifth of the total cases.

Refined case-based payment method: Case-based payment method enhanced to include patients from all age groups or from regions of the world with varying mixes of diseases and differing patterns of healthcare delivery.

Regression analysis: Statistical technique that uses an independent variable to predict the value of a dependent value. In the inpatient psychiatric facility prospective payment system (IPF PPS), patient demographics and length of stay (independent variables) were used to predict cost of care (dependent variable).

Rehabilitation facility: Facility specializing in the restorative processes and therapies that develop and maintain self-sufficient functioning consistent with individuals' capabilities. Rehabilitative services restore function after an illness or injury. Services are provided by physiatrists and nurses and physical, occupational, and speech therapists.

Rehabilitation impairment category (RIC): Clusters of impairment group codes (IGCs) that represent similar impairments and diagnoses. RICs are the larger umbrella division within the inpatient rehabilitation facility prospective payment system (IRF PPS). From the RICs, the case-mix groups (CMGs) are determined.

Reimbursement: Compensation or repayment for healthcare services already rendered.

Relative value scale (RVS): System designed to permit comparisons of the resources needed or appropriate prices for various units of service. It takes into account labor, skill, supplies, equipment, space, and other costs for each procedure or service.

Relative value unit (RVU): Unit of measure designed to permit comparison of the amount of resources required to perform various provider services by assigning weights to such factors as personnel time, level of skill, and sophistication of equipment required to render service. In the resource-based relative value scale (RBRVS), the RVU reflects national averages and is the sum of the physician work, practice expenses, and malpractice. RVUs are adjusted to local costs through the geographic practice cost indexes (GPCIs). *See also* Physician work, Practice expenses, Malpractice, *and* Geographic practice cost index.

Relative weight (RW): Assigned weight that reflects the relative resource consumption associating with a payment classification or group. Higher payments are associated with higher relative weights.

Remittance advice: Report sent by third party payer that outlines claim rejections, denials, and payments to the facility; sent via electronic data interchange.

Resource utilization group (RUG): Classification for resources used in nursing homes. Patients are classified into one of forty-four possible RUGs based on resident information collected in the minimum data set (MDS). The RUG subsequently classifies residents into seven payment categories.

Resource-based relative value scale (RBRVS): Type of retrospective fee-for-service payment method that classifies health services based on the cost of providing physician services in terms of effort, practice expense (overhead), and malpractice insurance.

Retrospective payment method: Type of fee-for-service reimbursement in which providers receive recompense after health services have been rendered.

Revenue cycle: The regularly repeating set of events that produces revenue.

Revenue cycle management: The supervision of all administrative and clinical functions that contribute to the capture, management, and collection of patient service revenue.

Rider: Document added to a healthcare insurance policy that provides details about coverage or lack of coverage for special situations that are not usually included in standard policies. May function as an exclusion or limitation.

Risk: Probability of incurring loss.

Risk pool: Group of people who will be covered by the healthcare insurance plan.

Rural area: Geographic area outside an urban area and its constituent counties or county equivalents. *See also* Core-based statistical area (CBSA) *and* Metropolitan statistical area (MSA).

Scope of Work: The contract specifications for quality improvement organizations (QIOs) to complete during their three-year contract period.

Second opinion: Cost containment measure to prevent unnecessary tests, treatments, medical devices, or surgical procedures.

Secondary insurer (payer): Entity responsible for the remainder of the healthcare expenses after the primary insurer pays. *See* Primary insurer.

Self-insured plan: Method of insurance in which the employer or other association itself administers the health insurance benefits for its employees or their dependents, thereby assuming the risks for the costs of healthcare for the group.

Self-pay: Type of fee-for-service reimbursement in which the patients or their guarantors pay for a specific amount for each service received.

Short-stay outlier: Hospitalization that is five-sixths of the geometric length of stay for the long-term care diagnosis related group (LTC-DRG).

Social Security Act: Federal legislation providing support for state public health activities and healthcare services for mothers and children; amended in 1965 to establish the Medicare and Medicaid programs.

Sole community hospital: Hospital that, by reason of factors such as isolated location, weather conditions, travel conditions, or absence of other hospitals (as determined by the Secretary of the Department of Health and Human Services [DHHS]), is the sole source of patient hospital services reasonably available to individuals in a geographical area who are entitled to benefits.

Staff model: Type of health maintenance organization (HMO) that provides hospitalization and physicians' services through its own staff and facilities (also known as closed panel).

Standard federal rate: National base payment amount in the prospective payment system for long-term care hospitals (PPS for LTC). This amount is multiplied with the relative weight of the long-term care diagnosis related group (LTC-DRG) to calculate the unadjusted payment. Published annually in the *Federal Register.*

Standardized payment: National base amount in the inpatient rehabilitation facility prospective payment system (IRF PPS). This amount is multiplied with the relative weight of the case mix group to calculate the unadjusted payment. Published annually in the *Federal Register.*

State Children's Health Insurance Program (SCHIP): A state–federal partnership created by the Balanced Budget Act of 1997 that provides health insurance to children of families whose income level is too high to qualify for Medicaid but too low to purchase healthcare insurance.

Stop-loss benefit: Specific amount, in a certain time frame such as one year, beyond which all covered healthcare services for that policyholder or dependent are paid at 100 percent by the healthcare insurance plan. *See also* Maximum out-of-pocket cost *and* Catastrophic expense limit.

Subscriber: Individual or entity that purchases healthcare insurance coverage. *See also* Certificate holder, Insured, Member, *and* Policyholder.

Teaching hospital: Hospital engaged in an approved graduate medical education residency program in medicine, osteopathy, dentistry, or podiatry.

Temporary Assistance for Needy Families Program (TANF): Replaced the Aid to Families with Dependent Children program; this program provides states with grant money designated to provide low-income families with assistance.

Third opinion: Cost containment measure to prevent unnecessary tests, treatments, medical devices, or surgical procedures.

Third party payer: Insurance company or health agency that pays the physician, clinic, or other healthcare provider (second party) for the care or services to the patient (first party). An insurance company or healthcare benefits program that reimburses healthcare providers and/or patient for covered medical services.

Third party payment: Payments for healthcare services made by an insurance company or health agency on behalf of the insured.

Title: Short name of a diagnosis related group (DRG), such as DRG 1, Craniotomy Age >17 Except for Trauma.

Transfer: Discharge of a patient from a hospital and readmission to postacute care or another acute care hospital on the same day.

TRICARE: The healthcare program for active duty and retired members of one of the seven uniformed services administered by the Department of Defense; formerly known as Civilian Health and Medical Program of the Uniformed Services (CHAMPUS).

TRICARE Extra: A healthcare program available for active duty family members (ADFM) that requires an annual deductible and a 20 percent copayment for services rendered by a TRICARE network provider.

TRICARE for Life (TFL): Secondary coverage for TRICARE beneficiaries who become entitled to Medicare Part A.

TRICARE Prime: The managed care option for the TRICARE program available for active duty family members (ADFM) who live or work within fifty miles or an hours drive of a military treatment facility.

TRICARE Prime Remote: The managed care option for the TRICARE program available for active duty family members (ADFM) who live or work in remote areas.

TRICARE Standard: A healthcare program available for active duty family members (ADFM) that requires an annual deductible plus 25 percent cost sharing of charges for services rendered by a TRICARE authorized provider.

Trim point: Numeric value that identifies atypically long lengths of stay (LOS) or high costs (long stay outliers and cost outliers, respectively). Commonly trim points are plus or minus three standard deviations from the mean. *See also* Outlier.

Unbundling: The fraudulent process in which individual component codes are submitted for reimbursement rather than one comprehensive code.

Upcoding: The fraudulent process of submitting codes for reimbursement that indicates a more complex or higher paying services than that which the patient actually received.

Urban area: Core-based statistical area (CBSA).

Usual, customary, and reasonable (UCR): Type of retrospective fee-for-service payment method in which the third party payer pays for fees that are usual, customary, and reasonable, wherein "usual" is for usual for the individual provider's practice; "customary" means customary for the community; and "reasonable" is reasonable for the situation.

Utilization review: The process of determining whether a patient's medical care is necessary according to established guidelines and regulations. Cost containment measure that assesses the appropriateness of the setting for the healthcare service in the continuum of care and the level of service.

Wage index: Ratio that represents the relationship between the average wages in a healthcare setting's geographic area and the national average for that healthcare setting. Wage indexes are adjusted annually and published in the *Federal Register.*

Waiting period: Time between the effective date of a healthcare insurance policy and the date the healthcare insurance plan will assume liability for expenses related to certain health services, such as those related to preexisting conditions.

Withhold: Portion of providers' capitated payments that managed care organizations deduct and hold in order to create an incentive for efficient or reduced use of healthcare services (also known as physician contingency reserve [PCR]).

Withhold pool: Aggregate amount withheld from all providers' capitation payments as an amount to cover expenditures in excess of targets.

Workers' Compensation: Medical and income insurance coverage for employees who suffer from a work-related injury or illness.

World Health Organization (WHO): Organization that created and maintains the International Classification of Diseases (ICD) used throughout the world to collect morbidity and mortality information.

Appendix B
Additional Readings and Resources

Coding Ethically

June Bronnert, RHIA, CCS

With the many reimbursement issues and regulatory requirements surrounding coding, it is sometimes necessary for coders to refamiliarize themselves with what it means to code ethically. AHIMA's Coding Policy and Strategy Committee developed the Standards of Ethical Coding, which were approved by AHIMA's Board of Directors in 2000.[1] The standards were developed to help coders address these issues.

While it is recommended that all those performing coding functions follow the standards, credentialed coders are required to follow this code in order to maintain their credentials. Coders sometimes take for granted the ethical decisions they face on a daily basis. What are the standards and how should coders follow them? This article will present various situations and potential action items coders may engage in to abide by the Standards of Ethical Coding.

The Standards

1. Coding professionals are expected to support the importance of accurate, complete, and consistent coding practices for the production of quality healthcare data.

2. Coding professionals in all healthcare settings should adhere to the ICD-9-CM (International Classification of Diseases, 9th revision, Clinical Modification) coding conventions, official coding guidelines approved by the Cooperating Parties, the CPT (Current Procedural Terminology) rules established by the American Medical Association, and any other official coding rules and guidelines established for use with mandated standard code sets. Selection and sequencing of diagnoses and procedures must meet the definitions of required data sets for applicable healthcare settings.

3. Coding professionals should use their skills, their knowledge of currently mandated coding and classification systems, and official resources to select the appropriate diagnostic and procedural codes.

4. Coding professionals should only assign and report codes that are clearly and consistently supported by physician documentation in the health record.

5. Coding professionals should consult physicians for clarification and additional documentation prior to code assignment when there is conflicting or ambiguous data in the health record.

6. Coding professionals should not change codes or the narratives of codes on the billing abstract so that meanings are misrepresented. Diagnoses or procedures should not be inappropriately included or excluded because payment or insurance policy coverage requirements will be affected. When individual payer policies conflict with official coding rules and guidelines, these policies should be obtained in writing whenever possible. Reasonable efforts should be made to educate the payer on proper coding practices in order to influence a change in the payer's policy.

7. Coding professionals, as members of the healthcare team, should assist and educate physicians and other clinicians by advocating proper documentation practices, further specificity, and resequencing or inclusion of diagnoses or procedures when needed to more accurately reflect the acuity, severity, and the occurrence of events.

8. Coding professionals should participate in the development of institutional coding policies and should ensure that coding policies complement, not conflict with, official coding rules and guidelines.

9. Coding professionals should maintain and continually enhance their coding skills, as they have a professional responsibility to stay abreast of changes in codes, coding guidelines, and regulations.

10. Coding professionals should strive for optimal payment to which the facility is legally entitled, remembering that it is unethical and illegal to maximize payment by means that contradict regulatory guidelines.[2]

Coding compliance plans usually include AHIMA's standards, and coders agree that coding behaviors should follow accordingly. However, what does this mean when performing the day-to-day coding tasks, when records are on your desk waiting to be coded? You know that a coding backlog is building due to various open positions, and your supervisor informs you that the current productivity standards are being reviewed for a potential increase. You have just received the latest edition of *CPT Assistant*, but it, along with the previous issue, remains unopened and unread on your desk.

The ethical standards are a part of these everyday situations and should provide a guide when making decisions on how to handle these events. Assessment of coder performance should take into account adherence to each of these standards.

Case Study

A Medicare patient presents to the laboratory for a complete blood count but forgets to bring the physician's order. Registration calls the physician's office, and they fax over the physician's order. However a diagnosis is not present on the order. When the encounter is ready for coding, the coder must query the physician for more documentation. The coder also knows that the test is covered by a local coverage determination, so the coder asks the physician to provide a medically necessary diagnosis. What standards does this violate?

The coder in this situation violates multiple standards:

Standard 4. Coding professionals should only assign and report codes that are clearly and consistently supported by physician documentation. It is not appropriate to refer to coverage determinations to pinpoint diagnoses that support medical necessity, nor is it acceptable to pick up diagnoses from prior records if they are not documented in the current visit record. This would be an example of a leading query. All HIM departments should carefully review their physician query forms to ensure that they comply with AHIMA's practice brief "Developing a Physician Query Process," which can be found online in the FORE Library: HIM Body of Knowledge at www.ahima.org.

Standard 5. Coding professionals should consult physicians for clarification of conflicting or ambiguous data.

Standard 6. Diagnoses or procedures should not be inappropriately included or excluded because payment or insurance policy coverage requirements will be affected.

Out of Compliance?

The second standard states that coding professionals in all settings should adhere to the ICD-9-CM and CPT coding conventions as published by the cooperating parties for ICD-9-CM and American Medical Association, respectively. While this appears to be basic, coders may often be out of compliance with this standard, which occurs in the following situations:

- Misidentification of the principal diagnosis that results in an inaccurate Diagnosis Related Group (DRG) assignment

- Misassignment of a CPT code that reports a procedure more complex than actually performed, resulting in a higher-weighted Ambulatory Payment Classification (APC)

- Assignment of multiple CPT codes when only one is necessary to obtain higher APC reimbursement

Coding professionals are also responsible for maintaining continuing education through a variety of methods, the most common being seminars, audio seminars, or quizzes. However, coding professionals need to be responsible for reviewing the official sources of coding advice, *Coding Clinic for ICD-9-CM* and *CPT Assistant*. The department management is responsible for making these resources available to all coders, but coders are responsible for reading them. The "Minutes of the Coordination and Maintenance Committee for

ICD-9-CM" and the book *CPT Update: An Insider's View* are excellent resources to understand the rationales behind the coding changes. If a coder does not comply with the above, he or she would be violating both standards 3 and 9.

The final standard of ethical coding states that coding professionals should strive for optimal payment to which the facility is legally entitled. This means the appropriate reimbursement for the services rendered, paid as expeditiously as feasible. Acute care inpatient facilities failing to validate DRG assignments are not only demonstrating poor revenue cycle management but also violating this standard by not verifying proper reimbursement.

Potential Violations

Pamela R. Yokubaitis's article "Are Ethics Guiding Your Workplace?" quotes Michael Daigneault's eight "reasons" that people give for ethical lapses:

- I have to cut corners to meet my goals.

- I lack the time or resources to do what is right.

- My peers expect me to act this way.

- My superiors want results, not excuses.

- I don't think it is really wrong or illegal.

- Others would think it is a good choice.

- No one will ever know the difference.

- I am afraid to do what I know is right. [3]

Do not let yourself fall into one of these categories. Be knowledgeable of the standards and how they influence your professional career. If a violation of these standards occurs, AHIMA has a process for reporting the allegations. A completed and signed form is submitted to AHIMA by either another AHIMA member, HIM professional, employer, or regulatory agency representative within one year of the alleged violation. A professional conduct committee has a complaint review subcommittee review the allegation. This subcommittee may either dismiss the case, proceed with an additional investigation, or proceed with a formal hearing. Various disciplinary actions could occur ranging from a letter of complaint dismissal to revocation of certification.

Coders will be faced with ethical challenges most days, and it is important to know the standards and how they apply in order to make the best decisions possible when solving your ethical dilemmas.

Notes

1. AHIMA. "Standards of Ethical Coding." *Journal of AHIMA* 71, no. 3 (2000): insert.

2. Ibid.

3. Yokubaitis, Pamela R. "Are Ethics Guiding Your Workplace?" *Journal of AHIMA* 74, no. 8 (2003): 66–68.

Developing a Coding Compliance Policy Document

Organizations using diagnosis and procedure codes for reporting healthcare services must have formal policies and corresponding procedures in place that provide instruction on the entire process—from the point of service to the billing statement or claim form. Coding compliance policies serve as a guide to performing coding and billing functions and provide documentation of the organization's intent to correctly report services. The policies should include facility-specific documentation requirements, payer regulations and policies, and contractual arrangements for coding consultants and outsourcing services. This information may be covered in payer/provider contracts or found in Medicare and Medicaid manuals and bulletins.

Following are selected tenets that address the process of code selection and reporting. These tenets may be referred to as coding protocols, a coding compliance program, organizational coding guidelines, or a similar name. These tenets are an important part of any organization's compliance plan and the key to preventing coding errors and resulting reimbursement problems. Examples are taken from both outpatient and inpatient coding processes for illustration purposes only. This document cannot serve as a complete coding compliance plan, but will be useful as a guide for creating a more comprehensive resource to meet individual organizational needs.

A coding compliance plan should include the following components:

- A general policy statement about the commitment of the organization to correctly assign and report codes

Example: Memorial Medical Center is committed to establishing and maintaining clinical coding and insurance claims processing procedures to ensure that reported codes reflect actual services provided, through accurate information system entries.

- The source of the official coding guidelines used to direct code selection

Example: ICD-9-CM code selection follows the Official Guidelines for Coding and Reporting, developed by the cooperating parties and documented in *Coding Clinic for ICD-9-CM*, published by the American Hospital Association.

Example: CPT code selection follows the guidelines set forth in the CPT manual and in *CPT Assistant*, published by the American Medical Association.

- The parties responsible for code assignment. The ultimate responsibility for code assignment lies with the physician (provider). However, policies and procedures may document instances where codes may be selected or modified by authorized individuals

Example: For inpatient records, medical record analyst I staff are responsible for analysis of records and assignment of the correct ICD-9-CM codes based on documentation by the attending physician.

Example: Emergency department evaluation and management levels for physician services will be selected by the physician and validated by outpatient record analysts using the HCFA/AMA documentation guidelines. When a variance occurs, the following steps are taken for resolution (The actual document should follow with procedure details).

- The procedure to follow when the clinical information is not clear enough to assign the correct code

Example: When the documentation used to assign codes is ambiguous or incomplete, the physician must be contacted to clarify the information and complete/amend the record, if necessary. (The actual document should follow with details of how the medical staff would like this to occur, e.g., by phone call, by note on the record, etc.). Standard protocols for adding documentation to a record must be followed, in accordance with the applicable laws and regulations.

- Specify the policies and procedures that apply to specific locations and care settings. Official coding guidelines for inpatient reporting and outpatient/physician reporting are different. This means that if you are developing a facility-specific coding guideline for emergency department services, designate that the coding rules or guidelines only apply in this setting

Example: When reporting an injection of a drug provided in the emergency department to a Medicare beneficiary, the appropriate CPT code for the administration of the injection is reported in addition to the evaluation and management service code and drug code. CPT codes are reported whether a physician provides the injection personally or a nurse is carrying out a physician's order. This instruction does not always apply for reporting of professional services in the clinics, because administration of medication is considered bundled with the corresponding evaluation and management service for Medicare patients.

Example: Diagnoses that are documented as "probable," "suspected," "questionable," "rule-out," or "working diagnosis" are not to have a code assigned as a confirmed diagnosis. Instead, the code for the condition established at the close of the encounter should be assigned, such as a symptom, sign, abnormal test result, or clinical finding. This guideline applies only to outpatient services.

- Applicable reporting requirements required by specific agencies. The document should include where instructions on payer-specific requirements may be accessed

Example: For patients with XYZ care plan, report code S0800 for patients having a LASIK procedure rather than an unlisted CPT code.

Example: For Medicare patients receiving a wound closure by tissue adhesive only, report HCPCS Level II code G0168 rather than a CPT code.

Many of these procedures will be put into software databases and would not be written as a specific policy. This is true with most billing software, whether for physician services or through the charge description master used by many hospitals.

- Procedures for correction of inaccurate code assignments in the clinical database and to the agencies where the codes have been reported

Example: When an error in code assignment is discovered after bill release and the claim has already been submitted, this is the process required to update and correct the information system and facilitate claim amendment or correction (The actual document should follow with appropriate details).

- Areas of risk that have been identified through audits or monitoring. Each organization should have a defined audit plan for code accuracy and consistency review and corrective actions should be outlined for problems that are identified

Example: A hospital might identify that acute respiratory failure is being assigned as the principal diagnosis with congestive heart failure as a secondary diagnosis. The specific reference to *Coding Clinic* could be listed with instructions about correct coding of these conditions and the process to be used to correct the deficiency.

- Identification of essential coding resources available to and used by the coding professionals

Example: Updated ICD-9-CM, CPT, and HCPCS Level II code books are used by all coding professionals. Even if the hospital uses automated encoding software, at least one printed copy of the coding manuals should be available for reference.

Example: Updated encoder software, including the appropriate version of the NCCI edits and DRG and APC grouper software, is available to the appropriate personnel.

Example: *Coding Clinic* and *CPT Assistant* are available to all coding professionals.

- A process for coding new procedures or unusual diagnoses

Example: When the coding professional encounters an unusual diagnosis, the coding supervisor or the attending physician is consulted. If, after research, a code cannot be identified, the documentation is submitted to the AHA for clarification.

- A procedure to identify any optional codes gathered for statistical purposes by the facility and clarification of the appropriate use of E codes

Example: All ICD-9-CM procedure codes in the surgical range (ICD-9-CM Volume III codes 01.01–86.99) shall be reported for inpatients. In addition, codes reported from the non-surgical section include the following (Completed document should list the actual codes to be reported).

Example: All appropriate E codes for adverse effects of drugs must be reported. In addition, this facility reports all E codes, including the place of injury for poisonings, all cases of abuse, and all accidents on the initial visit for both inpatient and outpatient services.

- Appropriate methods for resolving coding or documentation disputes with physicians

Example: When the physician disagrees with official coding guidelines, the case is referred to the medical records committee following review by the designated physician liaison from that group.

- A procedure for processing claim rejections

Example: All rejected claims pertaining to diagnosis and procedure codes should be returned to coding staff for review or correction. Any chargemaster issues should be forwarded to appropriate departmental staff for corrections. All clinical codes, including modifiers, must never be changed or added without review by coding staff with access to the appropriate documentation.

Example: If a claim is rejected due to the codes provided in the medical record abstract, the billing department notifies the supervisor of coding for a review rather than changing the code to a payable code and resubmitting the claim.

- A statement clarifying that codes will not be assigned, modified, or excluded solely for the purpose of maximizing reimbursement. Clinical codes will not be changed or amended merely due to either physicians' or patients' request to have the service in question covered by insurance. If the initial code assignment did not reflect the actual services, codes may be revised based on supporting documentation. Disputes with either physicians or patients are handled only by the coding supervisor and are appropriately logged for review

Example: A patient calls the business office saying that her insurance carrier did not pay for her mammogram. After investigating, the HIM coding staff discover that the coding was appropriate for a screening mammogram and that this is a non-covered service with the insurance provider. The code is not changed and the matter is referred back to the business office for explanation to the patient that she should contact her insurance provider with any dispute over coverage of service.

Example: Part of a payment is denied and after review, the supervisor discovers that a modifier should have been appended to the CPT code to denote a separately identifiable service. Modifier -25 is added to the code set and the corrected claim is resubmitted.

Example: A physician approaches the coding supervisor with a request to change the diagnosis codes for his patient because what she currently has is a pre-existing condition that is not covered by her current health plan. The coding supervisor must explain to the physician that falsification of insurance claims is illegal. If the physician insists, the physician liaison for the medical record committee is contacted and the matter is turned over to that committee for resolution if necessary.

- The use of and reliance on encoders within the organization. Coding staff cannot rely solely on computerized encoders. Current coding manuals must be readily accessible and the staff must be educated appropriately to detect inappropriate logic or errors in encoding software. When errors in logic or code crosswalks are discovered, they are reported to the vendor immediately by the coding supervisor

Example: During the coding process, an error is identified in the crosswalk between the ICD-9-CM Volume III code and the CPT code. This error is reported to the software vendor, with proper documentation and notification of all staff using the encoder to not rely on the encoder for code selection.

- Medical records are analyzed and codes selected only with complete and appropriate documentation by the physician available. According to coding guidelines, codes are not assigned without physician documentation. If records are coded without the discharge summary or final diagnostic statements available, processes are in place for review after the summary is added to the record

Example: When records are coded without a discharge summary, they are flagged in the computer system. When the summaries are added to the record, the record is returned to the coding professional for review of codes. If there are any inconsistencies, appropriate steps are taken for review of the changes.

Additional Elements

A coding compliance document should include a reference to the AHIMA Standards of Ethical Coding, which can be downloaded from AHIMA's Web site at www.ahima.org. Reference to the data quality assessment procedures must be included in a coding compliance plan to establish the mechanism for determining areas of risk. Reviews will identify the need for further education and increased monitoring for those areas where either coding variances or documentation deficiencies are identified.

Specific and detailed coding guidelines that cover the reporting of typical services provided by a facility or organization create tools for data consistency and reliability by ensuring that all coders interpret clinical documentation and apply coding principles in the same manner. The appropriate medical staff committee should give final approval of any coding guidelines that involve clinical criteria to assure appropriateness and physician consensus on the process.

The format is most useful when organized by patient or service type and easily referenced by using a table of contents. If the facility-specific guidelines are maintained electronically, they should be searchable by key terms. Placing the coding guidelines on a facility Intranet or internal computer network is a very efficient way to ensure their use and it also enables timely and efficient updating and distribution. Inclusion of references to or live links should be provided to supporting documents such as Uniform Hospital Discharge Data Sets or other regulatory requirements outlining reporting procedures or code assignments.

Prepared by

AHIMA's Coding Practice Team and reviewed by the Coding Policy and Strategy Committee and the Society for Clinical Coding Data Quality Committee

The Codes to Watch: Identifying the DRGs Most Prone to Payment Error

Kimberly Hrehor, MHA, RHIA, CHE

Monitoring codes prone to payment error is an important part of an organization's ongoing efforts to verify coding accuracy. Data from the Hospital Payment Monitoring Program (HPMP) helps identify codes most prone to errors such as over- and undercoding. Organizations can use these data to strengthen their compliance programs.

Collecting Random Samples from the States

The Centers for Medicare and Medicaid Services (CMS) has monitored Medicare inpatient payment error rates for inpatient prospective payment system (PPS) services since the Payment Error Prevention Program (PEPP) was initiated in the fall of 1999. In fall 2001 PEPP was renamed the Hospital Payment Monitoring Program. The purpose of the program remained the same: to measure, monitor, and reduce the incidence of improper payments for Medicare inpatient PPS-reimbursed services. Under this contract activity, quality improvement organizations (QIOs, formerly known as peer review organizations, or PROs) work with hospitals to identify and prevent payment errors. As a payment efficiency program, HPMP serves to protect the Medicare Trust Fund. The calculated payment error rates are also a crucial contributor to the annual fiscal statements for the agency.

To measure and monitor inpatient payment error rates, in 2001 CMS began randomly sampling final action reimbursed claims from each state, Puerto Rico, and the District of Columbia. The corresponding medical records are screened for medical necessity and validated for Diagnosis Related Group (DRG) coding errors by the clinical data abstraction centers. All records failing the screening are referred to the QIOs for full case review. An internal quality-control sample of 10 percent of records that did not fail screening is also sent for review, but error rates determined from the sample are not included in the calculated payment error rates.

In fiscal years 2000 and 2001 the sample included approximately 58,000 cases; in fiscal year 2002 the sample contained approximately 53,000 cases. Currently CMS is sampling 62 cases per state per month (except for Alaska, where 48 records are sampled monthly), an annual total of approximately 38,500 cases. At the time of this article, the latest data analyzed was from fiscal year 2002. Data for 2003 is now available for analysis, and data for 2004 is expected next year.

How Payment Errors Are Calculated

Payment errors identified in the reviews are categorized into six types:

- DRG coding errors

- Admission denials (medical necessity and appropriateness of setting)

- Billing errors

- Technical denials (recoupment of hospital reimbursement for failure to submit a medical record or for submitting a medical record that lacks necessary documentation)

- Combined DRG coding errors and admission denials

- Maryland length-of-stay errors (Maryland is a non-PPS state, and providers in the state are not reimbursed by Medicare under a DRG system.)

Payment errors are measured by dollars in error, which are calculated by determining the difference between what the hospital was paid on the originally sampled claim and what the correct payment should have been. Thus, for unnecessary admissions the dollars in error are equal to the entire reimbursement for the claim and represent an overpayment. For DRG changes, the dollars in error are equal to the difference between what the hospital was paid and the correct DRG payment. This could result in an overpayment to the hospital (in cases of overcoding) or in an underpayment to the hospital (in cases of undercoding).

The absolute value of dollars in error represents the total dollars in error, regardless of whether the hospital was overpaid or underpaid. The net dollars in error represent the net amount of dollars in error, taking into account overpayments and underpayments.

Of the six error types, DRG coding errors have not comprised a large proportion of overall dollars in error. In fiscal year 2002 DRG errors comprised 2.9 percent of the net dollars in error and 30.1 percent of the absolute value of dollars in error nationwide (see "Payment Error Snapshot," below). However, the trend over fiscal years 2000, 2001, and 2002 indicates an increase in net dollars in error for DRG changes, while the absolute value of dollars in error decreased from fiscal years 2000 to 2001 and increased from 2001 to 2002.[1] What does this mean? In essence, the net dollars in error for the nation reflected more undercoding than overcoding in 2000, which remained true, though to a lesser extent, in 2001. However, in 2002 the statistics paint a different picture: hospitals were, overall, overcoding.

Payment Error Snapshot

A national sample of DRG codes in fiscal year 2002 shows $4.8 million in overall error (absolute value of error). The positive net error amount of $330,110 indicates that more errors among the sample resulted from overpayments than underpayments.

Error Type	Description	Claims	Net Error Amount	% of Total Payment*	% of Total Net Error Amount	Absolute Value of Error Amount†	% of Total Payment*	% of Total Absolute Value of Error Amount
1	DRG Change	2,090	$330,110	0.1%	2.9%	$4,805,624	1.3%	30.1%
2, 5	Admission Denials‡	2,293	$8,806,431	2.3%	76.7%	$8,806,431	2.3%	55.2%
3	Billing Errors	293	$1,126,099	0.3%	9.8%	$1,126,099	0.3%	7.1%
4	Technical Denials	132	$1,057,941	0.3%	9.2%	$1,057,941	0.3%	6.6%
6	Maryland LOS Error	136	$166,134	0%	1.4%	$166,134	0%	1.0%
	Total	4,944	$11,486,715	3.1%		$15,962,229	4.2%	

* Total sample was 52,728 claims and total payment was $376,322,491.

† The absolute value of the error amount is the positive value of the error amount and is calculated claim by claim.

‡ Error type 2 = admission/prohibited action denial and error type 5 = admission denial and DRG change.

Overcoding: Top DRGs for Net Dollars in Error

The top 10 DRGs for net dollars in error due to overcoding in fiscal year 2002 are shown in the table below. Note that in some cases the net amount is equal to the absolute value amount. This occurs when all cases for that particular DRG were overcoded. Where these values differ, it indicates that one or more claims for that DRG were undercoded.

Many of the DRGs in this figure are familiar in terms of payment errors. Several have been studied by the Office of the Inspector General.[2-5] Many QIOs also have conducted PEPP or HPMP projects related to these DRGs. For the most part, these are high-paying DRGs.

Original DRG		Claims	Net Error Amount	Absolute Value of Error Amount
468	Extensive OR procedure unrelated to principal diagnosis	31	$233,946	$234,953
475	Respiratory system diagnosis with ventilator support	10	$127,912	$127,912
415	OR procedure for infectious & parasitic diseases	11	$113,665	$113,665
416	Septicemia age >17	32	$103,342	$107,333
014	Specific cerebrovascular disorders except TIA	44	$76,437	$78,128
483	Tracheostomy except for face, mouth & neck diagnoses	2	$63,876	$63,876
316	Renal failure	34	$62,192	$82,743
514	Cardiac defibrillator implant w/ cardiac cath	3	$49,694	$49,694
403	Lymphoma & non-acute leukemia w/ cc	14	$48,819	$48,819
076	Other resp system OR procedures w/ cc	6	$39,876	$39,876

Undercoding: Top DRGs for Net Dollars in Error

Sorting DRG errors by net dollars in error selects the top DRGs that were undercoded. A few of these DRGs may also be familiar as payment errors, as some QIOs may have conducted PEPP projects related to undercoding. Note that the net error amounts are for the most part lower than the amounts for overcoding shown above.

Original DRG	Claims	Net Error Amount	Absolute Value of Error Amount
109 Coronary bypass w/o PTCA or cardiac cath	7	-$54,404	$54,404
088 Chronic obstructive pulmonary disease	36	-$47,595	$69,467
149 Major small & large bowel procedures w/o cc	4	-$42,666	$42,666
090 Simple pneumonia & pleurisy age >17 w/o cc	25	-$39,515	$40,856
143 Chest pain	35	-$35,119	$35,404
175 GI hemorrhage w/o cc	21	-$32,885	$32,885
320 Kidney & urinary tract infections age >17 w cc	47	-$31,885	$54,660
094 Pneumothorax w/ cc	3	-$31,540	$33,337
479 Other vascular procedures w/o cc	10	-$29,101	$39,648
116 Other permanent cardiac pacemaker implant	7	-$28,337	$66,610

Top DRGs for Absolute Value of Dollars in Error

Ranking the results by absolute value of dollars in error provides another way to identify DRGs prone to payment errors. Seven of these DRGs make the top-10 overcoding or undercoding lists. Some, like DRG 079 (Respiratory infections and inflammations age >17 w/ cc), have a small net error amount but a large absolute value error amount. This indicates that both overcoding and undercoding occur, and hospitals are encouraged to focus on making sure the DRG is correct so that payment is correct.

Original DRG	Claims	Net Error Amount	Absolute Value of Error Amount
468 Extensive OR procedure unrelated to principal diagnosis	31	$233,946	$234,953
475 Respiratory system diagnosis with ventilator support	10	$127,912	$127,912
415 OR procedure for infectious & parasitic diseases	11	$113,665	$113,665
416 Septicemia age >17	32	$103,342	$107,333
079 Respiratory infections & inflammations age >17 w/ cc	23	$1,670	$106,752
089 Simple pneumonia & pleurisy age >17 w/ cc	65	-$5,643	$97,432
144 Other circulatory system diagnoses w/ cc	37	$11,755	$84,907
316 Renal failure	34	$62,192	$82,743
014 Specific cerebrovascular disorders except TIA	44	$76,437	$78,128
088 Chronic obstructive pulmonary disease	36	-$47,595	$69,467

Top DRGs for Frequency

DRGs associated with the highest dollars in error are not necessarily the errors that occur the most frequently. The top DRGs by volume of claims in error are identified below. Al- though the dollars associated with these errors may not be as great, they are worth watching simply due to their volume.

Original DRG	Claims	Net Error Amount	Absolute Value of Error Amount
089 Simple pneumonia & pleurisy age >17 w/ cc	65	-$5,643	$97,432
296 Nutritional & misc. metabolic disorders age >17 w/ cc	65	-$10,396	$61,184
182 Esophagitis, gastroent & misc digest disorders age >17 w/ cc	60	-$900	$57,203
140 Angina pectoris	53	-$27,737	$28,423
127 Heart failure & shock	52	-$5,142	$65,597
320 Kidney & urinary tract infections age >17 w cc	47	-$31,885	$54,660
014 Specific cerebrovascular disorders except TIA	44	$76,437	$78,128
144 Other circulatory system diagnoses w/ cc	37	$11,755	$84,907
088 Chronic obstructive pulmonary disease	36	-$47,595	$69,467
143 Chest pain	35	-$35,119	$35,404

Top Change Pairs by Volume

Lastly, there are some DRGs that have a tendency to be changed to another DRG. These have been identified as "DRG change pairs," and the top 10 by volume of claims are listed here. Of the 10 pairs, only two (DRGs 014-015 and 089-088) are changes to lower-paying DRGs.

Original DRG	Revised DRG	Claims	Net Error Amount	Absolute Value of Error Amount	Change
140 Angina pectoris	132 Atherosclerosis w/ cc	39	-$14,089	$14,089	Higher
090 Simple pneumonia & pleurisy age >17 w/o cc	089 Simple pneumonia & pleurisy age >17 w/ cc	20	-$32,254	$32,254	Higher
175 GI hemorrhage w/o cc	174 GI hemorrhage w/ cc	20	-$32,242	$32,242	Higher
014 Specific cerebrovascular disorders except TIA	015 Transient ischemic attack & precerebral occlusions	16	$30,791	$30,791	Lower
089 Simple pneumonia & pleurisy age >17 w/ cc	079 Respiratory infections & inflammations age >17 w/ cc	13	-$38,862	$38,862	Higher
183 Esophagitis, gastroent. & misc. digest disorders age >17 w/o cc	182 Esophagitis, gastroent & misc. digest disorders age >17 w/ cc	12	-$10,007	$10,007	Higher
125 Circulatory disorders except AMI, w/ card cath. w/o complex diag.	124 Circulatory disorders except AMI, w/ card cath & complex diag	12	-$16,936	$16,936	Higher
089 Simple pneumonia & pleurisy age >17 w/ cc	088 Chronic obstructive pulmonary disease	11	$6,561	$6,561	Lower
143 Chest pain	132 Atherosclerosis w/ cc	11	-$5,818	$5,818	Higher
096 Bronchitis & asthma age >17 w/ cc	088 Chronic obstructive pulmonary disease	11	-$4,989	$4,989	Higher

Monitoring Coding Accuracy

How can HIM coding professionals use this information? First, hospitals should ensure they have a strong coding compliance program.[6,7] HIM coding professionals should ensure that there is a process to randomly verify coding accuracy. They should also be aware of the error-prone DRGs identified in these tables. However, they should not limit their monitoring to these DRGs alone. HIM professionals are encouraged to review DRGs that are high in volume within their facility as well as others that have been associated with a high rate of payment errors or involve high reimbursement, such as DRG 475.

HIM professionals can also contact the HPMP department in their state's QIO. The QIO may be able to share data analysis related to DRG errors within the state and provide tools to assist hospitals with the identification and prevention of DRG errors. To locate state QIOs, visit the American Health Quality Association's Web site at www.ahqa.org and click on the "QIO Locator" link.

Notes

1. Centers for Medicare and Medicaid Services. "Fiscal Year 2002 Payment Error Cause Analysis." 2003. Unpublished data.

2. Office of the Inspector General, Office of Evaluations and Inspections. "DRG 79 Validation Study Update: Respiratory Infections and Inflammations." 1993. Available online at http://oig.hhs.gov/oei/reports/oei-12-89-00193.pdf.

3. Office of the Inspector General, Office of Evaluations and Inspections. "Medicare Payments for DRG 296: Nutritional and Miscellaneous Metabolic Disorders." 1999. Available online at http://oig.hhs.gov/oei/reports/oei-03-98-00490.pdf.

4. Office of the Inspector General, Office of Evaluations and Inspections. "Medicare Payments for Septicemia." 1999. Available online at http://oig.hhs.gov/oei/reports/oei-03-98-00370.pdf.

5. Office of the Inspector General, Office of Evaluations and Inspections. "Medicare Payments for DRG 475: Respiratory System Diagnosis with Ventilator Support." 1999. Available online at http://oig.hhs.gov/oei/reports/oei-03-98-00560.pdf.

6. Hanna, Joette. "Constructing a Coding Compliance Plan." *Journal of AHIMA* 73, no. 7 (2002): 48–56.

7. Office of the Inspector General. "The Office of Inspector General's Compliance Program Guidance for Hospitals." 1998. Available online at http://oig.hhs.gov/authorities/docs/cpghosp.pdf.

The analysis upon which this publication is based were performed under Contract Number 500-02-TX03, funded by the Centers for Medicare and Medicaid Services, an agency of the US Department of Health and Human Services. The content of this publication does not necessarily reflect the views or policies of theßer-cial products, or organizations imply endorsement by the US government. The author assumes full responsibility for the accuracy and completeness of the ideas presented.

Diagnosis Coding and Medical Necessity: Rules and Reimbursement

Janis Cogley, RN, CPC, CCS-P, CHC

Introduction

The origins of using diagnosis codes in hospitals and other healthcare settings goes back to the early 1950s when the US Public Health Service and the Veterans Administration extended the concept of using the International Classification of Diseases to hospital indexing of medical record storage and retrieval. However, the linkage of diagnosis codes to the concept of medical necessity did not occur until 1965 when Title XVIII and IX were added to the Social Security Act, the Medicare and Medicaid programs. The foundation of the Medicare and Medicaid programs is the concept of medical necessity and thus, the importance of diagnosis coding was elevated beyond a mere indexing of data.

The focus of my presentation is on how the bond between diagnosis coding and medical necessity impacts reimbursement of healthcare services. The presentation will explore the various rules in place for diagnosis coding and its importance in supporting the medical necessity of the services performed. The intent of this paper is to provide background information regarding the International Classification of Diseases and a discussion of the importance of medical necessity to the Medicare and Medicaid programs.

Background Information Regarding ICD-9-CM Coding

In 1968, the US Public Health Service published a product, the *Eighth Revision International Classification of Diseases, Adapted for Use in the United States*. This publication became commonly known as ICDA-8, and, beginning in 1968, it served as the basis for coding diagnostic data for both official morbidity and mortality statistics in the US. The current *International Classification of Diseases, Ninth Revision, Clinical Modification (ICD-9-CM)* is based on the official version of the World Health Organization's Ninth Revision, Internal Classification of Diseases (ICD-9).[1]

The term "clinical" is used to emphasize the modification's intent: to serve as a useful tool to classify morbidity data for indexing medical records, medical care review, and ambulatory and other medical care programs, as well as for basic health statistics. To describe the clinical picture of the patient, the codes must be more precise than those needed only for statistical groups and trend analysis. In January 1979, ICD-9-CM was made the single classification system intended primarily for use in the US.

Physicians have been required by law to submit diagnosis codes for Medicare reimbursement since the passage of the Medicare Catastrophic Coverage Act of 1988. This Act requires physician offices to include the appropriate diagnosis codes when billing for services provided to Medicare or Medicaid beneficiaries on or after April 1, 1989. At that time, the Centers for Medicare and Medicaid Services (CMS, formerly HCFA) designated ICD-9-CM as the coding system that physicians must use.

CMS considers *Coding Clinic*, published quarterly by the American Hospital Association, to be the official source for coding guidelines. Hospitals should follow the *Coding Clinic* guidelines to assure accuracy in ICD-9-CM coding and DRG assignment. Obviously, the guidelines are far too lengthy to include here, but every hospital, physician practice, and other healthcare organization should maintain current versions of the guidelines applicable to their healthcare system. For example, the *Coding Clinic* defines certain terms as follows:

Principal Procedure is the diagnosis that was performed for definitive treatment rather than one performed for diagnostic or exploratory purposes, or was necessary to take care of a complication. If two procedures appear to meet this definition, then the one most related to the principal diagnosis should be selected as the principal procedure.

Significant Procedure is a significant procedure as defined by the Uniform Hospital Discharge Data Set—one that is surgical in nature, carries a procedural or anesthetic risk or requires specialized training.

Documentation means the documentation that must be present in the medical record to substantiate a procedure was medically necessary and that it was performed. A procedure should not be coded from the title of a procedure; the narrative description of the procedure needs to be read and the correct codes need to be determined based on the narrative description. Procedures that are integral to another procedure are not coded separately, for example, the closure.[2]

General guidelines, coding conventions, and chapter-specific guidelines apply to all healthcare settings. Coding sequencing instructions in Volumes I, II, and III of ICD-9-CM take precedence over any guidelines. Each year, major additions and changes to the coding guidelines are published by the cooperating parties and are effective on October first of that year. The *Coding Clinic* purpose is to assist users in coding and reporting accurately when the ICD-9 manual itself does not provide clear direction.

The official guidelines have four sections. They may be generally described as:

- General coding guidelines
- Guidelines for reporting principal diagnosis for inpatient services
- Guidelines for reporting additional diagnosis codes for inpatient services
- Coding guidelines for outpatient services

The major distinctions between inpatient and outpatient reporting are:

- Definitions for principal versus "first listed" diagnosis codes

- The ability to code or not code "rule out" diagnoses

- More common application of V codes and signs/symptoms coding for outpatient services

The proper ICD-9-CM code is the highest level of detail according to the number of digits available. That is, if a code can be described by a four-digit code rather than a three-digit code, then the four-digit code should be selected; similarly, if a five-digit code is available, that code would represent the highest level of detail and should be selected. Codes that are not specified to the highest order possible are considered truncated and may result in a claim denial.

Several other common coding problem areas that may be confusing for physicians and facility coders are:

- The use of E codes. In the past, coders were advised by various payers not to use E codes. Worker's compensation and auto insurers usually require these codes because they provide more detailed information regarding the cause of an accident resulting in an injury. Coders should report E codes when the circumstances warrant it.

- The assignment of a "first listed" diagnosis in the outpatient setting. Often facility coders who are accustomed to applying inpatient coding guidelines for first listed and additional diagnosis code selections have a difficult time adapting to the diagnosis coding requirements for an outpatient setting. The outpatient coding guidelines state that, "For ambulatory surgery, code the diagnosis for which the surgery was performed. If the post-operative diagnosis is known to be different from the pre-operative diagnosis at the time the diagnosis is confirmed, select the post-operative diagnosis for coding since it is most definitive."[3]

- Coders fail to be as specific in their coding as the documentation supports. They select a generic or unlisted diagnosis when a more specific detailed one is available. This may be the result of relying exclusively on the diagnosis codes that are preprinted on an encounter form or another form. Often the forms are not updated to reflect additions, deletions, and description changes that occur at least once a year. The most applicable and specific diagnostic code must be selected when physicians are ordering diagnostic services (clinical diagnostic labs, radiology, and medicine diagnostic services).

- Diagnostic services are often subject to payment limitations based on medical necessity. The failure to provide the most applicable diagnoses may result in the service being denied. Physician practices as well as facilities should ensure that they have procedures in place to verify questionable and/or vague diagnosis codes. In addition, they need to tie in the diagnosis data to the completion of an Advance Beneficiary Notice (ABN) when the medical necessity is questionable and the patient is a Medicare beneficiary.

- Preventive services diagnosis coding also may present a unique challenge to coders. Medicare does not typically cover "preventive" services except under specific criteria and frequency limitations. Thus, it is important to report the applicable diagnosis codes to receive payment for medically necessary preventive services.

- When a psychiatric diagnosis is listed as the primary diagnosis for a Medicare patient, the services provided may be reduced as a result of the Outpatient Mental Health Treatment Limitation. Psychiatric diagnoses should be coded when they apply, but, if a medically indicated condition other than a psychiatric diagnosis is more appropriate, it should be coded first.

- Coders should assure that services requiring modifiers are properly supported with applicable diagnosis codes. For example, attaching of a "59" modifier to identify a separately excised lesion may require a separate diagnosis code for each excision and/or specimen obtained since the lesions may vary in tissue type. Providing distinct diagnoses for both services will support the necessity for performing and billing both services.

Selecting the correct diagnosis code based on the documentation requires an excellent understanding of the coding guidelines and good cooperation of the physician to provide a detailed description of why he/she provided certain services.

Background Information Regarding Medical Necessity

"Notwithstanding any other provision of this title, no payment may be made under part A or part B for any expenses incurred for items or services- (1)(A) which, except for items and services described in the succeeding subparagraph, are not reasonable and necessary for the diagnosis and treatment of illness or injury to improve the functioning of a malformed body member."

—Social Security Act Chapter XVIII, Section 1862(a) (1)

Some services that are covered under the Medicare program may be limited in coverage due to certain diagnoses, frequency parameters, etc. For example, the payment for a vitamin B-12 injection is limited to diagnoses such as pernicious anemia, gastrointestinal disorder, neuropathies, etc. Therefore, if the criteria are not met, the service will be denied. A procedure may be denied as not reasonable and necessary if it is considered investigational, experimental, or of questionable usefulness. A service may be denied as not reasonable and necessary if it is done more frequently than CMS' policy guidelines specify. When a facility or physician practice is aware of a situation, which Medicare may deny, and they give the Medicare beneficiary an ABN prior to the service and the service is denied, the full charge may be collected from the patient.

Medical necessity denials occur as a result of a National Coverage Determination (NCD) or a Local Coverage Determination (LCD). Between December 2003 and December 2005, Medicare carriers and fiscal intermediaries (FI) are converting their Local Medicare Review Policies (LMRPs) to LCDs.

NCDs and LCDs specify the clinical circumstances under which a service is covered (including whether the circumstances are considered reasonable and necessary). Local coverage decisions may vary in number and content from carrier to carrier and FI to FI.

For example, HGSA administrators, a Medicare carrier for Pennsylvania, has 18 policies under the category "surgical services." Trailblazer, a carrier covering several different states, has only seven LCDs under the surgical service category. Arkansas Blue Cross and Blue Shield, who also functions as a Medicare carrier for several states, has only eight policies under this category.

LCDs may be general, or more specific, and provide narrative descriptions of diagnoses that support the medical necessity of a specific service. In some cases, they may have a detailed list of ICD-9-CM codes under which the service will be considered as reasonable and necessary. The best reference for both NCDs and LCDs is the CMS Web site at www.cms.hhs.gov .

Another important section of the Social Security Act is 1842 (a) (2) (B), which requires Medicare carriers and FIs to apply "safeguards against unnecessary utilization of services furnished by providers." The safeguards may entitle prepayment screens, prepayment reviews, and postpayment reviews to identify inappropriate, medically unnecessary, or excessive services and to take actions where questionable practice patterns are found.

Both prepayment and postpayment reviews use the same set of medical policies. In general, claims received by carriers and FIs are processed on the assumption that providers have the integrity to submit correct information on claims. The claim information, however, must be supported by the medical documentation in the provider's file and must be made available upon request to a carrier or an FI.

The key elements of the medical review process are:

- Monitoring patterns of Medicare claim submissions to identify statistical deviations

- Identifying physicians and suppliers whose utilization patterns differ from medically recognized standards, criteria, and peer norms

- Recovering any inappropriate program expenditures resulting from abuse or overutilization of services

- Educating physicians and other healthcare providers to prevent future abuse of program funds

- Recommending administrative sanctions under 1128 (a) and 1826 (d) (2) of the Social Security Act when physicians and other healthcare providers fail to correct their inappropriate practices

CMS requires that before carriers and FIs assign significant resources to examine a provider claim to identify potential problems, that a probe audit be conducted. A probe review will be of a small number of claims and will not exceed 100 claims. Providers will be asked to submit any and all medical documentation applicable to the claims in question.

The probe review results may be classified as minor, moderate, or major. If a minor problem is detected, the carrier or FI will educate the provider on appropriate billing procedures, pursue recoupment of claims paid in error, and may conduct further analysis at a later date to ensure the problem was corrected. If a moderate problem is detected, additional action may be to place the provider under a prepayment review until they have demonstrated correction of the billing procedures. When a major problem is detected, in addition to a prepayment review, further sampling may be conducted, payment may be suspended, and a referral may be placed to the Benefit Integrity unit for investigation of fraud or abuse.

Fraud is the intentional deception or misrepresentation that an individual knows to be false, and knowing that the deception could result in some unauthorized benefit to himself/herself or some other person. Examples of fraud are:

- Billing for services and supplies that were not provided

- Misrepresenting the diagnosis for a patient to justify the services or equipment furnished

- Altering claim forms to obtain a high payment amount

- Unbundling (exploding) charges or upcoding

- Participating in schemes that involve collusion between a provider and a beneficiary, that result in higher costs or charges to the Medicare program (for example, kickbacks)

The term abuse describes incidents or practices of providers that are inconsistent with accepted sound medical practices. Abuse may directly or indirectly result in unnecessary costs to the program, improper reimbursement, or program reimbursement for services that fail to meet professionally recognized standards of care or which are medically unnecessary. CMS identifies the overutilization of medical and healthcare services, which occurs when a patient receives services that are not medically necessary or reasonable, as the leading type of abuse.

References

The Social Security Act
Medicare Program Integrity Manual, Chapter 13, Section 1
CMS Web site for NCDs and LCDs
Medicare Claims Processing Manual
ICD-9-CM Official Guidelines for Coding and Reporting, Effective October 1, 2003.
Coding Clinic , American Hospital Association

Endnotes

1. *2004 ICD-9-CM Expert for Physicians*, Volumes 1 and 2.

2. *Coding Clinic*, fourth quarter 1990, page 5.

3. *2004 ICD-9-CM Expert for Hospitals*.

Advance Beneficiary Notice

| Patient's Name: | Medicare # (HICN): |

ADVANCE BENEFICIARY NOTICE (ABN)

NOTE: You need to make a choice about receiving these health care items or services.

We expect that Medicare will not pay for the item(s) or service(s) that are described below. Medicare does not pay for all of your health care costs. Medicare only pays for covered items and services when Medicare rules are met. The fact that Medicare may not pay for a particular item or service does not mean that you should not receive it. There may be a good reason your doctor recommended it. Right now, in your case, **Medicare probably will not pay for –**

Items or Services:

Because:

The purpose of this form is to help you make an informed choice about whether or not you want to receive these items or services, knowing that you might have to pay for them yourself. Before you make a decision about your options, you should **read this entire notice carefully.**
x Ask us to explain, if you don't understand why Medicare probably won't pay.
x Ask us how much these items or services will cost you (**Estimated Cost: $**_____), in case you have to pay for them yourself or through other insurance.

PLEASE CHOOSE **ONE** OPTION. CHECK **ONE** BOX. **SIGN & DATE** YOUR CHOICE.

Option 1. YES.   I want to receive these items or services.

I understand that Medicare will not decide whether to pay unless I receive these items or services. Please submit my claim to Medicare. I understand that you may bill me for items or services and that I may have to pay the bill while Medicare is making its decision. If Medicare does pay, you will refund to me any payments I made to you that are due to me. If Medicare denies payment, I agree to be personally and fully responsible for payment. That is, I will pay personally, either out of pocket or through any other insurance that I have. I understand I can appeal Medicare's decision.

Option 2. NO.   I have decided not to receive these items or services.
I will not receive these items or services. I understand that you will not be able to submit a claim to Medicare and that I will not be able to appeal your opinion that Medicare won't pay.

_____   _____
Date   Signature of patient or person acting on patient's behalf

NOTE: Your health information will be kept confidential. Any information that we collect about you on this form will be kept confidential in our offices. If a claim is submitted to Medicare, your health information on this form may be shared with Medicare. Your health information which Medicare sees will be kept confidential by Medicare.

OMB Approval No. 0938-0566   Form No. CMS-R-131-G   (June 2002)

Internet Resources for Accurate Coding and Reimbursement Practices

The availability of valuable information on the Internet has a positive impact on how the health information coding profession meets todays codin g and reimbursement challenges. Coding professionals have access to Internet resources that assist with legislation, coding questions, coding education, payer policy, and clinical research. The Internet has also made it possible to network with coding professionals on a national level in virtual communities of practice.

This Internet resource guide was developed as a convenient resource for coding professionals in all settings. The list is not exhaustive, nor does inclusion on this list represent AHIMA's endorsement. All URLs were accurate at press time but keep in mind the dynamic nature of Web content.

Recommended Resources	Description	Sponsoring Organization	Web Site
Health Insurance Portability and Accountability Act (HIPAA) Administrative Simplification			
Standards for Code Sets	Under HIPAA, this is any set of codes used to encode data elements, such as tables of terms, medical concepts, medical diagnostic codes, or medical procedure codes.		
Current Dental Terminology (CDT)	The official code set used to report medical services and procedures performed by dental professionals.	American Dental Association	www.ada.org/prof/resources/topics/cdt/index.asp and www.ada.org
Healthcare Common Procedure Coding System (HCPCS) Level I — Current Procedural Terminology (CPT)	The official code set used to report procedures and services provided by healthcare professionals and outpatient institutions.	American Medical Association	www.ama-assn.org/ama/pub/category/3113.html and https://catalog.ama-assn.org/Catalog/home.jsp
Healthcare Common Procedure Coding System (HCPCS) Level II — HCPCS National Codes	The official code set used by healthcare professionals and outpatient institutions to report products, supplies, and services not included in the CPT code set.	Centers for Medicare and Medicaid Services	www.cms.hhs.gov/medicare/hcpcs/default.asp
International Classification of Diseases 9th Revision Clinical Modification (ICD-9-CM Volumes I and II)	The official coding classification system used by healthcare professionals and institutions to report morbidity and mortality information.	National Center for Health Statistics, Centers for Disease Control	www.cdc.gov/nchs/icd9.htm
International Classification of Diseases 9th Revision Clinical Modification (ICD-9-CM Volume III)	The official code set used by inpatient hospital institutions to report procedural information.	Centers for Medicare and Medicaid Services	www.cms.hhs.gov/payment systems/icd9/default.asp
National Drug Code (NDC)	A coding system for pharmacies to report services, supplies, drugs, and biologic information.	US Food and Drug Administration	www.fda.gov/cder/ndc/ preface.htm

Recommended Resources	Description	Sponsoring Organization	Web Site
Standards for Electronic Transactions	Under HIPAA, this is a transaction that complies with the applicable HIPAA standard.		
Designated Standard Maintenance Organization (DSMO)	The DSMO was established in the final HIPAA rule and is charged with maintaining the standards for electronic transactions, developing or modifying an adopted standard.	Secretary of the Department of Health and Human Services	www.hipaa-dsmo.org
Accredited Standards Committee X12 (ASC X12)	ASC X12 is a designated committee under the DSMO that develops uniform standards for cross-industry exchange of business transactions through electronic data interchange standards.	Secretary of the Department of Health and Human Services	www.x12.org
Dental Content Committee (DeCC) of the American Dental Association	DeCC is the designated committee under the DSMO responsible for addressing standard transaction content on behalf of the dental sector of the healthcare community.	Secretary of the Department of Health and Human Services	www.ada.org/prof/resources/ topics/dentalcontent.asp
Health Level Seven (HL7)	HL7 is a designated organization under the DSMO that addresses issues at the seventh, or application, level of healthcare systems interconnections.	Secretary of the Department of Health and Human Services	www.hl7.org
National Council for Prescription Drug Programs (NCDP)	A designated committee under the DSMO that specializes in developing standards for exchanging prescription and payment information.	Secretary of the Department of Health and Human Services	www.ncpdp.org
National Uniform Billing Committee (NUBC)	A designated committee under the DSMO that is responsible for identifying data elements and designing the CMS-1500.	Secretary of the Department of Health and Human Services	www.nubc.org
National Uniform Claim Committee (NUCC)	The national group that replaced the Uniform Claim Form Task Force in 1995 and developed a standard data set to be used in the transmission of noninstitutional provider claims to and from third-party payers.	Secretary of the Department of Health and Human Services	www.nucc.org
Other Electronic Transaction Resources			
Electronic Data Interchange (EDI)	A standard transmission format using strings of data for business information communicated among the computer systems of independent organizations.	Centers for Medicare and Medicaid Services	www.cms.hhs.gov/providers/ edi
National Provider Identifier (NPI)	An alphanumeric identifier used to identify individual healthcare providers for Medicare billing purposes and intended for use with all insurance plans.	Centers for Medicare and Medicaid Services	www.cms.hhs.gov/provider update/regs/cms0045f.pdf
Washington Publishing Company (WPC)	WPC manages and distributes EDI from organizations that develop, maintain, and implement EDI standards. The WPC home page provides implementation guides such as the X12N HIPAA Implementation Guide, educational resources, and additional HIPAA tools.	Washington Publishing Company	www.wpc-edi.com/ Default_ 40.asp
Workgroup for Electronic Data Interchange (WEDI)	A subgroup of Accreditation Standards Committee X12 that has been involved in developing electronic data interchange standards for billing transactions.	Centers for Medicare and Medicaid Services	www.wedi.org

Recommended Resources	Description	Sponsoring Organization	Web Site
Official ICD-9-CM Resources			
Coding Clinic for ICD-9-CM	Official publication for ICD-9-CM coding guidelines and coding advice as approved by the four cooperating parties.	American Hospital Association	www.hospitalconnect.com/ ahacentraloffice/coding/ icd-9-cm_prod.jsp
ICD-9-CM Guidelines for Coding and Reporting	Official coding guidelines developed to assist coding professionals in situations where the ICD-9-CM does not provide instruction.	National Center for Health Statistics, Centers for Disease Control	www.cdc.gov/nchs/datawh/ ftpserv/ftpicd9/ftpicd9. htm#guidelines
ICD-9-CM Volumes I and II Code Updates (Coordination and Maintenance Committee and addenda)	Addendum to the annual (biannual effective April 2005) diagnosis code updates and Coordination and Maintenance Committee reports.	National Center for Health Statistics, Centers for Disease Control	www.cdc.gov/nchs/about/ot heract/icd9/maint/maint.htm
ICD-9-CM Volume III Code Updates	Addendum to the annual (biannual effective April 2005) procedure code updates.	Centers for Medicare and Medicaid Services	www.cms.hhs.gov/payment systems/icd9/default.asp
HCPCS Level I CPT Resources			
Category I, II, III Updates	Category I CPT Codes: Code revisions are published annually and become effective at the beginning of each year. Category II CPT Codes: Code revisions are released electronically each July. The revisions are published in the CPT book and become effective at the beginning of the next year. Category III CPT Codes: New codes are distributed electronically on a semiannual basis and published in the CPT book annually.	American Medical Association	www.ama-assn.org/ama/pub/ category/3884.html
CPT Assistant	A monthly newsletter that provides official CPT coding advice.	American Medical Association	https://catalog.ama-assn.org/ Catalog/home.jsp
CPT Change Requests	CPT code modification process and request for changes.	American Medical Association	www.ama-assn.org/ama/pub/ category/3112.html
CPT Errata	Electronic list that provides corrections to the annual CPT category code changes.	American Medical Association	www.ama-assn.org/ama/pub/ category/3896.html
HCPCS Level II Resources			
Code Updates and Code Modification Process	National codes are published annually and go into effect at the beginning of each year. Temporary codes can be revised quarterly and the changes are made available electronically and published on an annual basis.	Centers for Medicare and Medicaid Services	www.cms.hhs.gov/medicare/ hcpcs
Coding Clinic on HCPCS	Coding resource newsletter that provides accurate coding advice for the users of HCPCS.	American Hospital Association	www.hospitalconnect.com/ ahacentraloffice/coding/ hcpcs_prod.jsp

Recommended Resources	Description	Sponsoring Organization	Web Site
CDT Resources			
CDT Updates	Code revisions are published and effective biannually at the beginning of odd-numbered years.	American Dental Association	www.ada.org/prof/resources/topics/cdt/index.asp
Additional Coding Classification Systems, Nomenclatures, and Vocabularies			
Diagnostic and Statistical Manual of Mental Disorders, Fourth Edition (DSM-IV)	A nomenclature to standardize the diagnostic process for patients with psychiatric disorders; includes codes that correspond to ICD-9-CM codes.	American Psychiatric Association	www.appi.org/dsm.cfx
Alternative Billing Concepts (ABC) Codes	Contains more than 4,000 codes that describe what is said, done, ordered, prescribed, or distributed by providers of alternative medicine. Disciplines covered by this system include acupuncture, holistic medicine, massage therapy, homeopathy, naturopathy, ayurvedic medicine, chiropractors, and midwifery.	Alternative Link	www.alternativelink.com/ali/home
Home Health Care Classification (HHCC) System	A taxonomy of nursing diagnoses and nursing interventions.	The HHCC System emerged from the federally funded Home Care Project conducted at Georgetown University School of Nursing.	www.sabacare.com
International Statistical Classification of Diseases and Related Health Problems, Tenth Revision (ICD-10)	The ICD-10 version of the disease classification system developed by the World Health Organization is used to report morbidity and mortality information worldwide. Effective with deaths occurring in 1999, the US replaced ICD-9 with ICD-10 for mortality reporting.	World Health Organization	www.cdc.gov/nchs/about/major/dvs/icd10des.htm
International Statistical Classification of Diseases, Tenth Revision, Clinical Modification (ICD-10-CM)	The future US coding classification system for healthcare professionals and institutions to report morbidity and mortality data.	National Center for Health Statistics, Centers for Disease Control	www.cdc.gov/nchs/about/otheract/icd9/abticd10.htm
International Statistical Classification of Diseases, Tenth Revision, Clinical Modification (ICD-10-CM)	The future US coding classification for institutions to report procedural information.	Developed by 3M Health Information Services under contract with the Centers for Medicare and Medicaid Services	www.cms.hhs.gov/providers/pufdownload/icd10.asp
International Classification of Primary Care (ICPC)	A reliable classification system for primary care physicians that enables the labeling of the most prevalent conditions that exist in the community as well as symptoms and complaints.	Published by the World Organization of Family Doctors	www.globalfamilydoctor.com

Recommended Resources	Description	Sponsoring Organization	Web Site
International Classification of Diseases for Oncology (ICD-O)	The standard tool for coding diagnoses of neoplasms in tumor and cancer registrars and in pathology laboratories. ICD-O is a dual classification with coding systems for both topography and morphology. The topography code describes the site of origin of the neoplasm and uses the same three-character and four-character categories as in the neoplasm section of Chapter II, ICD-10.	World Health Organization	www.who.int/bookorders/ anglais/detart1.jsp?sesslan =1&codlan=1&codcol=15& codcch=3350
International Classification of Functioning, Disability and Health (ICF)	The ICF is a health and health-related classification system that reports body functions and structures, activities, and participation.	World Health Organization	www3.who.int/icf/icftem plate.cfm?myurl=homepage. html&mytitle=Home%20Page
Logical Observation and Identifier Codes (LOINC)	The LOINC coding system electronically exchanges laboratory and clinical information.	The Regenstrief Institute maintains the LOINC database and its supporting documentation.	www.loinc.org
MEDCIN	MEDCIN is a terminology and presentation engine. It includes more than 250,000 clinical data elements encompassing symptoms, history, physical examination, tests, diagnoses, and therapy.	Medicomp Systems, Inc.	www.medicomp.com
Medical Dictionary for Regulatory Activities (MedDRA)	MedDRA is a global standard medical terminology and expected to supersede or replace terminologies currently in use with the medical product development process.	Maintenance and Support Services Organization	www.meddramsso.com/ NewWeb2003/medra_over view/index.htm
National Drug File Reference Terminology (NDF-RT)	The NDF-RT is being developed for the Veterans Administration as a reference standard for medications to support a variety of clinical, administrative, and analytical purposes.	Department of Veterans Affairs	www.va.gov/vdl/Clinical. asp?appID=89
RxNorm	RxNorm is a clinical drug nomenclature that provides standard names for clinical drugs (active ingredient, strength, and dose form) and for dose forms as administered.	National Library of Medicine	www.nlm.nih.gov/ research/ umls/rxnorm _main.html
North American Nursing Diagnosis Association (NANDA) International	Organization of the NANDA-International nursing diagnoses has evolved from an alphabetical listing in the mid-1980s to a conceptual system that guides the classification of nursing diagnoses in a taxonomy.	North American Nursing Diagnosis Association	www.nanda.org/html/ taxonomy.html
Nursing Intervention Classification (NIC)	NIC is a comprehensive, research-based, standardized classification of interventions that nurses perform.	University of Iowa College of Nursing	www.nursing.uiowa.edu/ centers/cncce/nic
Nursing Outcomes Classification (NOC)	NOC is a comprehensive, standardized classification of patient/client outcomes developed to evaluate the effects of nursing interventions.	University of Iowa College of Nursing	www.nursing.uiowa.edu/ centers/cncce/noc
Omaha System	The Omaha System is a research-based, comprehensive taxonomy designed to generate meaningful data following usual or routine documentation of client care.	Omaha System Advisory Committee	www.omahasystem.org

Recommended Resources	Description	Sponsoring Organization	Web Site
Systematized Nomenclature of Dentistry (SNODENT)	SNODENT is a systematized nomenclature of dentistry containing dental diagnoses, signs, symptoms, and complaints.	American Dental Association	www.ada.org
Systematized Nomenclature of Medicine Clinical Terms (SNOMED CT)	SNOMED CT is a comprehensive clinical terminology and infrastructure that enables a consistent way of capturing, sharing, and aggregating health data across specialties and sites of care.	SNOMED International, a division of the College of American Pathologists and the United Kingdom's National Health Service	www.snomed.org
Universal Medical Device Nomenclature System (UMDNS)	UMDNS is a standard international nomenclature and coding system used to facilitate identifying, processing, filing, storing, retrieving, transferring, and communicating data about medical devices.	ECRI (formerly the Emergency Care Research Institute)	www.ecri.org
Health, Research, and Comparative Data			
Unified Medical Language System (UMLS)	A program initiated by the National Library of Medicine to build an intelligent, automated system that can understand biomedical concepts, words, and expressions and their interrelationships.	National Library of Medicine	www.nlm.nih.gov/ research/ umls
Medical Literature, Analysis, and Retrieval System Online (MEDLINE)	MEDLINE is an online database that offers access to millions of clinical articles. The topic areas include medicine, dentistry, nursing, pharmacy, allied health, and veterinary medicine.	National Library of Medicine	http://medlineplus.gov
Agency for Healthcare Research and Quality (AHRQ)	AHRQ supports research and provides information on the quality of healthcare, patient safety issues, and healthcare costs.	Department of Health and Human Services	www.ahrq.gov
Medicare Provider Analysis and Review (MEDPAR)	The MEDPAR database is used for administrative purposes to collect information on Medicare claims and consists of data such as DRGs, ICD-9-CM codes, Medicare coverage information, and patient demographics.	Centers for Medicare and Medicaid Services	www.cms.hhs.gov/ statistics/ medpar/default.asp
American Hospital Directory (AHD)	The AHD provides an inpatient and outpatient Medicare claims database for more than 6,000 hospitals.	American Hospital Directory	www.ahd.com
Medstat	Medstat is a healthcare information company that provides market intelligence and benchmark databases, decision support solutions, and research services for managing the cost and quality of healthcare.	Thomson Corporation	www.medstat.com
Statistics			
National Committee on Vital Healthcare and Statistics (NCVHS)	NCVHS serves as a national advisory board to the public on health data, statistics, and information systems.	Department of Health and Human Services	www.ncvhs.hhs.gov

Recommended Resources	Description	Sponsoring Organization	Web Site
National Center for Health Statistics (NCHS)	NCHS is a public health statistics agency charged with collecting statistical information critical for improving public health in the US.	Department of Health and Human Services	www.cdc.gov/nchs
Centers for Disease Control and Prevention (CDC)	CDC includes federal agencies that oversee health promotion and disease control and prevention activities in the US.	Department of Health and Human Services	www.cdc.gov
National Center for Vital Statistics (NCVS)	NCVS provides statistical information compiled at the state level. Statistics include births, deaths, and fetal deaths.	Department of Health and Human Services	www.cdc.gov/nchs/nvss.htm
Clinical Resources			
National Institutes of Health (NIH)	NIH is the world's medical research organization, consisting of 18 separate health institutes, the National Center for Complementary and Alternative Medicine, and the National Library of Medicine.	Department of Health and Human Services	www.nih.gov
National Library of Medicine (NLM)	NLM is the national online library for biomedicine and health science information.	National Institutes of Health	www.nlm.nih.gov
The Visible Human Project	NLM's development of anatomically detailed and three-dimensional representations of normal human bodies.	National Institutes of Health	www.nlm.nih.gov/research/visible/visible_human.html
Virtual Hospital	Virtual Hospital is a digital health sciences library for healthcare providers and patients. It contains thousands of textbooks and booklets.	University of Iowa Health Care	www.vh.org
Compliance Resources			
Department of Health and Human Services (HHS) Office of Inspector General (OIG)	OIG protects the integrity of HHS programs, as well as the health and welfare of the beneficiaries of those programs.	Department of Health and Human Services	www.oig.hhs.gov
Fiscal Year OIG Work Plan	The focused CMS Work Plan assists OIG with the prevention of healthcare fraud, waste, and abuse.	Department of Health and Human Services	http://oig.hhs.gov/publications.html
Fraud Prevention and Detection	Resources including compliance programs, corporate integrity agreements, and exclusion programs.	Department of Health and Human Services	http://oig.hhs.gov/fraud.html
Fighting Fraud and Abuse	Resources to assist with the integrity of the Medicare program.	Centers for Medicare and Medicaid Services	www.cms.hhs.gov/providers/fraud/default.asp
Health Care Compliance Association	The Health Care Compliance Association is a professional association providing its members with compliance news, information, and a variety of related services.	Health Care Compliance Association	www.hcca-info.org
Medicare Reimbursement Resources			
Federal Register	The daily publication of the US Government Printing Office for proposed rules, rules, and notices of federal agencies and organizations, as well as executive orders and other presidential documents.	US Government	www.gpoaccess.gov/fr and www.access.gpo.gov/su_docs/fedreg/frcont04.html

Recommended Resources	Description	Sponsoring Organization	Web Site
Conditions of Participation and Conditions for Coverage	CMS develops Conditions of Participation (CoPs) and Conditions for Coverage (CfCs) that healthcare organizations must meet to participate in the Medicare and Medicaid programs.	Centers for Medicare and Medicaid Services	www.cms.hhs.gov/cop
Documentation Guidelines Evaluation and Management Services	Documentation guidelines developed to supplement the CPT Evaluation and Management service code definitions used for physician reporting.	Centers for Medicare and Medicaid Services	www.cms.hhs.gov/medlearn/ emdoc.asp
Electronic Code of Federal Regulations (e-CFR)	E-CFR is a sample model of a currently updated version of the Code of Federal Regulations (CFR). The CFR is the official compilation of federal rules and requirements.	National Archives and Records Administration's Office of the Federal Register and the Government Printing Office	www.gpoaccess.gov/ecfr
Intermediary-Carrier Contacts	A private company directory that contracts with CMS to pay Medicare Part A (Intermediary) and Part B (Carrier) claims.	Centers for Medicare and Medicaid Services	www.cms.hhs.gov/contacts/ incardir.asp
Internet Only Manuals (IOMs)	IOMs provide technical and professional information about the Medicare and Medicaid programs.	Centers for Medicare and Medicaid Services	www.cms.hhs.gov/manuals
Medicare Coverage Home Page	CMS develops coverage policies to indicate whether and under what circumstances certain services are covered under the Medicare program. The Medicare coverage home page provides access to coverage updates, coverage policies, and a Medicare coverage database.	Centers for Medicare and Medicaid Services	www.cms.hhs.gov/coverage
Medicare Learning Network (Medlearn)	The Medlearn site provides access to a variety of education products to assist providers and beneficiaries and their advocates in understanding the Medicare program.	Centers for Medicare and Medicaid Services	www.cms.hhs.gov/medlearn
Medlearn Matters	Medlearn Matters includes informational articles designed to help providers understand new or changed Medicare policy.	Centers for Medicare and Medicaid Services	www.cms.hhs.gov/medlearn/ matters
Medicare Payment Systems	This site provides valuable links to pages containing informational materials on Medicare payment systems and coding files.	Centers for Medicare and Medicaid Services	www.cms.hhs.gov/payment systems
Medicare Payment System Files	This site provides files for download for Medicare payment systems.	Centers for Medicare and Medicaid Services	www.cms.hhs.gov/providers/ pufdownload
Medicare Providers	This provider-specific home page is a one-stop resource focused on the informational needs and interests of Medicare providers, including physicians and other practitioners.	Centers for Medicare and Medicaid Services	www.cms.hhs.gov/providers
Paper Forms and Instructions	This link provides information on the CMS-1500, UB-92, CMS 1491, CMS 1490S, and EDI enrollment form.	Centers for Medicare and Medicaid Services	www.cms.hhs.gov/providers/ edi/edi5.asp

Recommended Resources	Description	Sponsoring Organization	Web Site
Medicare Preventive Services	Coding and reporting guidance for preventive services covered under the Medicare program.	Centers for Medicare and Medicaid Services	www.cms.hhs.gov/ preventiveservices
Health Information	This site provides Medicare beneficiaries with information about Medicare benefits, publications, and valuable Web sites.	Centers for Medicare and Medicaid Services	www.medicare.gov/Health/ Overview.asp
Quality Improvement Organizations (QIOs)	QIOs contract with CMS to ensure that Medicare beneficiaries receive high-quality healthcare that is medically necessary and appropriate and meets professionally recognized standards of care.	Centers for Medicare and Medicaid Services	www.cms.hhs.gov/qio
CMS Quarterly Provider Update	The update communicates current provider information on regulations, policies, and revisions made to the manual instructions.	Centers for Medicare and Medicaid Services	www.cms.hhs.gov/provider update

Governmental Data Sets

Data Elements for Emergency Department Systems (DEEDS)	Developed to create uniform specifications for data entered in emergency department patient records.	National Center for Injury Prevention and Control	www.cdc.gov/ncipc/pub-res/ deedspage.htm
Minimum Data Set for Long-Term Care (MDS 2.0)	A patient-centered assessment instrument that Medicare- and Medicaid-certified nursing facilities must use to conduct a comprehensive, accurate, standardized, reproducible assessment of each resident's functional capacity.	Centers for Medicare and Medicaid Services	www.cms.hhs.gov/medicaid/ mds20
Minimum Data Set for Post Acute Care (MDS-PAC)	A patient-centered assessment instrument that must be completed for every Medicare patient and emphasizes a patient's care needs instead of provider characteristics.	Centers for Medicare and Medicaid Services	www.cms.hhs.gov/review/ 03spring/default.asp
Nursing Minimum Data Set (NMDS)	This data set covers nursing diagnosis; nursing intervention; nursing outcome; intensity of nursing care; unique identifier of principal nurse provider; patient demographics; and service items from the uniform hospital data set.	NMDS Consortium	www.nursing.uiowa.edu/NI/ collabs_files/Synopsis%20 NMDS%20Nov%202003.pdf
Outcomes and Assessment Information Set (OASIS)	A standard core assessment data tool developed to measure the outcomes of adult patients receiving home health services under the Medicare and Medicaid programs.	Centers for Medicare and Medicaid Services	www.cms.hhs.gov/oasis/ oasisdat.asp
Uniform Hospital Discharge Data Set (UHDDS)	A core set of data elements adopted by the US Department of Health, Education, and Welfare in 1974 that are collected by hospitals on all discharges and all discharge abstract systems. The UHDDS definitions are used by acute care short-term hospitals to report inpatient data elements in a standardized manner.	Developed through NCVHS, required by HHS departmental policy	www.cms.hhs.gov/manuals/ 45_smm/sm_11_11375.asp
Uniform Ambulatory Care Data Set (UACDS)	A data set developed by the National Committee on Vital and Health Statistics consisting of a minimum set of patient/client-specific data elements to be collected in ambulatory care settings.	Recommended by NCVHS	www.ncvhs.hhs.gov/ncvhsr1. htm

Recommended Resources	Description	Sponsoring Organization	Web Site
Nongovernmental Data Sets			
Health Plan Employer Data and Information Set (HEDIS)	A set of performance measures designed to provide purchasers and consumers of healthcare with the information they need to compare the performance of managed care plans.	National Committee for Quality Assurance	www.ncqa.org/communi cations/publications/ hedispub. htm
ORYX	ORYX integrates outcomes and other performance measurement data into the accreditation process. Joint Commission–accredited hospitals collect data on standardized—or core—performance measures.	Joint Commission on Accreditation of Healthcare Organizations	www.jcaho.org/accredited +organizations/hospitals/ oryx/ oryx+facts.htm
AHIMA Member Resources			
Communities of Practice (CoP)	The CoP is an online member interaction tool providing up-to-date industry news, links to helpful resources, and, most importantly, solutions and ideas from peers. The monthly *CodeWrite* newsletters are contained in the Coding CoP.	AHIMA	https://www.ahimanet.org /COP
FORE Library: HIM Body of Knowledge	The FORE Library: HIM Body of Knowledge offers AHIMA-owned content and links to public material that encompass the theory and practice of health information management.	AHIMA	www.ahima.org, click on "Body of Knowledge"
HIM Productivity Standards	This site provides resources to locate productivity standards for health information management functions in an acute care facility	AHIMA	www.ahima.org, click on "Body of Knowledge"
HIM Resources: Coding	The AHIMA coding home page includes information on coding events, coding education, coding roundtables, and more.	AHIMA	www.ahima.org/coding
"Managing and Improving Data Quality"	This practice brief offers guidelines and recommendations for adhering to coding data quality mandates.	AHIMA	www.ahima.org, click on "Body of Knowledge"
Standards of Ethical Coding	The standard of professional ethics for health information coding professionals.	AHIMA	www.ahima.org/infocenter/ guidelines/standards.cfm
"Where to Find Answers to Your Coding Questions"	This article will help you find solutions to your toughest coding questions by using available guidelines and by leveraging the networking and resource-sharing capabilities of AHIMA's CoP.	AHIMA	www.ahima.org, click on "Body of Knowledge"
"Developing a Physician Query Process"	This practice brief provides information on developing a query to improve physician documentation and coding professionals' understanding of the unique clinical situation.	AHIMA	www.ahima.org, click on "Body of Knowledge"
"Regulatory Journey to Destination 10: Understanding the Process for Adoption of ICD-10-CM and ICD-10-PCS"	This article provides an understanding of the regulatory process for the adoption and implementation of ICD-10.	AHIMA	www.ahima.org, click on "Body of Knowledge"

Prepared by

AHIMA Coding Practice Team

Kathy Giannangelo, RHIA, CCS
Susan Hull, MPH, RHIA, CCS
Karen Kostick, RHIT, CCS, CCS-P
Rita Scichilone, MHSA, RHIA, CCS, CCS-P
Mary Stanfill, RHIA, CCS, CCS-P
Sarah Wills-Dubose, MA, MEd, RHIA
Ann Zeisset, RHIT, CCS, CCS-P

The Care and Maintenance of Charge Masters

Background

The various supplies and services listed on the charge master for the average facility drives reimbursement for approximately 73 percent of the UB-92 claims for outpatient services alone. The charge master—often called the master charge list or charge description list—is simply a computer file of charges for each item that may be used to treat the patient, as well as a select group of services.

A current and accurate charge master is vital to any healthcare provider seeking proper reimbursement. Without it, the facility would not receive proper reimbursement. Among the negative impacts that may result from an inaccurate charge master are:

- Overpayment
- Underpayment
- Undercharging for services
- Claims rejections
- Fines
- Penalties

Because a charge master is an automated process that results in billing numerous services for high volumes of patients—often without human intervention—there is a high risk that a single coding or mapping error could spawn error after error before it is identified and corrected.

Key Elements of a Charge Master List

The content and layout of a healthcare provider's charge master may vary from one organization to the next. However, one can expect to see the following data elements in the typical charge master file.

- Procedure description: This title describes the procedure to be performed. There is no set format or vocabulary for this description. Each description should be unique to your facility, yet comprehensible to all staff members who need to identify the procedure. Furthermore, each description should be separately identifiable. For example, no two line items should have the exact same description. Grouped under the heading of procedure might be surgery, laboratory, radiology, etc.

- Service description: This title describes the service to be performed. There is no set format or vocabulary for this description. As with procedure description, each service description should be unique to your facility, yet comprehensible to all staff members who need to identify the service. Again, each service description should be separately identifiable—no two line items should have the exact same description. Grouped under the heading of service might be evaluation and management, observation, emergency room visits, and clinical visits.

- CPT/HCPCS code: The corresponding CPT or HCPCS code that identifies the specific service or procedure. It is important to note that not all services and procedures listed on the charge master will have a corresponding code. Since all supplies and services may not require a code assignment and the use of unlisted or nonspecific codes is not desirable to the organization, it may be better to just leave this field blank in these instances.

- Revenue code: A three-digit code number representing a specific accommodation, ancillary service, or billing calculation required for Medicare billing. National and state uniform billing committees and HCFA update the list of acceptable revenue codes on an ongoing basis.

- Charge dollar amount: The specific amount charged by the facility for each procedure or service. This is not the actual amount that the facility will be reimbursed by a third-party payer. Instead, the charge dollar amount represents the standard charge for that item. The facility may want to compare the charge amount listed to the Medicare fee schedule to ensure that the charge amount is equal to or higher than the Medicare fee. Some facilities maintain unique charge dollar amount listings by payer.

- Department code number: A unique number assigned to each ancillary department by the facility.

- Charge description number: An internally assigned unique number that identifies each specific procedure or service listed on the charge master.

The Charge Master Committee

Ideally, charge master maintenance should not be the responsibility of one individual. Rather, it should be overseen by a committee composed of key facility representatives that will contribute to the accuracy and quality of both the document database and charge master review process. Proper charge master maintenance requires expertise in coding, billing regulations, clinical procedures, and health record documentation.

The charge master committee should include representation from:

- Health information management
- Ancillary departments
- The financial services/business office
- Information systems

Responsibilities of the charge master committee include:

- Develop policies and procedures for the charge master review process
- Perform an annual charge master review when new CPT/HCPCS codes are available
- Key elements of the annual charge master review, including:

> Review all CPT codes for accuracy, validity, and relationship to charge description number
>
> Review all procedure and service descriptions for accuracy and clinical appropriateness
>
> Review all revenue codes for accuracy and linkage to charge description numbers
>
> Ensure that the usage of all HCPCS, CPT, and revenue codes are in compliance with Medicare guidelines or other existing payer contracts
>
> Review all charge dollar amounts for appropriateness by payer
>
> Review all charge description numbers for uniqueness and validity
>
> Review all department code numbers for uniqueness and validity

- Perform ongoing charge master maintenance as the facility adds or deletes new procedures, updates technology, or changes services provided
- Establish a procedure to allow clinical department directors to submit charge master change requests for new, deleted, or revised procedures or services

- Make sure there is no duplication of code assignment by coders and charge master assigned codes in any department (e.g., GI endoscopy lab or cardiology cath lab)

- Review all charge ticket and order entry screens for accuracy against the charge master and appropriate mapping to CPT/HCPCS codes when required

- Review and comply with directives in Medicare bulletins, transmittals, Medicare manual updates, and official coding guidelines

- Comply with guidelines in the National Correct Coding Initiative or other known coding or bundling edits

- Carefully consider any application that involves one charge description number "exploding" into more than one CPT/HCPCS code to prevent inadvertent unbundling and unearned reimbursement for services

- Review and take action on all remittance advice denials involving HCPCS/CPT coding or HCFA coding guidelines

Charge Master Resources

- CPT-4 codes and guidelines: Contact the American Medical Association, 515 N. State St., Chicago, IL 60610, (312) 464-5000, http://www.ama-assn.org

- HCPCS codes and guidelines: Contact the US Government Printing Office, Superintendent of Documents, Washington, DC 20402, (202) 783-3232. For training and guidance, contact your regional Medicare fiscal intermediary

- National Correct Coding Initiative: Contact the National Technical Information Service (NTIS), Technology Administration, US Department of Commerce, 5285 Port Royal Rd., Springfield, VA 22161, (703) 605-6000, http://www.ntis.gov

Prepared by
Harry Rhodes, MBA, RHIA, CHPS, Director of Practice Leadership

Acknowledgments
Assistance from the following individuals is gratefully acknowledged:

Rita Scichilone, MHSA, RRA, CCS, CCS-P
Dianne Willard, MBA, RRA, CCS-P

References

Abdelhak, Mervat. *Health Information: Management of a Strategic Resource.* Philadelphia, PA: W. B. Saunders Company, 1996.

"Expert Advice on Preparing for the APCs." *Medical Record Briefing* 14, no. 4 (1999): 3.

Falconer, Carol. *St. Anthony's UB-92 Editor: A Guide to Medicare Billing.* Reston, VA: St. Anthony Publishing, 1994.

Prophet, Sue. *Health Information Management Compliance: A Model Program for Healthcare Compliance.* Chicago, IL: AHIMA, 1998.

Richard, Tricia. *The Hospital Chargemaster Guide.* Reston, VA: St. Anthony Publishing, 1999.

Coding Connections in Revenue Cycle Management

Ruth Cummins, RHIA, CCS, and Julie Waddell

Recently, there has been a significant amount of talk in the healthcare industry about revenue cycle improvement. So what is all of the excitement about? It is about the bottom line. Specifically, how we can improve our bottom line through more effective and efficient revenue cycle management. For hospitals to maintain financial viability under the pressures of the current healthcare environment, the revenue cycle must be a significant focal point, and HIM and coding professionals should play major roles in the process. This article will highlight many of the coding connections for the key revenue cycle processes within patient access, HIM, and patient financial services.

The Coding Connection in Patient Access Services

Critical revenue cycle processes that occur in the patient access department include initial data collection (e.g., name, date of birth, insurance information, reason for admission, patient type); medical record number (MRN) assignment; and medical necessity determination. Coding connects (or needs to connect) with patient access services in the following areas: MRN, patient type, source documentation, and medical necessity.

The MRN is vital in connecting the patient documentation to the services provided to the patient. If an inaccurate MRN is used, complete and historical clinical information may not be available, resulting in potentially incomplete or inaccurate code assignment. Regular communication and collaboration between HIM and patient access to maintain accurate MRN assignment is imperative.

The patient access department, in many facilities, is responsible for assigning the patient type (e.g., inpatient versus observation patient). It is very frustrating for the coding staff to have to alter a patient type post-service due to inappropriate assignment. This correction process slows down the revenue cycle. The coding staff should collaborate with patient access in identifying ways to resolve inaccurate patient type assignments.

During the scheduling and patient registration process, test order documentation, including reason for the test, should be presented. Source documentation is critical for the final code assignment. Coding professionals should be involved in educating front-line personnel (i.e., those registering patients) regarding appropriate test order requirements.

The coding staff should also have access to the source documentation when coding to ensure complete, accurate, and consistent coding.

Hospitals and healthcare providers must determine if services will be covered based on the reason for the test prior to services being rendered. In most healthcare organizations, this is left to the front-line staff in patient access. Often, these individuals are in entry-level positions with little or no healthcare background. Connecting the patient access department with coding professionals is critical in complying with medical necessity requirements and reducing the risk of denials on the back end.

Although it is not always feasible to employ a coding professional in patient access, healthcare providers should consider creating a coding liaison position to assist patient access in determining medical necessity and following up with physicians on proper test orders. Coding orientation courses should be provided as a requisite for patient access staff as well. The revenue cycle can be dramatically affected by connecting coding to the patient access process.

Documentation, HIM, Coding, and Chargemaster Services

Key focal points in documentation, HIM, coding, and chargemaster services that affect revenue cycle performance include who assigns the codes; source documentation; coding quality and productivity; and revenue integrity.

Healthcare providers must determine where CPT and HCPCS codes will originate, or "who codes for what." Information system requirements should be considered when determining whether a code will be generated with a charge (i.e., hard-coded in the chargemaster) or whether the code will be assigned by coding staff based on source documentation.

Typically, routine diagnostic services such as lab and radiology are hard-coded in the chargemaster while surgical interventions are normally assigned by a coder. Lack of coordination between coding and chargemaster staff can cause conflicts, duplicative coding, and billing errors.

When determining whether a code belongs in the chargemaster or if it should be coded by a coder, ask yourself the following questions: "Is the code always the same for the procedure or service provided?" If yes, then the code likely belongs in the chargemaster. "Is coding assignment variable, contingent upon site, method, or complication?" If yes, then the code should be assigned by a coder. "Are there variables inherent in the documentation that would modify the code?" If yes, then the code should be assigned by a coder.

Equally important as who codes for what is the source documentation a coder uses to assign the appropriate ICD-9-CM and CPT or HCPCS code. As we all know, if it was not documented, it was not done. Whether the code is hard-coded in the chargemaster or is assigned by a coder, the source documentation must paint a clear picture of the clinical condition of the patient and the services provided. Often clinicians will witness services being provided; however, final dictation or documentation may omit specifics, which allow additional codes or charges to be added. Coding plays a critical role in validating source documentation for coding and billing purposes.

Concurrent clinical documentation management programs and query processes should be implemented to ensure physician documentation appropriately reflects the clinical picture of the patient and the services provided so that accurate and complete coding and billing can be accomplished.

HIM departments should establish coding quality and productivity standards. Ongoing internal and external quality audits are essential to ensure both compliance with coding rules and regulations, and appropriate payment for services. Coders need to keep current on coding and payment guidelines through continuing education and regulatory alerts and updates. To improve the efficiency of the revenue cycle (specifically, to reduce the discharged not final billed cases), coding productivity standards should be in place with a tool to effectively monitor daily progress.

Revenue integrity is the process of validating documentation, charges, and codes to ensure complete, compliant, and accurate billing and coding processes. A good revenue integrity team, which includes coding professionals, identifies lost charges and coding issues along with providing education and the development of processes to improve this component of the revenue cycle.

The Coding Connection and Patient Financial Services

Of the many activities that occur in patient financial services (PFS), two key revenue cycle components are billing and denial management. Data collected from patient access, information from the chargemaster, and HIM coding all come together in the form of a bill. Sophisticated bill edit systems have the ability to apply Medicare medical necessity, Outpatient Code Edits (OCE), and Correct Coding Initiative (CCI) edits to the claim prior to submission. Once these edits are applied, someone knowledgeable in coding and clinical protocols must resolve the edits to try to avoid claim delays and denials.

Coding connects (or needs to connect) with PFS in the following areas: discharged not final billed (DNFB) monitoring; medical necessity; OCE and CCI edits; and payment verification.

Every HIM department should have an effective DNFB reporting tool. HIM staff should be able to quickly identify high-dollar cases and the oldest cases. A process should be in place to quickly address the cases identified. Goals should also be set (e.g., one day over the bill hold days), and aggressive monitoring should be done on a daily basis. Significant communication and collaboration among the entire revenue cycle team is required to maintain the DNFB at industry best-practice standards.

Medical necessity does not take place only in the patient access area. Most billing systems allow providers to check for medical necessity one last time prior to claim submission. Connecting the billing process to coding is critical in reducing the number of medical necessity denials. Coding professionals are key players in querying the physician a final time for additional documentation to support services ordered and performed.

Coders are also critical in resolving OCE and CCI edits. Edit conflicts may be caused by a number of reasons, including lack of knowledge by the clinician entering charges and codes coming from both the chargemaster and the coding process. Coders should be involved in the daily bill edit process in order to avoid delays in final billing and claim rejections. Coders can resolve difficult edits by removing an inappropriate charge, recommending a chargemaster change, or evaluating source documentation to ensure complete and accurate coding. Some bill edit systems allow specific edits to be driven or assigned to certain individuals or departments. Edits such as comprehensive, component, and mutually exclusive should be assigned to a coder for resolution.

Finally, a verification process should be in place to ensure expected payments are received on both the outpatient (APC) and inpatient (DRG) assignment.

For healthcare providers to survive under the surmounting financial and operational pressures in an ever-changing environment, the coding process must be connected to the key services within the revenue cycle. Ongoing teamwork between coding and the areas of patient access, chargemaster maintenance, and PFS creates an exciting opportunity for HIM and coding professionals to spotlight their leadership skills. Make sure you are connected!

How Does Your Coding Measure Up?: Analyzing Performance Data Gives HIM a Boost in Managing Revenue

Kurt Price, MS, and Dean Farley, PhD

Accurate and complete coding ensures that a hospital receives the reimbursement it deserves—full reimbursement that is fully compliant with coding and payment rules. As the payment environment grows more complex, HIM professionals are being asked to play a more active and formal role in their hospitals' revenue cycle management. Successfully assuming these new responsibilities includes employing a tool that may also be new to many HIM professionals—data analysis. Monitoring coding performance data is an important method for improving coding productivity and effectiveness and advancing the HIM role in revenue management.

Tracking HIM performance must go beyond typical operational measures that document performance in the narrow context of the hospital's own experience. To be an effective participant in revenue and compliance management, HIM professionals must have access to—and take advantage of—the information that allows them to answer the following questions:

- Does our coding appear out of compliance according to the Office of Inspector General's (OIG) upcoding measures?

- Do our complication and comorbidity (CC) coding rates appear overly aggressive compared to peer hospitals?

- Do our CC coding rates suggest a potential for improved reimbursement through more accurate and complete coding?

- Do our Ambulatory Payment Classification (APC) coding patterns suggest a compliance risk or revenue improvement opportunity?

- Do I know the financial risk and reimbursement impacts of these and other coding patterns at our hospital?

Using actual profiling results, this article illustrates how HIM professionals can incorporate coding, compliance, and reimbursement performance data into their monitoring and improvement efforts.

Evaluating Current Performance, Identifying Future Improvements

Profiling HIM performance allows hospitals to go beyond narrow operational metrics and evaluate themselves in a broad industry context, identifying areas where they appear to be out of alignment with industry averages. This focuses efforts on improving coding, compliance, and reimbursement management in areas where the hospital stands out as a compliance risk or where incomplete billing may be undermining reimbursement. By establishing a routine and replicable evaluation process, profiling can be used as a basis for evaluating current performance and future changes in performance.

Ideally then, HIM can become at least in part a data-driven process. Typical steps in this process should enable the HIM department to:

- Establish quantitative baseline performance levels for the hospital overall, as well as for specific clinical areas (e.g., CC coding rates for selected DRGs)

- Conduct qualitative documentation, coding, and billing audits to identify deficiencies and vulnerabilities

- Identify and implement remedial strategies

- Assess progress in quantitative terms

- Calculate financial implications of deficiencies and improvements

These steps can be repeated and expanded as necessary to provide an effective ongoing monitoring and improvement program.

The federal government's emphasis on compliance underscores the importance of profiling documentation and coding performance. Medicare compliance programs and directives of the Centers for Medicare and Medicaid Services (CMS) and OIG directly influence compliance monitoring in hospitals. OIG identifies benchmarking, longitudinal studies, and regular reporting as key elements of an effective compliance program.[1,2] CMS has incorporated these perspectives in its Medicare review programs managed by quality improvement organizations (QIOs), in particular, the Hospital Payment Monitoring Program (HPMP) implemented in 2003.

Both internal and external data are important for performance evaluation. External data, such as Medicare inpatient and outpatient claims data, ground the evaluation in measurable industry norms and force hospitals to evaluate performance beyond "local experience." These data establish what is typical and how much variation there is around normal performance. Further, external data encourages hospitals to assess how they differ from the norm and how those differences might affect performance.

Internal data provide other advantages and can add significant depth to a performance profiling program. Using a hospital's own historical data enables consistent comparison of performance measures over time and injects local factors into the evaluation process. It also gets around the typical limitations of external data: timeliness, uncertain data collection processes, and privacy considerations. In contrast with external data, using internal data encourages evaluators to ask and assess where the organization is now, how far it has come, and what else has changed that might affect results.

Profiling in Action

The following examples illustrate the process of performance profiling in the HIM professional's role of managing revenue and compliance. The process is one of discovery, investigation, and action: discovery of risk and opportunity areas through profiling are investigated using focused reviews, and appropriate corrective strategies can be developed and implemented. Industry coding guidelines and expertise (*Coding Clinic for ICD-9-CM*, for example) support this process.

Numerous documentation and coding areas, both inpatient and outpatient, should be incorporated in a performance profiling program, including:

- Key OIG and QIO/HPMP target areas
- CC coding rates (DRGs)
- Medicare casemix index (DRGs)
- Outpatient Code Editor failure rates
- Outpatient coding into APC levels
- Medicare Discounted Service Index (APCs)
- DRG and APC outlier payment rates

The examples provided here come from the first two areas comparing rates and historical trends and estimating the financial implications.

The performance results in these examples are derived from a commercially available profiling tool using publicly available data for all hospitals in the US. These analyses are for illustration purposes, and alternative profiling approaches or benchmark datasets are available or could be developed to serve this purpose.

The profiling examples present the actual findings for a large teaching hospital (fictitiously named Metro Medical Center [MMC] for purposes of this article), with its performance compared against the benchmark performance for all large teaching hospitals in the US. MMC's story for each example, however, is for illustration purposes only.

DRG 416

OIG has identified DRG 416 as one of the DRGs at high risk for upcoding, and CMS has included DRG 416 as one of its HPMP target areas. The compliance review method employed by CMS tabulates the frequency with which high-risk DRGs occur among a hospital's cases as a fraction of cases in DRGs with the potential to be grouped into the high risk category. As specified by CMS, this means the number of DRG 416 cases as a percentage of cases in DRGs 416, 320, and 321.

Distinguishing Septicemia (DRG 416) from Urinary Tract Infections (UTIs) with and without CCs (DRGs 320 and 321, respectively) has been a major issue for this hospital. The most recent profiling results (shown in figure 1) suggest that MMC codes cases into DRG 416 more frequently than benchmark hospitals: 52.5 percent of MMC cases in DRGs 416, 320, and 321 are coded into DRG 416, compared to 47.2 percent for benchmark hospitals, for a variance of 5.3 percentage points.

Figure 1. DRG 416 Snapshot: Above the Benchmark

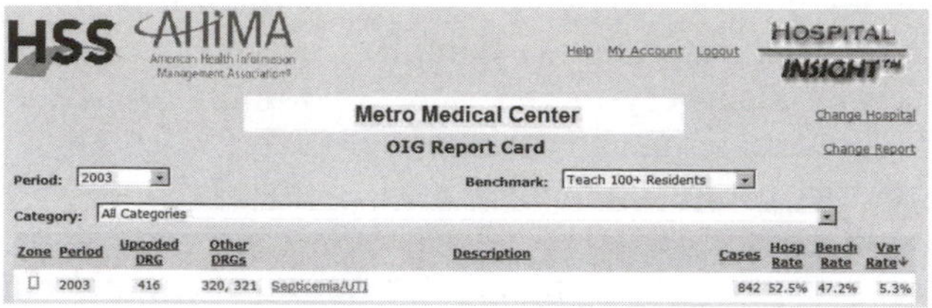

Several years ago, however, the same profiling analysis uncovered an even larger variance of more than 15 points. This represented a significant compliance risk, and MMC initiated focused coding and documentation reviews of septicemia and UTI cases. These reviews revealed that, for many physicians, urosepsis refers to a urinary tract infection only. The ICD-9-CM system similarly classifies urosepsis in this way, and code 599.0 (Urinary Tract Infection, NOS) was appropriately assigned. However, there was also a substantial proportion of physicians who believe that urosepsis means sepsis (a systemic infection that involves bacteria in the bloodstream) that originated in the urinary tract.

Coding issues resulted when MMC coders assumed that all physicians meant "sepsis" when they documented "urosepsis." The clinical presentation, treatment, and severity of the patient are very different between the two conditions, and the medical record documentation must support assignment of a code for sepsis (038.X, 995.91). The MMC HIM department implemented changes, working to improve the accuracy of coding for these DRGs.

The five-year trend shown in figure 2 illustrates that MMC's compliance risk for DRG 416 has decreased dramatically. In 2000 and 2001 the hospital's rate for DRG 416 was 15.2 points higher than the benchmark, and in these years MMC's rates were among the highest 10 percent of all benchmark hospitals (as indicated by the "Zone" flagged red for those years). The rate difference has decreased in the last two years to reach 5.3 points.

Figure 2. DRG 416 Trend: Decreasing Risk

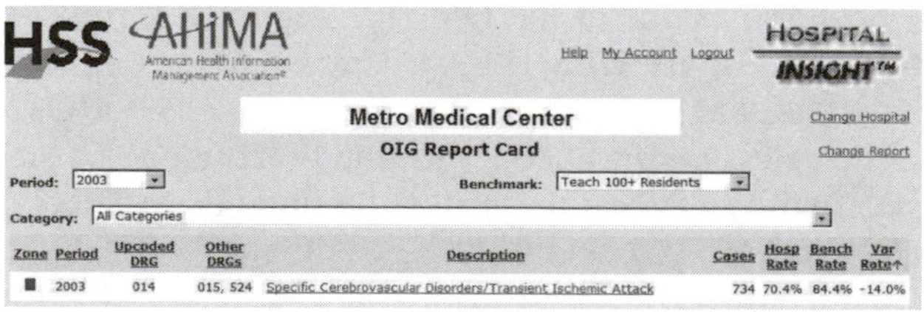

DRG 14

DRG 14 is another DRG identified by OIG as a high risk for upcoding; it is also targeted by HPMP. The example shown in figure 3 analyzes the frequency of DRG 14 cases as a percentage of cases in DRGs 14, 15, and 524. Rather than representing a compliance risk for MMC, this error-prone DRG may actually reflect an opportunity for improved revenues. The profiling results suggest that MMC codes cases into DRG 14 much less frequently than do benchmark hospitals: 70.4 percent of MMC cases compared to 84.4 percent for benchmark hospitals. MMC's rate for DRG 14 is among the lowest 10 percent of all benchmark hospitals, as indicated by the indicator flagged blue.

Figure 3. DRG 14 Snapshot: Lowest 10 Percent

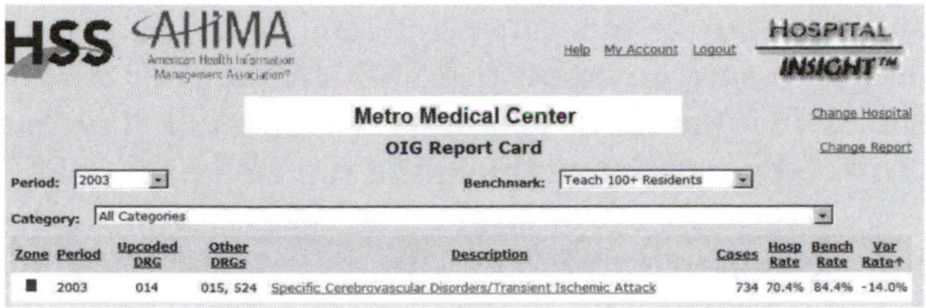

A documentation and coding review of these cases reveals that the issue for DRG 14 involves the appropriate coding of the term "stroke" as documented in a medical record without further physician substantiation of the presence of an infarction. For many years "stroke" was indexed in ICD-9-CM to code 436 (Acute, but ill-defined, cerebrovascular disease), which was grouped to DRG 14 (Intracranial Hemorrhage or Cerebral Infarction). Effective October 2002 (FY 2003), the DRG grouping method was changed so that if "stroke" only was documented without an infarction, code 436 was then regrouped to DRG 15 (Nonspecific CVA and Precerebral Occlusion without Infarction).

The five-year trend for MMC shown in figure 4 confirms a dramatic drop in DRG 14 cases in 2003 compared to previous years. Thus MMC suspected and confirmed with profiling data that beginning in 2003 many cases were grouped to DRG 15 that should have been grouped to DRG 14 if more complete documentation and coding had occurred for these cases.

Figure 4. DRG 14 Trend: Sudden Drop

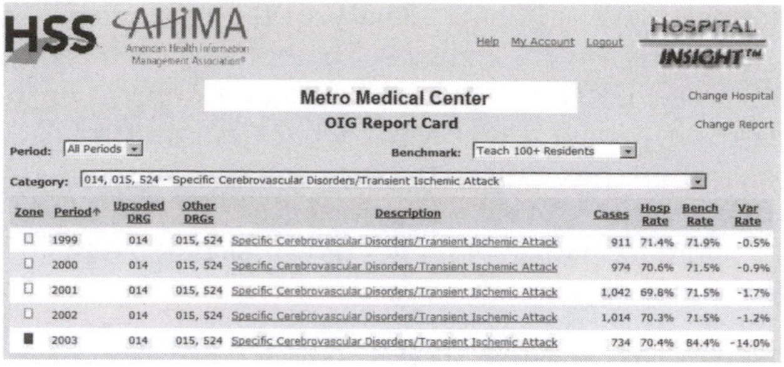
HSS AHIMA American Health Information Management Association®

Help My Account Logout

HOSPITAL INSIGHT™

Metro Medical Center

OIG Report Card

Change Hospital

Change Report

Period: All Periods

Benchmark: Teach 100+ Residents

Category: 014, 015, 524 - Specific Cerebrovascular Disorders/Transient Ischemic Attack

Zone	Period	Upcoded DRG	Other DRGs	Description	Cases	Hosp Rate	Bench Rate	Var Rate
☐	1999	014	015, 524	Specific Cerebrovascular Disorders/Transient Ischemic Attack	911	71.4%	71.9%	-0.5%
☐	2000	014	015, 524	Specific Cerebrovascular Disorders/Transient Ischemic Attack	974	70.6%	71.5%	-0.9%
☐	2001	014	015, 524	Specific Cerebrovascular Disorders/Transient Ischemic Attack	1,042	69.8%	71.5%	-1.7%
☐	2002	014	015, 524	Specific Cerebrovascular Disorders/Transient Ischemic Attack	1,014	70.3%	71.5%	-1.2%
■	2003	014	015, 524	Specific Cerebrovascular Disorders/Transient Ischemic Attack	734	70.4%	84.4%	-14.0%

Much public comment has since indicated that in many physicians' minds (and inherent in the documentation), a stroke was considered an infarction. As of October 2004 (FY 2005), the word "stroke" is now indexed in ICD-9-CM to code 434.91 (Cerebral artery occlusion, unspecified, with infarction). The same documentation of "stroke" that grouped cases to DRG 15 for two years will now group the same cases to DRG 14. Theoretically, this could be a continuing issue for hospitals if their coders are not using the updated index carefully. If they continue to assign code 436 whenever "acute CVA" is documented, they will continue to group an inappropriately high proportion of cases into DRG 15 that should be grouped into DRG 14.

If MMC completed similar hospital profiling analyses on a real-time basis using its own data, it could have identified this issue as it was occurring, thus preventing the hospital from losing reimbursement. For many of the cases during 2003 and 2004, patients did suffer a CVA, but the documentation may not have documented the word "infarction." With timely profiling results, coding and HIM department managers could have queried physicians and requested that this more specific information be added to the medical record in order that it be coded more appropriately to the CVA DRG 14.

CC Coding Rates

CC coding rates are analyzed for DRG combinations (or "DRG pairs") that are distinguished solely by the presence or absence of a CC. The analyses tabulate the number of cases assigned to DRGs requiring a CC as a percentage of discharges assigned to either DRG in the CC pair. These types of evaluations are used to identify DRGs with potential upcoding that could place the hospital at compliance risk or could suggest incomplete coding of CCs.

To analyze potential revenue opportunities in the documentation and coding of CCs, MMC focused on the top 10 DRG pairs where its CC coding rates were lower compared to benchmark hospitals (see figure 5). As shown, DRG pair 110-111 is the largest-volume pair, accounting for 1.4 percent of MMC's cases, and its CC coding rate is nearly 15 percentage points lower than benchmark hospitals—70.4 percent compared to 85.2 percent.

Figure 5. Top DRG Pairs below Benchmark

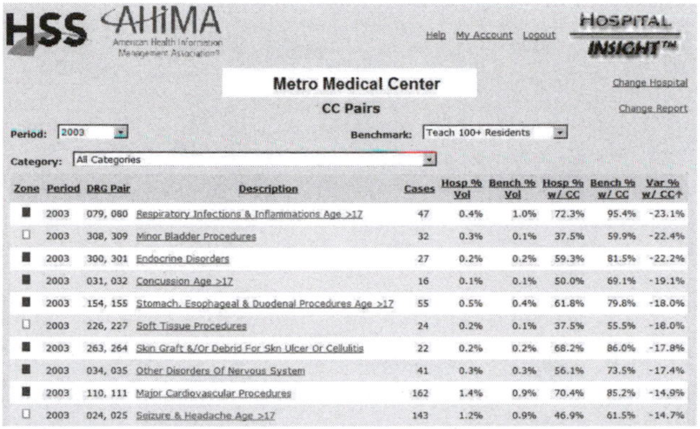
HSS AHIMA American Health Information Management Association
Help My Account Logout
HOSPITAL INSIGHT™
Metro Medical Center
Change Hospital
CC Pairs
Change Report
Period: 2003
Benchmark: Teach 100+ Residents
Category: All Categories

Zone	Period	DRG Pair	Description	Cases	Hosp % Vol	Bench % Vol	Hosp % w/ CC	Bench % w/ CC	Var % w/ CC↑
■	2003	079, 080	Respiratory Infections & Inflammations Age >17	47	0.4%	1.0%	72.3%	95.4%	-23.1%
□	2003	308, 309	Minor Bladder Procedures	32	0.3%	0.1%	37.5%	59.9%	-22.4%
■	2003	300, 301	Endocrine Disorders	27	0.2%	0.2%	59.3%	81.5%	-22.2%
■	2003	031, 032	Concussion Age >17	16	0.1%	0.1%	50.0%	69.1%	-19.1%
■	2003	154, 155	Stomach, Esophageal & Duodenal Procedures Age >17	55	0.5%	0.4%	61.8%	79.8%	-18.0%
□	2003	226, 227	Soft Tissue Procedures	24	0.2%	0.1%	37.5%	55.5%	-18.0%
■	2003	263, 264	Skin Graft &/Or Debrid For Skn Ulcer Or Cellulitis	22	0.2%	0.2%	68.2%	86.0%	-17.8%
■	2003	034, 035	Other Disorders Of Nervous System	41	0.3%	0.3%	56.1%	73.5%	-17.4%
■	2003	110, 111	Major Cardiovascular Procedures	162	1.4%	0.9%	70.4%	85.2%	-14.9%
□	2003	024, 025	Seizure & Headache Age >17	143	1.2%	0.9%	46.9%	61.5%	-14.7%

The five-year trend shown in figure 6 demonstrates that the lower CC coding rate for DRG pair 110-111 has been a consistent pattern for MMC. However, the disparity in CC rates has greatly increased over time and has remained among the lowest 10 percent of benchmark hospitals for the last three years.

Figure 6. DRG Pair 110-111 Trend: Increasing Disparity

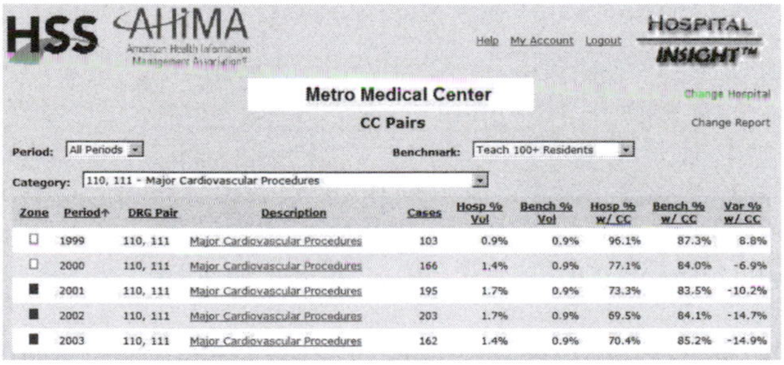
HSS AHIMA American Health Information Management Association
Help My Account Logout
HOSPITAL INSIGHT™
Metro Medical Center
Change Hospital
CC Pairs
Change Report
Period: All Periods
Benchmark: Teach 100+ Residents
Category: 110, 111 - Major Cardiovascular Procedures

Zone	Period↑	DRG Pair	Description	Cases	Hosp % Vol	Bench % Vol	Hosp % w/ CC	Bench % w/ CC	Var % w/ CC
□	1999	110, 111	Major Cardiovascular Procedures	103	0.9%	0.9%	96.1%	87.3%	8.8%
□	2000	110, 111	Major Cardiovascular Procedures	166	1.4%	0.9%	77.1%	84.0%	-6.9%
■	2001	110, 111	Major Cardiovascular Procedures	195	1.7%	0.9%	73.3%	83.5%	-10.2%
■	2002	110, 111	Major Cardiovascular Procedures	203	1.7%	0.9%	69.5%	84.1%	-14.7%
■	2003	110, 111	Major Cardiovascular Procedures	162	1.4%	0.9%	70.4%	85.2%	-14.9%

Thus MMC appears to have a persistent and growing undercoding problem for DRG pair 110-111. If further review reveals that there are true documentation and coding deficiencies, MMC has been losing revenue and corrective action is necessary. The revenue opportunity may indeed be significant. Figure 7 shows that if MMC's CC coding rate for DRG pair 110-111 matched the benchmark rate, its average reimbursement would increase by more than $1,300 per case, totaling roughly $215,000 for its 162 cases. The reimbursement implications of CC coding for DRG pair 110-111 identify it as a high-priority area.

Figure 7. DRG Pair 110-111: Potential Reimbursement Implications

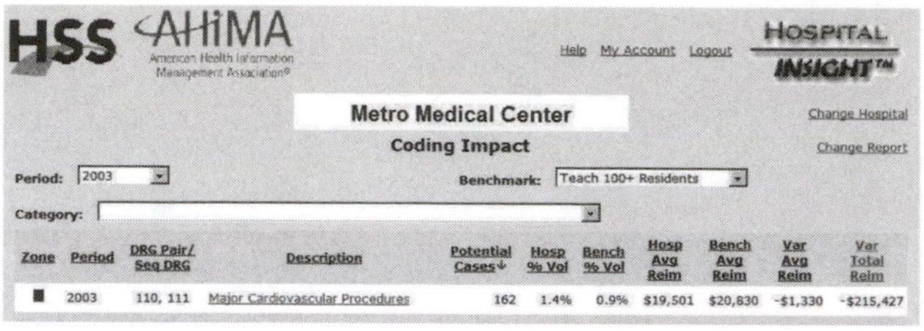

While profiling results for specific DRG pairs will identify specific areas that should be considered for review, the comparison of overall CC coding rates could point to more systematic documentation and coding concerns for the HIM department. For example, a major barrier to accurate and complete documentation for coding is the requirement that cases be coded within the "bill hold" period, which is typically three to five days after discharge. The accounts receivable report deadlines and goals drive HIM department managers to push coding as quickly as possible, sometimes with negative effects on optimal coding and corresponding reimbursement. In this situation, routine monitoring of CC coding rates would detect such a systematic pattern of undercoding and help HIM department managers identify the necessary remedial action.

Making It Happen

In spite of the advantages of employing performance profiling data in HIM, there can be barriers to doing so. From an institutional perspective, there are issues of ownership and control that may limit the HIM department's ability to define the types of management reporting and operating guidelines for the hospital. Obviously, the larger the role the HIM department plays in the compliance and revenue management processes, the more opportunity there is for the HIM department to bring about more effective use of performance data.

Given the opportunity, HIM professionals should be ready and willing to lead the way in using profiling data. HIM departments that perceive quantitative profiling measures as an opportunity, and whose goals and objectives support the use of the data, will do so.

HIM operational changes can promote more effective use of data. Management objectives and rewards can establish measurable performance standards relating to clinical data quality, even tying compensation and bonuses to performance. Providing adequate resources for data analysis and proper alignment of responsibilities is crucial. It is also crucial that HIM departments develop and articulate data-driven management strategies that include clear links between performance profiling data and existing monitoring and improvement activities (e.g., record reviews and audits).

In the end, successful use of performance profiling requires a long-term commitment to improve data quality throughout the organization. Just as data can be the source of problems, it can be a big part of the solution. The benefits of performance profiling encompass both improved data quality and stable and enhanced revenues with reduced compliance risk.

Notes

1. "Compliance Program Guidance for Hospitals." *Federal Register* 63, no. 35 (1998):8987–98.

2. "Supplemental Compliance Program Guidance for Hospitals." *Federal Register* 70, no. 19 (2005): 4858–76.

Charge Capture and the Physician Revenue Cycle

Susan M. Hull, MPH, RHIA, CCS, CCS-P

Poor charge capture processes are responsible for the loss of millions of dollars in revenue every year. Particularly in the area of inpatient services, loss of charges is a frequent occurrence. At Shands Healthcare in Florida, John Hajjar, MD, director of the urology practice group, found that 20 percent of all inpatient services rendered by the members of his group were not billed.[1] Among the process failures that may result in lost revenue are the following:

- Charges are not captured at all.

- Codes are incorrect or inappropriate for the patient and/or service.

- The order of codes is not optimal.

- ICD-9-CM diagnosis codes are not appropriately linked to CPT codes to assure documentation of medical necessity.

The revenue cycle in the typical physician's office setting differs from the hospital revenue cycle only in scope or size. The basic components are the same. In this presentation, we are going to primarily focus on the issue of charge capture and charge generation. I will begin with a brief overview of the entire revenue cycle and then focus on these topics.

The revenue cycle in the physician office setting has two basic components: front-end functions and back-end functions. The so-called front-end functions begin at the time of first encounter and continue through the provision of services and bill generation. The back-end functions begin with receipt of a remittance advice or equivalent and end at the time that the account is zero-balanced.

Overview of the Physician Practice Revenue Cycle

The basic elements in the physician practice revenue cycle include the following:

1. Initial contact. The initial contact may take any one of several forms. The most common are patient request for services, a request for consultation from another practitioner, or a referral from another service provider, either a physician, or the emergency department of a hospital on whose referral staff the physician serves. Other sources of first contact may include medicolegal referrals, such as from attorneys in personal injury suits or workers compensation cases. In addition, mandated second opinions from HMOs and PPOs may be a source of referrals.

In the hospital, initial contact may come from the emergency department or the admissions office, notifying the attending physician that a patient has been admitted.

At this stage of the cycle, obtaining accurate patient information is critical. The earlier in the process that essential data can be obtained, the greater the likelihood of preventing future errors. Staff should assure that the services are appropriate and covered as soon as possible, as well as assuring that the patient is appropriate for the practice.

2. Patient registration. At the time that the patient presents to the physician office, the process of patient registration begins. This process can be begun prior to the patient physically presenting at the office, of course. Included in the processes of patient registration are insurance verification and generation of the charging instrument.

The collection of complete and accurate demographic and insurance data at this point in the cycle is critical. Small errors made at the time of patient registration can become huge impediments later in the revenue cycle. Also at this point, the Advance Beneficiary Notice should be obtained for any services that will be rendered in the office that may not be covered by Medicare. These would include routine diagnostic assessments, screening tests (except in specific covered circumstances), questionably covered procedures, and any other services for which documentation of medical necessity is not present.

When a patient is admitted to the hospital, the office staff may not be aware of the admission for days. Most hospital data systems, however, now generate a notification message to the attending physician's office at the time of patient admission. If the patient does not have an existing office record, one should be begun at this time.

3. Provision of services and charge capture. At the point that services are provided, the process of charge capture begins. Among the issues that must be addressed to assure appropriate charge capture are the following:

- Identification of the person or persons responsible for charge capture in specific circumstances and at specific points during the provision of services

- Assuring the presence of appropriate, legible documentation of services

- Assuring the timeliness of charge capture

- Maintenance of a charging instrument that is complete, current, accurate, and does not tend to result in over-coding or under-coding

4. Charge reconciliation process. The charge reconciliation process is one of the most important and frequently over-looked aspects of the revenue cycle. Included in the charge reconciliation process are the following functions:

- Lost charge identification and entry

- Late charge identification

- Validation of charges by comparison with the physician documentation (Were the correct procedures billed?)

- Physician query process, often highly unsophisticated in physician office setting

- Making sure that the documentation matches the charge ticket (Do the notes support what was billed?)

- Process assessment to identify reasons for late and/or missed charges and corrective action

5. Coding. During the coding process, ICD-9-CM and CPT codes are assigned to report the services performed and the reasons for these services. Accuracy of CPT code assignment directly impacts reimbursement based upon the physician fee schedule; accuracy of ICD-9-CM codes indirectly impacts reimbursement. The function of the ICD-9-CM diagnosis codes is to substantiate and validate the CPT code assignment.

Issues addressed during the coding process, in addition to substantiation of the services billed, include documentation of medical necessity for additional services ordered and observance of the requirements of the National Correct Coding Initiative.

The adequacy of the coding process is a function of staffing and resources. A knowledgeable coding staff, with quality materials available for assistance, is necessary to assure appropriate code assignment. Care must be taken that the coding resources are complete and current. If electronic coding resources are used, they must be maintained.

The assignment of modifiers is also a part of the coding process. Inappropriate use of modifiers may result in over- or under-reporting of services and consequent inappropriate reimbursement.

6. Claim generation. Once the services have been rendered and codes assigned, the claim is generated. Our goal is always a clean claim the first time, every time.

A clean claim is one that accurately and completely reflects the circumstances of the visit and passes through all payer edits without delay. The demographics, ICD-9-CM codes, and CPT codes must all correlate. If additional documentation is needed to support a code assignment (such as an operative report), it should be obtained at this time.

At this time, too, coordination of benefits should be addressed. All payers have requirements for coordination of benefits. The Medicare Web site now contains a valuable resource for explaining coordination of Medicare benefits, which can be accessed at www.cms.hhs.gov/medicare/cob/.

The timeliness of claims submission is also important. Although Medicare allows the provider until the end of the calendar year following that in which the services were provided to file an initial claim, many managed care companies have very stringent requirements for claim submission, sometimes as short a time as thirty days following services. If the claim is not submitted within the contracted period of time, the practice will have no further recourse.

7. Notification of payment. The practice is notified of payment in various ways, depending upon the payer. At the time that payment is obtained, payments and adjustments must be posted. Good business practices are important in posting of payments and adjustments.

8. Reimbursement analysis. The reimbursement is virtually never the billed amount. The practice must review all denials or significant reductions in payment to determine the cause. If appropriate, claims should be resubmitted. In addition, all denials that can be appealed should be appealed. Only if the bill was clearly erroneous should denials be written off.

Of note, the identities of those who have authority to write off claims must be clearly stated and under what circumstances they can write off claims. A sampling of written off claims should be done by the practice manager on a regular basis.

The simple act of appealing a denial will usually result in improved reimbursement. Particularly with Medicare, an appeal to the area medical director, with appropriate supporting documentation, will usually result in reversal of the denial.

If significant numbers of claims are being reimbursed at lower than expected rates, a process review should be done and corrective action taken. The new process should then be tested to assure that it is having the desired effect. If training needs are identified as a part of the process review, the education should be provided to the appropriate staff. Money spent on education is always worth it.

9. Receivables analysis. The practice should conduct a periodic review of all pending claims and follow up as appropriate.

10. Credit/Collections. This is the last step in the revenue cycle. This process ends at the time that an account is zero-balanced. Return all credits promptly. Medicare regulations require that credits be returned within 60 days of receipt.

In addition, form CMS-838 must be completed and submitted quarterly, to report any credit balances. Follow established procedures for collection. An account cannot be written off to bad debt until the established processes of attempted collection have been completed. These processes should be the same for all patients, regardless of payer.

Charge Capture

The consequences of inadequate charge capture processes include the following:

- Lost billings due to process collapse

- Denied claims due to inadequate linkage of diagnosis and procedure codes

- Extension of the reimbursement cycle. Time is money.

- Excess administrative costs and reduction in time available for patient care

As noted above, the processes that must be addressed in evaluating the charge capture process include the following:

- Identifying the person or persons responsible for charge capture in specific circumstances and at specific points during the provision of services. The physician is ultimately responsible for all charging in his or her practice and is the most qualified to assign the evaluation and management level of service codes, whereas the radiologic technician is the appropriate staff to enter charges for imaging services.

- Assuring the presence of appropriate, legible documentation of services. Electronic health records may increase the legibility of documentation, but cannot automatically guarantee that the documentation is appropriate to the presenting problem. A possible advantage of having someone other than the physician enter the evaluation and management level of service codes is that that individual will be forced to rely upon the actual documentation, rather than a combination of the documentation in the record and that in the physician's head.

- Assuring the timeliness of charge capture. Charges should be captured as soon as possible after the services are delivered.

- Maintaining a charging instrument that is complete, current, accurate, and does not tend to result in over-coding or under-coding.

The goals of a good charge capture methodology should include the following:

- As much as possible, capture data one time, preferably in an electronic environment. Repeated episodes of data capture lead to increased opportunities for errors, duplications, and missed charges.

- Decrease the number of instances where data are entered manually by either the physician or other staff (for example, laboratory personnel, radiology technologist, and nurse). Physician practice data systems are currently available that will allow laboratory data to be downloaded directly into the patient's clinical record.

- Eliminate as much as possible the need for physically moving data from one place to another.

- Place the decision making for charging with the person who is performing the work. Wherever possible, the person who actually performed the service should be entering the charges.

Charge Ticket Design

The design of the charging instrument is critical to the charge capture process. Whether electronic or paper, the form must be designed in such a way as to assure that ICD-9-CM and CPT codes can be linked, that all charges can be captured, and that all possible charges are available for capture. There are currently countless electronic charge capture programs available for physician use. Several of these are listed in the "Endnotes" section of this paper. The level of sophistication of these systems varies widely. Some are essentially electronic notepads on which the physician makes notes that are later converted into charges. Others incorporate prescription pads in the charging form and may include electronic calculation of evaluation and management level of service based upon interface with the documentation in the electronic record.

The minimum required information for inclusion on charge ticket is the following:

- Patient identification, including a secondary identifier, such as date of birth or Social Security number, to assure that the proper patient account is charged.

- Date of service

- Treating physician if a multi-physician practice

- Services or procedures rendered (for example, CPT code)

- Reason for each service (for example, ICD-9-CM diagnosis)

- Place that service or procedure was rendered if several sites

Additional data elements that might be appropriate include time of service and the name of the referring physician if this is a consultation. A few payers will reimburse additional for services rendered after-hours and on an emergency basis.

Devising an effective charge ticket for hospital services has been a challenge for practices forever. Typically, the hospital charge ticket contains room for an inadequate number of diagnoses to support varying levels of hospital visits. The most effective charging instrument for recording hospital visits, in the absence of a fully electronic, fully integrated system with capability for bedside data entry by all practitioners, is the classic 3 x 5 card. These 3 x 5 cards generally work better than 8-1/2 x 11-inch pages, as they fit into the pocket of the rounds coat and can be easily accessed without repeated folding and unfolding. The format of the card should be such that the physician can easily add all the above pieces of data. Each service code (whether evaluation and management level of service or interventional procedure) should have a matching diagnosis code box. Physicians should be encouraged to vary the levels of evaluation and management codes assigned, in accordance with the CPT guidelines. In addition, if highest-level services are being charged, there may be need for a more "intense" ICD-9-CM diagnosis code for that particular day's service. For example, a patient who enters the hospital with an acute myocardial infarction and improves steadily would be coded as a level 1 subsequent hospital visit on the days he is improving. If, however, the patient develops cardiogenic shock, for that day a higher-level evaluation and management code would be assigned; the diagnosis for that visit would not be AMI, but rather cardiogenic shock.

Some practices opt for cards that allow recording of multiple days' visits. Such a system, however, makes it more difficult to link services and diagnoses (such as in the above example) and makes it more likely that the card (and its charges) will be lost. Ideally, charges for hospital visits should be entered on a daily basis, rather than at the end of the admission.

If the office is linked to the hospital data system, the day's cards can be printed up in the morning and provided to the physician prior to rounds. At the end of the day, a reconciliation record should be maintained to assure that all cards have been returned.

Whether an electronic or paper format is used, the most important functions are the appropriate linking of ICD-9-CM and CPT codes and the availability of all possible procedure codes.

It is extremely important that the charge capture instrument offer the physician the opportunity to charge all levels of service. A University of Chicago physician practice group was found to be billing only the two highest levels of evaluation and management codes, and review of their charge ticket showed that only these levels were available for charging.[3] It is essential that all five levels of evaluation and management codes be present on the charge ticket. Inappropriate charging can result in severe penalties to the practice, including potential prosecution under Medicare for fraud and abuse and even exclusion from the Medicare program (and other programs).

The issue of whether to include ICD-9-CM diagnosis codes on the superbill has long been debated. Assigning a non-specific code when a more specific and more accurate one exists is not appropriate. Program Memorandum AB-01-144, issued September 26, 2001 (available for review at http://cms.hhs.gov/manuals/pm_trans/ab01144.pdf) defines the outpatient coding guidelines, which also apply to physicians' offices. The guidelines clearly state that the condition that was responsible for the services rendered must be reported to the highest degree of specificity possible and with the correct number of digits. Inclusion of ICD-9-CM codes on superbills requires that the number of codes be severely restricted. Even a practice that sees a well-defined patient population may need to report hundreds of ICD-9-CM codes at one time or another.

There are several options for addressing the issue of ICD-9-CM code assignment. These include:

- Include no diagnosis codes on the superbill, but have professional coding staff assign the codes based upon the physician documentation in the health record. Advantages of this option include high quality coding, assigned in accordance with the most current guidelines. Disadvantages include the need for access to the dictated (or written) visit report. Electronic records, which allow access by multiple staff members concurrently, may address this issue, but the need for very rapid transcription of dictated reports may be an issue.

- Attempt to include all possible diagnosis codes on the superbill, complete to the required fourth or fifth digits. Advantages of this option include rapid turn-around of the charges. Disadvantages include the need for an extensive document, the possibility for errors from checking the wrong box, and the need for frequent review and updating.

- Include truncated ICD-9-CM diagnosis codes and provide blanks for the entry of additional diagnostic descriptors, then have trained staff assign the most accurate code. Advantages of this option include the need for fewer diagnosis codes on the charge ticket, but disadvantages include the need for additional physician input to assure appropriate coding, which may not be easy to obtain.

Linkage of ICD-9-CM and CPT Codes

Linkage of ICD-9-CM and CPT codes is critical to reimbursement. The physician billing form (CMS-1500) contains spaces for only four diagnosis codes. Thus, the diagnoses selected must be those that are most supportive of the services performed. The first-listed diagnosis should be that which is the reason for the visit, per outpatient (physician) coding guidelines. The first-listed procedure code should be that with the highest relative weight. This may or may not be the evaluation and management visit code. Each CPT code should be linked to that ICD-9-CM diagnosis code that is most supportive of the service.

The easiest way to link diagnosis and procedure codes is to encourage physicians to number diagnoses rather than to simply check them off on a list. If a coding professional receives a diagnosis sheet with four check-marks on it, she is forced to make a clinical judgment about sequencing and linkage, a decision which she is not professionally qualified to make. Only the practitioner can link the procedures and diagnoses, as this is a part of the medical decision-making process. Many electronic charging programs require the physician to number the diagnoses and to provide the linkages.

Physician Query Process

If the charge ticket does not contain adequate documentation to assign ICD-9-CM diagnosis codes, the physician must be queried. This should be a written process, not relying upon additional information provided verbally. If the physician states that an additional diagnosis may be listed, the diagnosis should be added to the visit record by the physician and authenticated by him or her.

All diagnoses addressed during a visit should be documented in the visit record. Simply noting the diagnosis on the charge ticket is not sufficient. The charge ticket is not a part of the official visit record, and the information included in it is not part of the documentation that will be assessed if the practice is ever audited. If no diagnoses are recorded in the visit record, there is no documented basis for medical decision making, and an auditor would give no "credit" for medical decision making.

Summary

The creation of an effective charge capture mechanism requires attention to the financial needs of the practice, as well as compliance issues. A charging instrument that fulfills all important functions will allow for complete and accurate assignment of both ICD-9-CM diagnosis and CPT procedural codes, facilitate linkage between the code sets, and assure that all compliance guidelines are met. Whether a paper or an electronic format is used, the charge ticket is the most important element in the creation of an optimal charge capture system and must be tailored to the particular practice. Any expense incurred in developing the appropriate instrument will be more than equaled in reduction of lost or late charges, improvement in timeliness and appropriateness of reimbursement, and reduced exposure under Medicare compliance guidelines.

Endnotes

1 Pamela L. Moore. "Improving Charge Capture: Lost Charges Can Really Add Up," *PhysiciansPractice*, 2002. Available at www.shands.org/professional/ppd/practice/ finance/lostcharges.asp.

2 http://cms.hhs.gov/forms/cms838a.pdf

3 "Whistleblower, charge ticket, and upcoding spell trouble for U of Chicago Hospitals," hcPro Compliance Info.com.

Appendix B References

AHIMA Coding Practice Team. "Developing a Coding Compliance Policy Document (AHIMA Practice Brief)." *Journal of AHIMA* 72, no.7 (2001): 88A-C.

AHIMA Coding Practice Team. "Internet Resources for Accurate Coding and Reimbursement Practices." (AHIMA Practice Brief) *Journal of AHIMA* 75, no.7 (July-August 2004): 48A-G.

Bronnert, June. "Coding Ethically." *Journal of AHIMA* 76, no.9 (October 2005): 108,110,112.

The Care and Maintenance of Charge Masters. Issued July/August 1999 by the American Health Information Management Association.

CMS. 2005. Advance Beneficiary Notice (ABN). Available online from http://cms.hhs.gov/medicare/bni/default.asp?

Cogley, Janis. "Diagnosis Coding and Medical Necessity: Rules and Reimbursement." 2004 IFHRO Congress & AHIMA Convention Proceedings, October 2004

Cummins, Ruth, and Julie Waddell. "Coding Connections in Revenue Cycle Management." *Journal of AHIMA* 76, no.7 (July-August 2005): 72-74.

Hrehor, Kimberly. "The Codes to Watch: Identifying the DRGs Most Prone to Payment Error." *Journal of AHIMA* 76, no.7 (July-August 2005): 36-40.

Hull, Susan M. "Charge Capture and the Physician Revenue Cycle." AHIMA's 75th Anniversary National Convention and Exhibit Proceedings, October 2003

Price, Kurt, and Dean Farley. "How Does your Coding Measure Up? : Analyzing Performance Data Gives HIM a Boost in Managing Revenue." *Journal of AHIMA* 76, no.7 (July-August 2005): 26-31.

Appendix C
Answer Key for "Check Your Understanding" Questions

Check Your Understanding 1.1

1. B

2. 1929 in Texas, when Blue Cross first created a plan for school teachers

3. D

4. Resource-based relative value scale (RBRVS)

5. Global surgical package, including the procedure, local/topical anesthesia, preoperative visit, and postoperative care/follow-up; special-procedure package, including costs associated with a diagnostic or therapeutic procedure; ambulatory-visit package, including physicians' charges, laboratory tests, and x-rays

Check Your Understanding 2.1

1. The Health Insurance Portability and Accountability Act of 1996 (HIPAA)

2. C

3. National Center for Health Statistics (NCHS) and the Centers for Medicare and Medicaid Services (CMS), which together compose the ICD-9-CM Coordination and Maintenance Committee

4. *Coding Clinic for ICD-9-CM*

5. CPT

Check Your Understanding 2.2

1. Abuse, the submission of unintentionally inaccurate charges on a claim for reimbursement

2. C

3. Policies and procedures, education and training, and auditing and monitoring

4. False

5. Listings of diagnoses are the same but the presence or absence of complication or comorbidity diagnoses prompts assignment of cases to higher or lower DRGs.

Check Your Understanding 3.1

1. A healthcare plan offering dependent coverage includes benefits for spouses and family members of the insured individual.

2. Comprehensive policies provide coverage for most healthcare services but may have deductibles that must be met before the insurance company pays expenses, and the insured must also pay coinsurance for all covered expenses until the maximum out-of-pocket cost is reached.

3. C

4. Credited coverage

5. Prior approval is typically required for outpatient surgeries; diagnostic, interventional, and therapeutic outpatient procedures; physical, occupational, and speech therapies; mental health and dependency care; inpatient care including surgery, home health, private nurses, and nursing homes; and organ transplants.

Check Your Understanding 4.1

1. a. Inpatient hospital services
    b. Supplemental medical insurance
    c. Medicare Advantage
    d. Medicare drug benefit

2. Medigap policies offer supplemental insurance covering the cost-shared expenses such as the deductibles and 20 percent of durable medical equipment costs that patients otherwise pay.

3. Coverage differs among the states because Medicaid allows states to maintain a unique program adapted to state residents' needs and average incomes. Although state programs must meet coverage requirements for groups such as recipients of adoption assistance and foster care, other types of coverage, such as vision and dental services, are determined by the states' Medicaid agencies.

Check Your Understanding 4.2

1. a. TRICARE Extra
    b. TRICARE Standard
    c. TRICARE Prime
    d. TRICARE for Life (TFL)

2. True; CHAMPVA becomes a secondary payer when another health insurance benefit is available.

3. B

Check Your Understanding 5.1

1. To have visits to an oncologist—or any other specialist—an MCO member obtains a referral from his or her primary care provider.

2. Types are preventive, wellness-oriented, acute, and chronic.

3. Wellness programs

Check Your Understanding 5.2

1. The hospital-led IDS is the most common type of IDS and may include group practices; home health agencies; hospices; nursing homes; ambulatory surgery, outpatient care centers, and urgicenters; and ancillary providers.

2. The four types are: group practice without walls, physician-hospital organization, management service organization, and the medical foundation.

3. Group practices without walls (PWWs) or clinics without walls (CWWs) share administrative systems and have greater leverage in negotiating reimbursement with MCOs. Management service organizations (MSOs) provide management services and administrative and information systems to multiple group practices or small hospitals, thereby distributing overhead costs.

Check Your Understanding 6.1

1. Yale University in the late 1960s and early 1970s

2. Ignored

3. Is a CC present? Is a major complication or complex diagnosis present? Is the patient's age greater or less than seventeen years? What is the patient's sex? What is the patient's discharge disposition? For neonates, what is the birth weight of the baby?

4. The base-year payment rate is updated using an update factor established by Congress to account for inflation. Also, the labor-related share is adjusted by the wage index for the hospital's geographic area.

5. The market basket index, which is based on the mix of goods and services included in the PPS

Check Your Understanding 6.2

1. An inpatient deductible must be paid for the ninety-day benefit period, plus a daily coinsurance payment applies for the sixty-first through ninetieth day.

2. True

3. Standard federal rate

4. Inpatient rehabilitation facility patient assessment instrument (IRF PAI)

5. False; staff members do not enter RICs; the pricer (grouper) calculates the appropriate categories from the impairment group codes (IGC) entered on the PAI.

Check Your Understanding 7.1

1. CPT codes

2. Physician work (WORK), physician practice expenses (PE), and malpractice (MP)

3. Levels are dependent on the complexity of service performed (basic versus specialty care), the EMT's level of training required to perform the service, and the type of transport involved (land vehicle versus helicopter).

4. False; Medicare-certified ASCs must maintain their own administrative functions, record keeping, and financial and accounting systems

5. The ASC list

Check Your Understanding 7.2

1. The ambulatory payment group (APG) system developed by 3M HIS

2. Fee schedules and a PPS

3. True

4. The low-utilization payment adjustment (LUPA) is applied when an agency provides four or fewer visits in an episode; reimbursement in this case is made for each visit rather than for the sixty-day episode.

5. Clinical severity, functional status, and service utilization

Check Your Understanding 8.1

1. Preclaims submission activities such as collecting responsible parties' information, educating patients about their ultimate financial responsibility for services rendered, collecting appropriate waivers, and verifying data about procedures before they are performed and their charges submitted.

2. Electronic order entry systems help to capture charges at their point of service delivery. If facilities lack electronic systems, staff collect paper-based charges on charge tickets, superbills, or encounter forms to be entered by billing staff into the patient accounting system.

3. Scrubbers edit claims to locate and flag for correction any data that may contain errors, such as dates of service that are incompatible, inaccurate diagnosis and procedure codes, no substantiation of medical necessity, and inaccurate assignment of revenue codes.

Check Your Understanding 8.2

1. Can be measured to gauge performance improvement

2. The Medicare Outpatient Code Editor (OCE)

3. The CDM stored several incorrect codes and retained a previous code after it was updated; training in updated codes was not conducted for everyone who used them; and the chart flow process bypassed the staff who would have coded and reported use of supplies on claims.

Index

(continued)